BLOOD CELLS IN NUCLEAR MEDICINE, PART I

DEVELOPMENTS IN NUCLEAR MEDICINE
Series editor Peter H. Cox

Cox, P.H. (ed.): Cholescintigraphy. 1981. ISBN 90-247-2524-0

Cox, P.H. (ed.): Progress in radiopharmacology 3. Selected Topics. 1982. ISBN 90-247-2768-5

Jonckheer, M.H. and Deconinck, F. (eds.): X-ray fluorescent scanning of the thyroid. 1983. ISBN 0-89838-561-X

Kristensen, K. and Nørbygaard, E. (eds.): Safety and efficacy of radiopharmaceuticals. 1984. ISBN 0-89838-609-8

Bossuyt, A. and Deconinck, F.: Amplitude/phase patterns in dynamic scintigraphic imaging. 1984. ISBN 0-89838-641-1

Hardeman, M.R. and Najean, Y. (eds.): Blood cells in nuclear medicine I. Cell kinetics and bio-distribution. 1984. ISBN 0-89838-653-5

Fueger, G.F. (ed.): Blood cells in nuclear medicine II. Migratory blood cells. 1984. ISBN 0-89838-654-3

Blood cells in nuclear medicine, part I

Cell kinetics and bio-distribution

edited by

MAX R. HARDEMAN, PhD

Department of Internal Medicine
Academic Medical Center
University of Amsterdam
Amsterdam, The Netherlands

YVES NAJEAN, MD

Department of Nuclear Medicine
Hôpital Saint Louis
Paris, France

1984 **MARTINUS NIJHOFF PUBLISHERS**
a member of the KLUWER ACADEMIC PUBLISHERS GROUP
BOSTON / THE HAGUE / DORDRECHT / LANCASTER

Distributors

for the United States and Canada: Kluwer Academic Publishers, 190 Old Derby Street, Hingham, MA 02043, USA
for the UK and Ireland: Kluwer Academic Publishers, MTP Press Limited, Falcon House, Queen Square, Lancaster LA1 1RN, England
for all other countries: Kluwer Academic Publishers Group, Distribution Center, P.O. Box 322, 3300 AH Dordrecht, The Netherlands

Library of Congress Cataloging in Publication Data

Main entry under title:

Blood cells in nuclear medicine, Part I, Cell kinetics and bio-distribution.

(Developments in nuclear medicine)
Based on two meetings held in 1982 in Amsterdam and Paris.
Includes index.
1. Radiolabeled blood cells--Diagnostic use--Congresses 2. Blood cells--Radiolabeling--Congresses. 3. Indium--Isotopes--Diagnostic use--Congresses. 4. Radioisotope scanning--Congresses. 5. Nuclear medicine--Technique--Congresses. I. Hardeman, Max R. II. Najean, Yves. III. Title: Cell kinetics and bio-distribution.
IV. Series: Developments in nuclear medicine (1984)
[DNLM: 1. Blood Cells--physiology--congresses. 2. Cell Movement--congresses. 3. Indium--diagnostic use--congresses. 4. Radioisotopes--diagnostic use--congresses. W1 DE998KF / WH 140 B655 1982]
RC78.7.R43B56 1984 616.07'57 84-8100

ISBN-13: 978-94-009-6029-9 e-ISBN-13: 978-94-009-6027-5
DOI: 10.1007/978-94-009-6027-5

Copyright

CONTENTS

LABELLED PLATELETS: SCINTIGRAPHIC STUDIES

ERYTHROCYTES

FOREWORD

The labelling and in vivo use of blood-cells is not new; in 1940 Hahn and Hevesy measured the blood-volume in a rabbit by labelling the animal erythrocytes with radioactive phosphorus. Since then, many experimental and clinical investigations using radiolabelled cellular blood-elements have been described in literature. However, during the past few years, their use has become increasingly popular due to the development of efficient labelling techniques involving radionuclides suitable for gamma scintigraphy.

Indium-111 labelling, following the techniques as described in the first chapter of this book, not only allows the visualization of sites with active cell accumulation, but by virtue of the high labelling efficiency, also permits the labelling of autologous cells even in the case of severe cytopenia.

The following three chapters are dealing with platelets. Platelet production in man is more difficult to analyse from a quantitative and qualitative point of view, than the red cell and granulocyte production; we do not presently have for the platelet series a specific tracer like iron 59 for hemoglobin synthesis, nor a precise and reproducible method for quantifying stem cells, as for CFU/GM, BFU and CFU/E. However, some recent advances have increased our understanding of megakaryocyte production and the subsequent release of platelets for the identification and quantification of human megakaryocytic stem cells and for a better use of seleno-methionine as marker of platelet protein synthesis. The simultaneous study of autologous and homologous platelet lifespan is possible. Analysis of the survival curves may, however, not be easy when survival is not clearly different from normal values, e.g. in vascular diseases; controversies on the published results of a prognostic significance of shortened platelet lifespan and of normalization following anti-aggregating drugs may be due to the methods used for calculating platelet renewal. Chapter II is devoted to a critical analysis of methods in use for platelet production- and survival calculations. Some recent results of kinetic studies are also presented. From a theoretical point of view, progress of our knowledge on platelet-vascular wall interactions makes clinical studies of in vivo platelet function and kinetics very important for patho- physiological analysis. And, from a practical point of view, early detection of platelet deposits, evidence of platelet activation, could have clinical consequences for diagnosis, prognosis and choice of treatment in venous and arterial diseases as well as kidney-graft rejection (chapter III). In vivo platelet studies are, however, heavy methods, for the laboratory as well as for the patient. In practice, it is difficult to repeat this test before and after clinical change surgical procedures or anti-aggregant therapy. Hence the reason why the development of radio-immunological assay-methods for beta-thromboglobulin and platelet factor 4, two witnesses of platelet activation give hope of a more easy insight on platelet function in disease states. Chapter IV summarizes our knowledge concerning the physiological basis of these tests as well as the results obtained in several pathological situations.

The clinical application of Indium-111 labelled leukocytes is mainly dealing with granulocytes in use for the scintigraphic detection of various inflammatory processes as can be read in chapter V which is concluded with a paper on radiation dosimetry.

For immunologists and oncologists the use of Indium-111 labelled lymphocytes is of great interest. There may be, however, ethical restrictions against the use of these long-lived cells in normal individuals due to the chromosome damaging effect of the high-energy Auger electrons from Indium-111 (chapter VI). As long as the consequences i.e. the long term effect of this radiation-injury is not substantiated any further, a risk-benefit analysis for the use of Indium-111 lymphocytes in patients, other than terminal cases, might be difficult. In the final chapter the labelling and clinical application of erythrocytes is discussed.

Since this book gives a comprehensive review of the state of the art, both regarding methodology and clinical applications, it is of use for scientists of various disciplines working in the isotope laboratory as well as in the clinic.

M.R. Hardeman
Y. Najean

April 1984

LIST OF FIRST AUTHORS

Berge ten, R.J.M. - Central Laboratory of the Netherlands Red Cross Blood Transfusion Service and Laboratory for Experimental and Clinical Immunology of the University of Amsterdam, Amsterdam, The Netherlands

Boneu, A. - Centre Claudius Regaud, Hôpital La Grave, Service de Médecine Nucléaire, Toulouse, France

Breton-Gorius, J. - Hôpital Henri Moudor, Creteil, France

Buseman-Sokole, E. - Academic Medical Centre, University of Amsterdam, Department of Nuclear Medicine, Amsterdam, The Netherlands

Cardinaud, R. - CEN Saclay, Service de Biophysique Gif-sur-Yvette, France

Dewanjee, M.K. - Mayo Clinic, Radiopharmaceutical Laboratory, Missesota, USA

Eber, M. - Centre Paul Strauss, Service de Médecine Nucléaire, Strasbourg Cedex, France

Guillausseau, P.J. - Hôpital Lariboisière, Service de Médecine Interne et Diabètologie Paris, France

Hardeman, M.R. - Academic Medical Centre, University of Amsterdam, Department of Internal Medicine, Amsterdam, The Netherlands

Hawker, R.J. - Queen Elizabeth Medical Centre, University of Birmingham, Department of Surgery, Birmingham, U.K.

DuP Heyns, A. - South African Medical Research Council, University of the Orange Free State, Blood Platelet Research Unit, Bloemfontein, South Africa

Hill-Zobel, R.L. - The Johns Hopkins University, Department of Radiology, Baltimore, USA

Lötter, M.G. - South African Medical Research Council, University of the Orange Free State, Blood Platelet Research Unit, Bloemfontein, South Africa

Ludlam, C.A. - Royal Infirmary, Department of Haematology, Edinburgh, U.K.

Najean, Y. - Hôpital Saint-Louis, Service Central de Médecine Nucléaire, Paris Cedex

Paulus, J.M. - Hôpital de Bicêtre, Institute de Pathologie Cellulaire, Le Kremlin-Bicêtre, France

Pelissier, E. - Hôpital Broussais, Centre de Transfusion, Paris, France

Peters, A.M. - Hammersmith Hospital, Department of Diagnostic Radiology, London, U.K.

Rövekamp, M.H. - Wilhelmina Children Hospital, Department of Surgery, Utrecht, The Netherlands

Royen van, E.A. - Academic Medical Centre, University of Amsterdam, Department of Nuclear Medicine, Amsterdam, The Netherlands

Saverymuttu, S.H. - Hammersmith Hospital, Department of Medicine, London, U.K.

Schbath, J. - Hôpital Neuro-Cardiologique, Unité de Pharmacologie Clinique, Lyon, France

Schmidt, K.G. - Odense University Hospital, Department of Radiophysics, Odense, Denmark

Schoot van der, J.B. - Academic Medical Centre, University of Amsterdam, Department of Nuclear Medicine, Amsterdam, The Netherlands

Sinzinger, H. - University of Vienna, Department of Nuclear Medicine at the 2nd Department of Internal Medicine, Vienna, Austria

Thakur, M.L. - Thomas Jefferson University, Department of Nuclear Medicine, Philadelphia, USA

Vigneron, N. - Hôpital Saint-Louis, Service Central de Médecine Nucléaire, Paris Cedex, France

Voisin, Ph. - Centre Régional de Transfusion Sanguine, Groupe d'hémorhéologie, Vandoeuvre les Nancy, France

Vreeken, J. - Academic Medical Centre, University of Amsterdam, Department of Internal Medicine, Amsterdam, The Netherlands

Wagstaff, J. - Cancer Research Campaign, Christie Hospital, Department of Medical Oncology, Manchester, U.K.

Wahner, H.W. - Mayo Clinic, Section of Diagnostic Nuclear Medicine, Rochester, USA

ACKNOWLEDGEMENTS

After a first Symposium on Radio-labelled Blood-cells, which was held in New York (1979), two others were held in Amsterdam and Paris in 1982.

Presentations from participants in the latter two meetings have been used as a basis to produce this book. Several chapters are modified versions of presentations published in the "Nucleair Geneeskundig Bulletin", Supplement no. 1 (1982).

As neither of the editors have English as their mother language, they would like to thank Dr P.H. Cox, the series editor, for his help in this respect. Furthermore, the editors are grateful to Mrs. M.J.M.C. Busker who prepared the bulk of the manuscript as camera-ready copy.

INTRODUCTION

1 APPROACHES TO RADIOLABELLING BLOOD-CELLS: PAST, PRESENT AND FUTURE

M.L. THAKUR

INTRODUCTION

The importance of cellular blood-elements in health and disease can never be overemphasized. Associated with every organic illness there is an involvement of blood-cells. The view that disturbances in structure or functions of individual cells form the basis of disease was first put forth by Rudolph Virchow in 1858 (1). For decades thereafter our understanding of cellular involvement was limited to the data derived from fixed images of cells under the light microscope. Over the past 25 years interest in blood-cells has intensified and a new and multidisciplinary science of cell pathology has emerged. Advances in optical and cell separation techniques, tissue culture, and in the knowledge of cell function have made it possible to categorize diseases and identify the type of blood-cells involved. These have provided a sound basis for studies with radiolabelled blood-cells, a technique that has become increasingly popular and has served as an effective research tool.

Using radiolabelled blood-cells, researchers have made fundamental contributions in the basic knowledge of cell kinetics and physiology. Further development in cell labelling techniques, in conjunction with the advancements in nuclear imaging have made it possible to use radiolabelled blood-cells as a noninvasive means of diagnosing diseases. Useful as it may be, we have become increasingly aware of the current limitations in the cell labelling technique.

The object of this article is to highlight the past and present approaches to the technique, emphasize the current problems and discuss future directions that might help to provide solutions.

The early approach

Most of the early work with radiolabelled cellular blood-elements was aimed at labelling cells in vivo and determining the cell origin, kinetics and intravascular survival time. Several radioactive chemicals and biochemicals were employed. Broadly these have been classified as a) DNA or cohort labels and b) non-DNA or random labels (2).

Phosphorus-32 ($t_{\frac{1}{2}}$-14.5 d, β^{-}max 1.67 MeV) as sodium phosphate and carbon-14 ($t_{\frac{1}{2}}$-5500Y, β^{-}max 156 keV) labelled nucleic acid precursors such as adenine, guanine, and orotic acid were made available to bone marrow stem cells. The radioactivity thus became an integral part of DNA during maturation of the cell cycle. This provided a true cohort cell label (3). Rubini et al administered tritiated thymidine to humans. They observed that nearly 90% of the radioactivity cleared rapidly from plasma and was associated with the thymidine in the newly formed DNA of proliferating cells. The technique again provided a true cohort cell label. The remaining 10% radioactivity was excreted in the urine (4). This efficient incorporation of thymidine into DNA provides the possibility of labelling cells of uniform age in vivo with a gamma emitting tracer, and using them effectively in noninvasive imaging studies. However, in such an approach cells would be labelled non specifically. Furthermore, the risk of the DNA transformation due to radiation and subsequent genetic consequences may be high.

The biologically active selenium-75 (^{75}Se, $t_{\frac{1}{2}}$-120 d, 265 keV-60% selenomethionine, given intravenously, was reported to label cohort leukocytes, erythrocytes and platelets (4,5,6). Following this work, the agent was given intravenously to 10 health volunteers. Several blood-samples were drawn and erythrocytes, leukocytes and platelets were isolated. The measurement of concomitant radioactivity strongly indicated that there was a considerably reutilization of the radioactivity by the blood-cells. Therefore, although the approach provided a gamma emitting radionuclide as a true cohort cell tracer, ^{75}Se-selenomethionine could not be used reliably (7).

Probably the most reliable and widely used in vivo cell

tracer has been ^{32}P-diisopropylfluorophosphate (DFP-32). Seven years following a report by Grobb et al, that DFP given in vivo binds to erythrocytes, Cohen and Warringa employed DFP-32 as a potential in vivo cell tracer (8,9). When the agent diluted in oil, was administered to humans intramuscularly, the radioactivity appeared in blood within 90 min (9). Approximately 30% of the administered radioactivity was associated with the plasma proteins, erythrocytes, leukocytes and platelets (10). Extensive work, leading to the contribution of the most fundamental information in neutrophil and platelet kinetics has been reported with the use of DFP-32, despite the difficulties associated with the non-specificity, the cell isolation and the ^{32}P-β^-counting (10,11-14). The subsequent reports, however, dealt with the reutilization of the tracer and toxicity of the compound (8,15).

Current approach

Interestingly enough all radioactive compounds explored thereafter were aimed at labelling cellular blood-elements in vitro. These agents were all non-DNA, nonspecific and associated with gamma emitting radionuclides. These include primarily ^{51}Cr ($t_{\frac{1}{2}}$-27d, 320 keV-7% sodium chromate, Tc^{99m} ($t_{\frac{1}{2}}$-6 hour, 140 keV-90%) pertechnetate, other Tc^{99m}-labelled compounds, ^{67}Ga ($t_{\frac{1}{2}}$-78 hour, 93 keV-40%, 184 keV-24%, 296 keV-94%) citrate and ^{111}In ($t_{\frac{1}{2}}$-67 hour, 173 keV-89%, 247 keV-94%) labelled compounds.

The one exception to the in vitro labelling is the in vivo use of Tc^{99m}-pertechnetate. This radionuclide is routinely employed as an efficient erythrocyte tracer, in vivo (16). This provides an excellent tool for gated cardiac blood-pool studies (17). Greater than 90% radioactivity binds to erythrocytes. The percentage of radioactivity associated with other cells such as leukocytes and platelets is not determined. For labelling platelets and leukocytes, however, the cells must be isolated in vitro, and incubated with stannous chloride before Tc^{99m}-pertechnetate is added to the cell suspension (17,18). Tc^{99m} is a short-lived, the least expensive radionuclide, and is available worldwide. It also emits gamma photons, highly efficient for external detection by a gamma camera. For certain applications, involving the use of platelets where serial gamma camera imaging for several days is required, the half-life of Tc^{99m} is considered to be too short. However, for abscess localization studies which have been shown to be feasible between 4 to 18 hours after administration of labelled leukocytes, the use of Tc^{99m} as a tracer should be much prefered. However, a high percentage of spontaneous release of Tc^{99m} activity from labelled cells has withheld the use of this radionuclide for such studies (19).

Considering this spontaneous release of radioactivity may be due to the cell surface labelling, neutrophil labelling by phagocytosis has been investigated. In this technique Tc^{99m}-sulfur colloid or Tc^{99m}-phytate which forms a colloid in the presence of plasma calcium is incubated with a neutrophil suspension (20). The technique was successful in principle but met with several practical difficulties. Unengulfed radioactive particles could not be easily isolated without causing loss of cell viability. Many particles apparently considered engulfed, remained on the cell surface and released radioactivity upon the addition of "cold" colloid particles. A full preservation of the physiologic functions of neutrophils, subsequent to this stimulation remained doubtful. 50 to 80% of cells labelled with Sn-colloid in whole blood, in vitro, and given to patients for example were rapidly accumulated in the liver and spleen (21). This quantity accumulated in these organs is much higher than the quantity of cells labelled with ^{111}In-oxine. This may present cells with altered physiologic functions after phagocytosis. The authors have, however, reported that on 85% of the occasions, diagnosis made using cells labelled by phagocytosis was accurate.

The recent additions of lipid soluble ^{111}In-agents have added a new impetus to the field of radiolabelled blood-cells. One of the agents, namely ^{111}In-8-hydroxy quinoline (^{111}In-oxine), when incubated with a cell suspension in vitro, diffuses passively through the cell membranes and transfers the radioactivity to cyto plasmic components (22). This prevents the spontaneous elution of radioactivity from labelled cells. This, together with the suitability of ^{111}In for external detection have, thus far, made ^{111}In as an indispensable radionuclide in radiolabelled cell imaging studies.

Much has been achieved with platelets, neutrophils and lymphocytes labelled with ^{111}In-oxine (23-25). These studies include locating inflammatory lesions and sites of vascular abnormalities deep in the body. Furthermore, determination of cell kinetics and quantifications of in vivo cell distribution by gamma camera imaging have been also possible (26). However, the fact remains that ^{111}In-oxine cell labelling technique is nonspecific. It requires isolating the desired types of cells from whole blood, in vitro. Also, the compound allows efficient labelling of cells only when suspended in nonplasma media (27). The adverse reactions of these procedures, particularly on human platelets, have been evident (28). These disadvantages of ^{111}In-oxine have lead to the generation of many new ^{111}In-agents such as water soluble ^{111}In-oxinate, ^{111}In-acetyl acetone, and recently ^{111}In-tropolone (29-32). These have been shown to label isolated blood-cells presumably by the same mechanism. Besides limited advantages over each other, however, the agents have been unable to resolve the fundamental problems in today's art of cell labelling.

Future directions

How can the present problems be solved? Shall we a) develop newer and better cell separation techniques and b) design agents that will efficiently label cells in plasma? or c) shall we divert our energy and design agents that will selectively and efficiently label cells in whole blood?

The currently employed cell separation techniques such as sedimentation for harvesting leukocytes, gradient centrifugation for separating lymphocytes, and selective centrifugation for obtaining platelets are all time consuming and inefficient. The sedimentation method for example produces a mixed population of leukocytes, invariably contamined with 5-25% erythrocytes (33). Mixed leukocytes cannot be used for kinetic studies. If such studies are to be performed then neutrophils or lymphocytes must be separated by the density gradient method (24). This exposes neutrophils as well as lymphocytes, for an extended period of time, to a nonphysiologic and nonisotonic medium and still fails to isolate them free of other cells. The subsequent purification steps such as lysis of red cells from a neutrophil preparation and centrifugation have been shown to reduce cell viability (33).

Platelet population in human blood is highly heterogeneous (35). It consists of the young-denser platelets, intermediates, and the old-lighter platelets. The lighter platelets have been shown to have considerably shorter survival (74.6±15.3 hours) than that of younger and denser platelets (313.6±45.3 hours). The centrifugation method probably eliminates the denser, and physiologically more active platelets. Improper centrifugation can cause degranulation and result in obtaining less aggregable platelets (28)

Fluoroscence-activated cell separation techniques designed to isolate pure cells without trauma may be the answer to these problems. Unfortunately, the low rate (approximately 10^4 cells/min) at which the cells can be currently separated, would require 8 to 16 hours to separate $5x10^7$ to 10^8 cells. A number of cells smaller than this will not permit a commonly desired, 60% or higher labelling efficiency. The lengthy period of cell separation, precludes the use of this otherwise excellent cell separation device.

An ability to label cells selectively in whole blood would eliminate most of the problems currently faced in the cell labelling techniques. With a careful combination of cell biology and chemistry, selective cell labelling in whole blood may be feasible Our preliminary investigations in using neutrophil receptors as labelling sites have produced encouraging results (37). Receptor mediated chemoattractivity of certain synthetic peptides is well established (38). Among these, formyl-methionyl-leucyl-phenylalanine (FMLP) was regarded as a most potent agent. We have covalently attached FMLP to plasma transferrin which in turn has served as a strong chelating agent for ^{111}In. The entire molecule remains chemoattractive and labels neutrophils selectively. Previous data have demonstrated the ability of neutrophils to internalize such molecules and yet to respond normally to other chemotactic stimuli (39). This will allow the FMLP^{111}In-transferrin molecule to be a nonsurface, truly internalized, specific tracer for neutrophils, without impairing the cell function. The currently achieved 60% labelling efficiency is far from ideal. However,

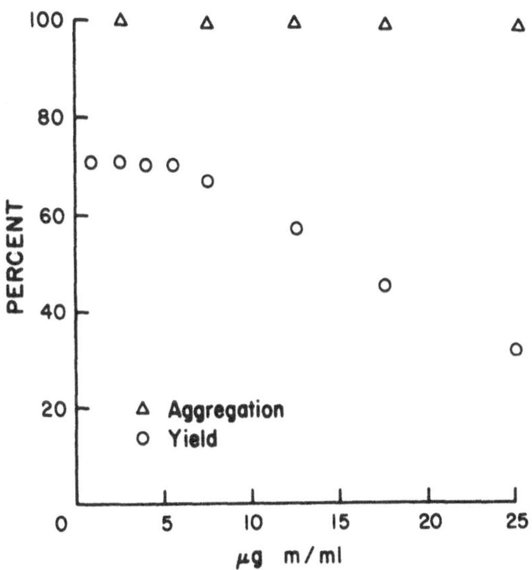

Fig. 1. The figure demonstrates that when $4x10^8$ platelets are suspended in 1 ml plasma and incubated at 37°C for 10 min, with the new ^{111}In-agent, 70% radioactivity is incorporated with the platelets. (Average of 3 experiments). As the concentration of Merc increased beyond 7 µg/ml, the labelling efficiency decreased. However, the aggregability of labelled platelets in relation to the unlabelled control platelets remained unchanged. Labelling efficiencies of up to 90% have been achieved with higher platelet concentration in plasma. Cells such as neutrophils and lymphocytes can also be efficiently labelled in plasma with this agent. This is regarded as an improvement over the currently used ^{111}In-chelates, which do not permit such a high incorporation of radioactivity into cells suspended in plasma.

if enhanced to 90 or higher percent, it would lead to a kit method for labelling neutrophils with ^{111}In, selectively in whole blood. Such labelling of lymphocytes and platelets may be feasible in the future.

In the meantime we have been engaged in developing a new agent that chelates with ^{111}In in aqueous media and labels cells efficiently in plasma (40). In an aqueous medium, the agent chelates ^{111}In almost quantitatively and obviates the need for extracting the radioactive compound free of unbound radioactivity. When incubated with cells in plasma, 70%-90% radioactivity is associated with cells in 15 min. This development has a special importance in the case of labelling human platelets where a variety of salt balanced media are currently used and preservation of platelet physiologic function is constantly questioned. The new agent labels platelets without loss of in vitro aggregability (fig 1) and in vivo survival (7-8 days). The agent, thus warrants further work and promises important improvement in cell labelling techniques.

REFERENCES

1. Virchow R, Die celluläre Pathologie in ihrer Begründung auf physiologische und pathologische Gewebelehre, Berlin 1958.
2. Thakur ML, Gottschalk A, Role of radiopharmaceuticals in Nuclear Hematology. Radiopharmaceuticals II, Soc. of Nucl. Med. New York, pp 349-359, 1979.
3. Perry S, Goodwin HA, Zimmerman TS, Physiology of Granulocytes, part I, Jama 203:937, 1968.
4. Rubini JR, Westcott E, Keller S, In vitro DNA labelling of bone-marrow and leukemia blood leukocytes with tritiated thymidine-II. H-3 thymidine biochemistry, in vitro. J. Lab. clin. Med. 68:566, 1966.
5. Cooley H, Gardner FH, The use of selenomethionine (se-75) as a label for canine and human platelets. Amer. Soc. Clin. Inv. 44:1036, 1965 (abstract).
6. Penner JA, Meyers MC, Methionine-^{75}Se uptake in circulating blood cells and plasma proteins. J. Lab. clin. Med. 68:1005, 1966, (abstract).
7. McIntyre PA, Evatt B, Hodkinson BA et al, Selenium-75, selenomethionine as a label for erythrocytes, leukocytes and platelets in man, J. Lab. clin. Med. 74:472, 1980.
8. Grobb D, Lilienthal JL jr, Harvey AM et al, The administration of Di-isopropyl fluorophosphate (DFP) to man, Bull. Johns Hopk. Hosp. 81:217, 1947.
9. Cohen JA, Warringa MGPJ, The effect of P^{32} labelled diisopropylfluorophosphate in the human body and its use as labelling agent in the study of the turnover of blood plasma and red cells, J. clin. Invest. 33:459, 1954.
10. Leeksma CHW, Cohen JA, Determination of the life span of human platelets using labelled DFP. J. clin. Invest. 35: 964, 1956.
11. Athens JW, Mauer AM, Ashenbrucker H et al, Leukokinetic Studies I, A method for labelling leukocytes with $DF^{32}P$. Blood 14:303, 1959.
12. Mauer AM, Athens JW, Ashenbrucker H et al, Leukocyte kinetics II, a method for labelling granulocytes in vitro with radioactive DFP^{32}. J. clin. Invest. 39:1681, 1960.
13. Athens JW, Haab OP, Raab SO et al, Leukocykinetic studies IV. The total blood, circulating and marginal granulocytes, turnover rate in normal subjects. J. clin. Invest. 40:989, 1961.
14. Raab SO, Athens JW, Haab OP et al, Granulokinetics in normal dogs, Amer. J. Path. 206:83, 1964.
15. Mizuno NS, Perman V, Bates FW et al, Lifespan of thrombocytes and erythrocytes in normal and thrombopenic calves. Blood, 14:708, 1959.

16. Callahan RJ, Froelich JW, McKusick KA et al, A modified method for the in vivo labelling of red blood cells with Tc-99m: concise communication. J. nucl. Med. 23:315, 1982.

17. Berger HJ, Matthay RA, Pytlik LM et al, First-pass radionuclide assessment of right and left ventricular performance in patients with cardiac and pulmonary disease. Semin. Nucl. Med. 9:275, 1979.

18. Uchida T, Tasunaga K, Kaniyone S et al, Survival and sequestration of ^{51}Cr and $^{99m}TcO_4$-labelled platelets. J. nucl. Med. 15:801, 1974.

19. Linhart N, Bok B, Mergman M et al, Technetium-99m labeled human leukocytes: in vitro and animal studies. In: Indium-111 labeled neutrophils, platelets and lymphocytes. Thakur ML, Gottschalk A (eds), Trivirum Pub. Co., New York, pp 69-78, 1980.

20. McAfee J, Thakur ML, Survey of radioactive agents for in vitro labelling of phagocytic leukocytes, II, Particles 488:292, 1976.

21. Oberhausen E, Schroth HJ, Phagocytosis labelling of migratory blood cells and its applications. Labelled migratory blood cells. Third World Congress, Post Congress Symposium, Graz, 1982.

22. Thakur ML, Segal AW, Louis L et al, Indium-111 labelled cellular blood components, Mechanism of labelling and intracellular location in human neutrophils. J. nucl. Med. 18:1020, 1977.

23. Thakur ML, Gottschalk A (eds), Indium-111 labeled neutrophils, platelets and lymphocytes, Trivirum Pub. Co. New York, 1980.

24. Cell labelling with gamma emitting radionuclide for in vivo study, Proc. Brit. Inst. of Radiol. Brit. J. Radiol. 53:922, 1980.

25. This volume.

26. Klonizakis I, Peters AM, Fitzpatrick ML et al, Radionuclide distribution following injection of ^{111}In-labelled platelets. Brit. J. Haemat. 46:595, 1980.

27. Thakur ML, Coleman RE, Welch MJ, Indium-111 labelled human leukocytes for abscess localization; preparation, analysis, tissue distribution and comparison with Ga-67 citrate in dogs. J. Lab. clin. Med. 89:217, 1977.

28. Thakur ML, Walsh L, Malech HL et al, Indium-111 labelled human platelets; improved method, efficacy and evaluation. J. nucl. Med. 22:381, 1981.

29. Goedemans WTH, Simplified cell labelling with In-111 acetylacetone and Indium-111 oxinate. Brit. J. Radiol. 54:636, 1981.

30. Sinn H, Silvester DJ, Simplified cell labelling with In-111 acetylacetone. Brit. J. Radiol. 52:758, 1979.

31. Dewanjee MK, Rao SH, Didisheim P, Indium-111 tropolone, a new high affinity platelet label; preparation and evaluation of labelling parameters. J. nucl. Med. 22:981, 1981.

32. Danpure HJ, Osman S, Brady F, The labelling of blood cells in plasma with ^{111}In-tropolonate. Brit. J. Radiol. 543-247, 1982.

33. Thakur ML, Lavender JP, Arnot RN et al, Indium-111 labeled leukocytes in man. J. nucl. Med. 18:1012, 1977.

34. Boyum A, Isolation of mononuclear cells from granulocytes from human blood. Scan. J. clin. Invest. 21:97, suppl. 1968.

35. Corash L, Shafer B, Perlow M, Heterogeneity of human whole blood platelet subpopupations II. Use of subhuman primate model tot analyze the relationship between density and platelet age. Blood 52:726, 1978.

36. Herzenberg LA, Sweet RG, Fluorescence-activated cell sorting. Scientific American 232:108, 1978.

37. Zoghbi SS, Thakur ML, Gottschalk A et al, Selective cell labelling; a potential radioactive agent for labelling of human neutrophils. J. nucl. Med. 22:32, 1981 (abstract).

38. Schiffman E, Corioran BA, Wahl SM, Formylmethionyl peptides as chemoattractants for leukocytes. Proc. Nat. Acad. Sci. USA 72:1059, 1975.

39. Goldstein IM, Chemotactic factor receptors on leukocytes; scratching the surface (editorial). J. Lab. clin. Med. 97:599, 1981.

40. Thakur ML, Barry MJ, Preparation and evaluation of a new indium-111 agent for efficient labelling of human platelets in plasma. 4th Internat. Symp. on Radiopharm. Chem. pp 140-142, Jülich, 1982.

CELL LABELLING TECHNIQUES

2 LABELLING TECHNIQUES OF GRANULOCYTES AND PLATELETS WITH ^{111}IN-OXINATE

M.R. HARDEMAN, E.G.J. EITJES-VAN OVERBEEK, A.J.M. VAN VELZEN, M.H. RÖVEKAMP

INTRODUCTION

In principle, with the ^{111}In-oxinate method as described here all types of cells present in the incubation mixture are labelled. The non-specific labelling can impede a sensitive detection due to a high background, in spite of the fact that the body will select the correct cell type from the labelled mixture by using specific cell functions in certain pathological processes (e.g. the chemotaxis of granulocytes into an abscess). It is clear that among the cells present in whole blood the erythrocytes by virtue of their numerical abundance bind the major part of the radioactivity present, so that they give a high background compared with the thrombocytes and/or leukocytes. In order to make the investigation more efficient, one should therefore enrich the preparation with the cell type concerned, e.g. a thrombocyte suspension for the detection of (arterial) thromboses, aneurysms, or the rejections of kidney transplants, a granulocyte suspension for the localization of abscesses and inflammatory reactions, and an erythrocyte suspension for the determination of the blood volume and localization of gastro-intestinal hemorrhage. Depending on the type of study, single or multiple centrifuging is often sufficient for the separation. There is a danger that further separation steps may damage the cells, whereby a relatively pure cell preparation is obtained, but one that, because of the loss of a relevant cell function, is of little value for in-vivo use. For example, defibrination of blood for the selective elimination of thrombocytes is a very harsh process, which may also affect the function and/or the viability and yield of other types of cells. The selective hypotonic lysis of erythrocytes also appears not to be all that selective: the granulocytes contained in the mixture remain present (i.e. microscopically discernible), but their phagocytosis capacity is considerable, reduced (1).

Generally speaking, therefore, one must compromise between a minimum handling of the cells required for the in-vivo investigation and the purity of the final cell suspension, and the cell-separation methods described below must be viewed in this light.

Further diagnostic possibilities include in-vivo cell-survival investigations. Theoretically, this kind of in-vivo study in particular requires pure preparations in order not to complicate the kinetics, but in practice the life-times of erythrocytes (120 days), thrombocytes (8-10 days) and granulocytes (half-life 5-6 h) differ so widely that any effect e.g. on the thrombocyte kinetics due to a small admixture of erythrocytes in the preparation to be labelled will be limited to a minor residual activity after 8-10 days, which will run approximately parallel to the time base and on which the thrombocyte survival curve will be superimposed. In contrast, any admixture of labelled granulocytes would especially affect the initial phase of the thrombocyte survival curve. This should be borne in mind when one is particularly interested in the kinetics of reversible storage in the spleen undergone by many thrombocytes during the first few hours after the injection. Regarding erythrocytes, the relative short half-life of ^{111}In, compared to the life-span of these cells, makes this nuclide less suitable for red cell survival studies; in this case it is advisable to use the "classical" cell label ^{51}Cr.

Apart from the presence of competing cell types, the plasma proteins (mainly transferrin) give rise to high (non-specific) background activity. Some workers accept this, but in our experience it was necessary to centrifuge and resuspend the cells in a protein free physiological saline prior to labelling. In particular, thrombocytes can present problems through the appearance aggregation if particular steps of the procedure have been omitted (see below).

During the entire procedure from blood collection until the injection of the preparation, three sets of safety criteria must be satisfied:

a) Radiation protection: this involves to the normal safety precautions for the handling of radioactive materials.

b) Sterility: this means that all the procedures must be conducted in a closed system unless a laminar-flow cabinet is available. All surfaces, including the skin of the patient, to be pierced by needles must be sterilized beforehand. Each cell preparation should be sampled for a microbiological check.

c) Cell viability: care should be taken to prevent cell damage as much as possible, such as might occur as a result of the isolation technique. Rapid collection through thin needles may place severe shear stress on the cells, leading to irreversible damage. The use of whirl mixers for resuspending the packed cells has also been known to be detrimental. The final preparation should not contain any aggregated cells.

The procedure that will be discussed below, applies to work carried out in a closed system. The facility of a laminar flow cabinet is not a necessity but if available, some parts of the procedure can be conducted more easily. Unless otherwise stated, all procedures are carried out at roomtemperature.

Materials

ACD-A

PBS

Methylcellulose, BDH, high substitution, 2% solution in physiological saline filtered cold (3 μm) and sterilized ^{111}In-oxinate, Byk-Mallinckrodt CIL B.V., Petten, The Netherlands.

Tris buffer, 0.2 M, pH 8.0.

Vials with screw-cap and rubber septum, 30 ml, sterile.

Blood collection set, 1.2 mm diameter needle.

Short air outlets.

Abbreviations:

ACD acid citrate dextrose
PPP platelet-poor plasma
PRP platelet-rich plasma
PLRP platelet-leukocyte-rich plasma
PBS phosphate-buffered saline (pH 7,4) consisting of an aqueous solution of: 0,82% NaCl, 0,16 Na_2HPO_4, 0,02% $NaH_2PO_4 \cdot 2H_2O$.

Spinal needles (B-D, needle 75-12 18G3).
Syringes, tuberculin and 2-5-10 ml.
Culture and counting tubes.
Dose calibrator.
Micro-hematocrit centrifuge, capillaries and sealing wax.
Glassware, sterilized, free from grease and non-siliconized.

Collection of blood

This is done with the aid of blood collection set including a needle with a diameter of 1.2 mm; closed sterile 30 ml vials, containing 5 ml of ACD and provided with an air outlet are used. 25 ml blood is collected into each of these vials and mixed gently during and after collection.

In view of the optimal maintenance of cell viability, ACD is the preferred anticoagulant for subsequent in-vivo studies. Where an additional in-vitro examination is required (cell count, blank radioactivity measurement, haematocrit determination, etc.), the contents of the collection tubing can be collected in a vial with EDTA.

Thrombocyte isolation

The procedure is depicted in fig. 1. Collect 2 x 30 ml of ACD-blood from the patient, remove the air traps and centrifuge both vials with ACD-blood for 20 min at 130 g; for a normal clinical bench centrifuge with a radius of approximately 13 cm (centre of tube to spindle) this corresponds to about 800 rpm. Allow the centrifuge to come to rest without the use of a brake and carefull introduce new air outlets. Remove the supernatant PRP with the aid of 10 ml syringes with spinal needles and place into 2 new vials provided with air outlets. Using ACD, adjust the pH of the PRP to 6.5. This step is fairly critical; under normal conditions 0.7-0.9 ml of ACD is required for every 10 ml of PRP. 1 ml of the acidifie PRP is transferred to a small counting tube which can be used to test the pH and the thrombocyte count. If required, the pH can be further adjusted with more ACD. The viability of the thrombocytes decreases rapidly at pH values lower than 6.5. Centrifuge the cell for 10 min at 500 g (approximately 2000 rpm). After the vials have

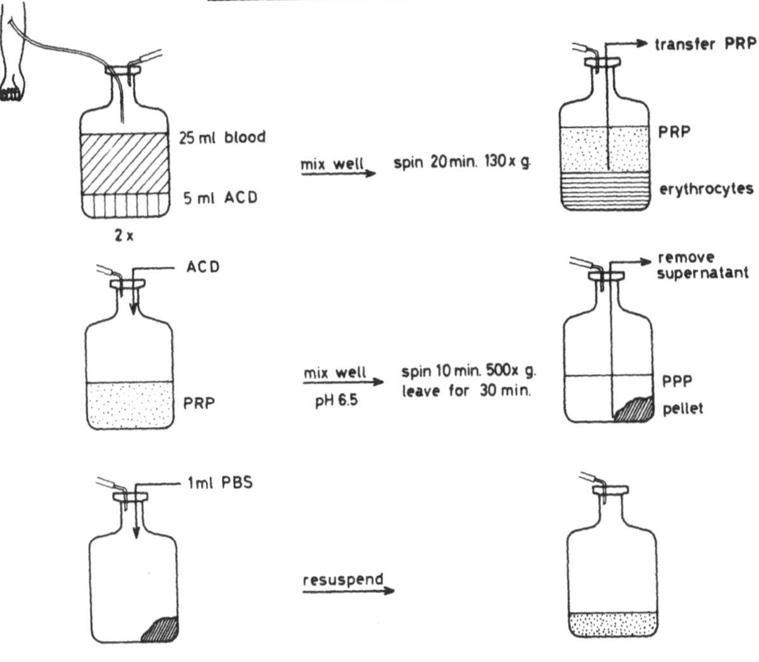
ISOLATION PROCEDURE FOR PLATELETS
transfer PRP
25 ml blood
PRP
mix well
spin 20 min. 130 x g.
5 ml ACD
erythrocytes
2 x
ACD
remove
supernatant
mix well
pH 6.5
spin 10 min. 500x g.
leave for 30 min.
PPP
PRP
pellet
1ml PBS
resuspend

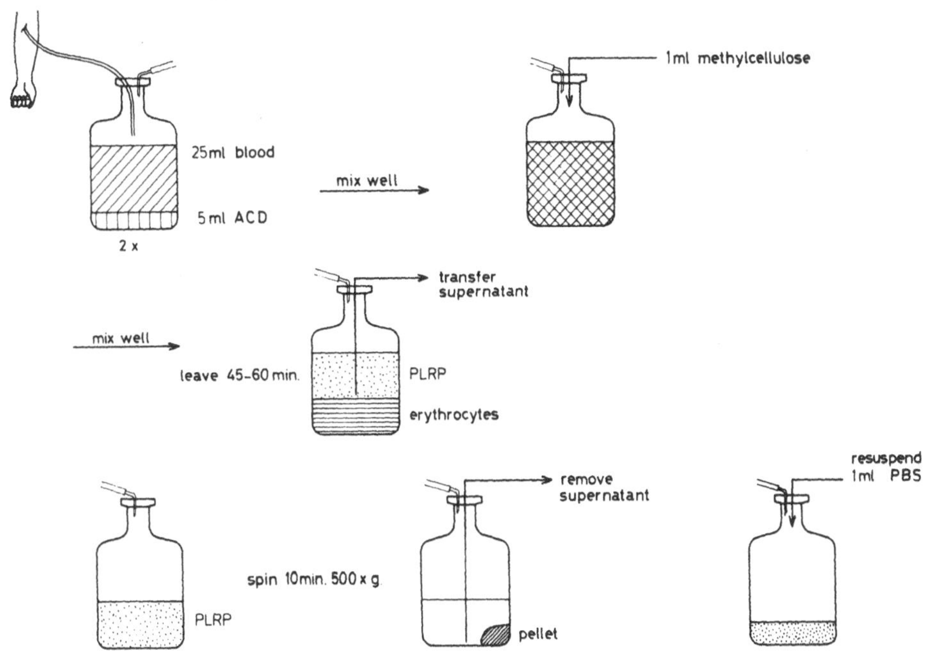
ISOLATION PROCEDURE FOR GRANULOCYTES
1ml methylcellulose
25ml blood
mix well
5ml ACD
2 x
transfer
supernatant
mix well
leave 45-60 min.
PLRP
erythrocytes
resuspend
1ml PBS
remove
supernatant
spin 10min. 500 x g.
PLRP
pellet

come to rest, without using the brake, they should be left to stand for 30-45 min. Although not fully understood, this rest phase, which may involve an enzymatic breakdown of ADP, has been shown in practice to facilitate resuspension of the thrombocytes and gives rise to less irreversible aggregation. The next step is removal of the supernatant PPP with a spinal needle, so that a virtually dry pellet remains at the bottom of the vial. A small quantity of the PPP from both vial in transferred into one culture tube for a sterility check, while the remainder of the PPP is kept in another sterile vial in case it proves necessary to resuspend the cells if the labelling efficiency is low (see under Quality Control). Both thrombocyte pellets are resuspended in 1.0 ml of PBS by gentle shaking. In this way a thrombocyte suspension can be prepared that is rather pure i.e. with a negligable contamination of erythrocytes and leukocytes. The final cell concentration is important for adequate labelling efficiency. With this protocol th final platelet concentration (using normal blood) is about $10^{12}/1$, which may yield an ultimate labelling efficiency of 90% (2) when other incubation conditions are also optimal (see under "labelling").

Leukocyte (granulocyte) isolation

The procedure is depicted in fig. 2. Collect 2 x 30 ml of ACD-blood from the patient and add 1 ml of methylcellulose solution to each vial. Mix gently with a minimum formation of froth, and leave the vials to stand for 45-60 min, allowing the bulk of the aggregated erythrocytes to precipitate. Aspirate the major part of the supernatant (granulocyte- and thrombocyte-rich plasma) from both vials with the aid of syringe and a spinal needle, and transfer it to one new 30 ml vial provided with an air trap.

After removing the air trap, centrifuge the vial for 10 min at 500 g. For a normal clinical bench centrifuge with a radius of approximately 13 cm (centre of tube to spindle), this corresponds to some 1800 rpm. After the centrifuge has stopped without the use of a brake, a new air outlet is carefully connected and the maximum amount of plasma is aspirated, again using a syringe and spinal needle. This plasma is sampled for a bacterial culture. The cell pallet containing granulocytes and a number of erythrocytes and thrombocytes is then carefully resuspended in 2 ml of PBS. There will be almost none residual methylcellulose left in the final preparation, however, since this component might provoke allergic reactions, it is recommended not to use it in cases where is known on forehand that the blood has a high erythrocyte sedimentation rate. Alternatively, similar substances like dextran or hydroxyethyl starch (3) could be used.

With this procedure a mixed cell preparation is obtained; the cellular composition as well as the percentage of total radioactivity bound to each cell type are shown in table 1. Further purification is possible, however, the risk for additional mechanical and/or chemical damage of the cells will, as has been stated before, also increase. Moreover, the active involvement of platelets in abscesses, using pure ^{111}In-oxinate labelled platelets, has been demonstrated (4). Finally, the suitability of mixed cell preparations, prepared according to this protocol, has been demonstrated recently for the clinical detection of inflammatory processes (5).

Table 1. Cell type bound activity in relation to the cellular composition of 10 consecutive cell suspension

	% of total cell bound activity (mean ± s.d.)	% of total cell count (mean ± s.d.)
leucocytes	64.1 ± 20.2*	21.9 ± 8.8
red blood cells	24.1 ± 16.4	28.0 ± 6.8
platelets	11.8 ± 6.0	50.3 ± 12.0

*Granulocytes 37.4 ± 12.3; Lymphocytes 24.8 ± 13.5

Labelling

To obtain a final pH 7.0, shortly before use, 0.35 ml sterile Tris-buffer is added to the ^{111}In-oxinate solution which is now ready for use. A quantity of the lipophylic oxinate complex, corresponding to the required dose of radioactivity (normally between 100-500 μCi) is transferred with the aid of a tuberculin syringe to the vial with the cell suspension and mixed carefully. After 20-30 min samples are taken from the vial, using a tuberculin syringe and a spinal needle (+ air outlet):

- about 0.05 ml into a culture tube from bacteriological testing,
- about 0.15 ml into a counting tube for cell counts and determination of the labelling percentage.

Determination of the percentage labelling

This is done by the micro-haematocrit method. The labelled cell suspension is introduced into 3 haematocrit capillaries which are then closed on one side with sealing wax. To avoid contamination of the sealing wax with the radioactivity adhering to the outside of the capillaries, the end of the capillary that has not been in contact with the cell suspension is pushed into the sealing wax whereafter the outside of the capillaries is cleaned with paper tissue moistened with a decontaminant liquid. After centrifuging for 3 min in a haematocrit centrifuge, the capillaries are cut with a glass-saw just above the packed cells, and the separated end are placed in counting tubes. The percentage labelling can be estimated in the dose calibrator, to be repeated more accurately in a later stage with the aid of a gamma counter.

$$\text{Percentage of labelling} = \frac{\text{activity in cell-fraction}}{\text{activity in cell-fraction} + \text{activity in supernatant}} \times 100$$

Quality control of the cell preparation

Beside cell labelling efficiency, sterility testing should also be performed, although the results will be known after the event. In addition to a macroscopic inspection for aggregates, a cell count and eventually also the leukocyte differential count may be performed. If the labelling efficiency for some reason or the other is found to be low e.g. 65%, resulting in a diminished sensitivity of the subsequent scintigraphy due to background activity, the incubation could be prolonged for a while at room-temperature or at 37°C. If this does not increase the amount of cell bound activity, a final wash step, risking additional cell damage, can be considered. If aggregates remain visible macroscopically, also after prolonged incubation with gentle shaking, the preparation should be discarded. A very serious problem is the lack of relevant and suitable in-vitro viability and/or functionality tests for the various cell types. One ought to have information about these parameters for a proper interpretation of the scintigraphic results e.g. a negative scan could mean either non-adequate functioning labelled cells that do not recognise a certain pathological site or well-functioning cells but no pathological region. Dealing with granulocytes, the in-vitro measurement of chemotaxis has been shown to correlate with the in-vivo behaviour of these cells (6,7) (fig. 3). The technique, however, is cumbersome and thus not suitable for routine application in these studies, although it has been very valuable in the evaluation of various

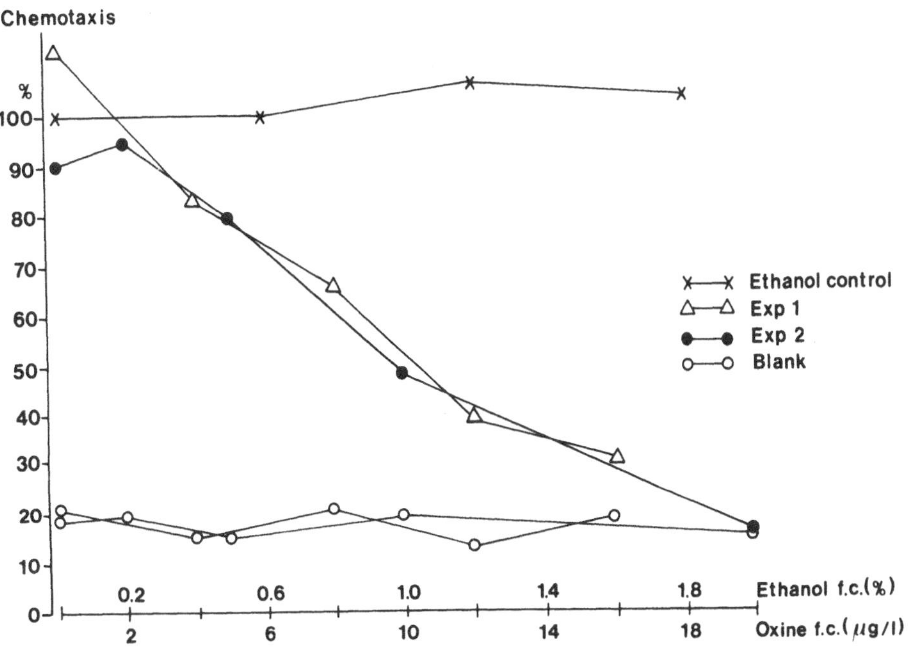

Fig. 3. The influence of different oxine- and/or ethanol concentrations on granulocyte chemotaxis. Due to the fact that these experiments date back to the time when "home-made" ^{111}In-oxinate complexes were used, an ethanol-control experiment, without oxine, was also included. The experiments were performed in co-operation with Dr D. Roos, Dept. of Cell Biochemistry, Central Lab. of the Bloodtransfusion Service, Amsterdam.

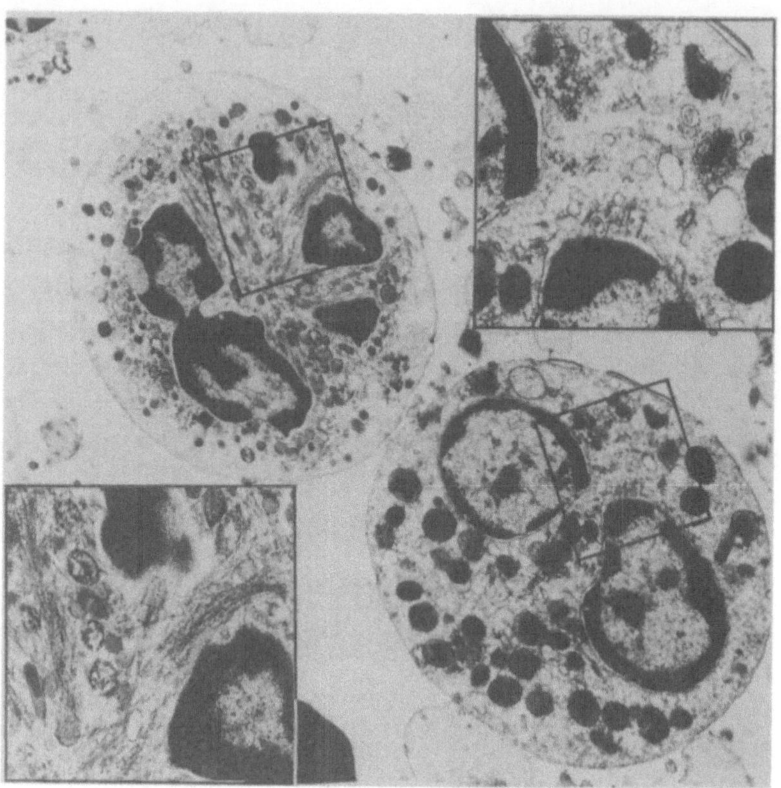

Fig. 4. Electron-micrograph of a neutrophilic (top, left and eosinophilic granulocyte (below, right), taken from a granulocyte suspension, treated with 20 µg/ml oxinate and fixed with glutaraldehyde. "Needle"-like structures can be seen in the neutrophilic granulocyte (see also insert, below left) Magn. 9700.

methodological variations. For the moment no other in-vitro granulocyte function test has been proven to be of value in predicting a potential successful abscess detection.

At final oxinate concentration of 20 µg/ml cell suspension, chemotaxis was inhibited completely; electron micrographs of these cells demonstrated the existence of some kind of needles inside the ^{111}In-oxinate labelled neutro-philic granulocytes (fig. 4). Control preparations, treated in the same way, but without oxine, did not show this phenomenon. It is still an intriguing question whether these needles have something to do with the impaired chemotaxis!

Regarding thrombocytes, the situation is even worse. In many studies the maintenance of their capacity to aggregate in-vitro has been used as a measure for their in-vivo function and/or viability. There are, however, several objections against the relevancy of this parameter, regarding the predictive value for the in-vivo behaviour of these cells. In the first place it has to be recalled that the aggregation response is strongly dependent upon the concentration of the applied stimulating agent e.g. ADP. Apart from the possible influence of the various substances used in platelet labelling, the procedure as such, involving pletting and resuspension considerably impairs the aggregation sensitivity. By increasing the amount of stimilus up to unphysiological amounts, platelets can often be brought to aggregation again; it is, however, questionable whether this has any significance in the evaluation of the in-vivo behaviour of these cells. Another indication that in-vitro aggregation does not necessarily reflect in-vivo survival is the fact that in platelet-storage experiments, the optimal storage temperature for the maintenance of their aggregability, viz. 4°C (8) is not the same as that required for the best survival of the infused platelets, 22°C (9). Moreover, platelets that had completely lost their aggregation response to ADP, recovered the ability to aggregate (in-vitro) in the same way as fresh platelets, 8 hours after transfusion (into a patient with aplastic anemia). Most convincing, however, are the positive scans, found by us and others (10) in patients with active thrombotic processes, like aneurysms aortae treated with aspirine before and injected with ^{111}In-labelled platelets, showing a completely blocked in-vitro secondary aggregation (tested before the labelling procedure). Fortunately, in-vivo recovery and survival measurements have proven that it is possible, using a strict protocol, to isolate and label blood cells with ^{111}In-oxinate without the introduction of important defects. Nevertheless, new relevant and suitable in-vitro tests for both granulocytes and platelets are urgently needed!

REFERENCES

1. Thakur ML, Lavender JP, Arnot RN, Silvester DJ, Segal AW, J. nucl. Med. 18: 1014, 1977.
2. Schmidt KG, Rasmussen JW, Scand. J. Haemat. 23:97, 1979.
3. Weiblen BJ, Forstrom L, McCullough J, J. Lab. clin. Med. 94:246, 1979.
4. Hawker RJ, Hall CE, Thromb. Haemost. 46:433, 1981.
5. Rövekamp MH,Thesis, University of Amsterdam, 1982.
6. Hardeman MR, In: Disease Evaluation and Patient Assessment in Rheumatoid Arthritis, Stafleu's Scientific Publ. Co. Alphen ad Rijn, Brussels, 1979.
7. Hardeman MR, Brit. J. Radiol. 53:927, 1980.
8. Murphy S, Gardner FH, New Engl. J. Med. 280:1094, 1969.
9. Shively JA, Gott CL, De Jongh SD, Vox Sang. Basel, 18:204, 1970.
10. Vreeken J et al, This volume.

3 ^{111}INDIUM LABELLING OF HUMAN WASHED PLATELETS; KINETICS AND IN VIVO SEQUESTRATION SITES

M. EBER, J.P. CAZENAVE, J.C. GROB, J. ABECASSIS, G. METHLIN

INTRODUCTION

The measurement of survival, tissue distribution and sites of destruction of human platelets is considered to be of some use to differentiate platelet disorders, to understand thrombosis and to evaluate the effects of drugs on platelets (1). The introduction of ^{111}Indium (2) as a radioactive platelet label was a major improvement in comparison to the generally used ^{51}Chromium (3). ^{111}Indium is a gamma emitter with an energy favorable for external detection by a gamma camera. Furthermore, in the absence of transferrin, ^{111}Indium complexed to 8-hydroxyquinoline provides a very high efficiency labelling of about 80 to 90% (4). The labelling in nonplasmatic medium makes it necessary to wash platelets in conditions such that their discoid shape and their functions are not lost. Mustard's technique for washing human platelets is known to fulfil these conditions (5). Joist and Thakur (4) demonstrated that rabbit platelets, washed with a similar technique and labelled with ^{111}Indium-oxine remain non activated and survive normally when reinjected to the animals.

We have modified Mustard's method for labelling human platelets using prostacyclin as a platelet inhibitor instead of apyrase (6). The influence of oxine concentration on platelet function, the labelling efficiency and the in vivo kinetics of labelled platelets in normal subjects and in asplenic patients has been studied. The results and their comparison with other published data suggest that the in vivo behaviour, recirculation, organ distribution and survival of ^{111}Indium-labelled platelets is related to the shape and function of the injected platelets.

Materials and methods

A. Materials

1. Sterile plastics. All manipulations of blood-plasma and platelets are done with sterile plastic materials: 50 ml conical Corning tubes (Ref. 11134); 15 ml conical Corning tubes (Ref. 11132); plastic pipets Pastette (Ref. 4504175, Biolyon, France); Eppendorf tips; 18/10 gauge needle fitted to plastic tubing.

2. Centrifuge. Centrifuges (Jouan or Sorvall RC-3B) are pre-warmed at 37° C.

3. Aggregometer. A two-channel Payton aggregometer (Ref. 207-10001, Dade, France) connected to a two-channel recorder is used.

4. Radioactivity measurement. A well type automatic gamma camera (Ultrogamma II, LKB). Multi crystals external counting system with a magnetic tape recorder (Cardio 4, SAIP, France). Gamma camera (Picker, France) fitted with a high energy collimator and connected to an one line computer (Informatek, France) was used.

B. Reagents

1. Reagents to prepare washed human platelets.

a) Anticoagulant. Acid citrate dextrose (ACD) solution is prepared sterile and apyrogen according to the formula of Aster and Jandl (7): trisodium citrate, 2 H_2O 2.5 g; citric acid, H_2O 1.4 g; D(+)-glucose anhydrous 2 g; H_2O q.s. 100 ml (pH 4.5; 250 mOsm). To collect blood, use 1 vol of ACD to 6 vols of blood (final pH is 6.5, citrate 22 mM).

b) Tyrode-albumine solution. Tyrode solution is prepared sterile and apyrogen from stock solutions.

Stock I : NaCl 16 g; Kcl 0.4 g; $NaHCO_3$ 2 g; NaH_2PO_4, H_2O 0.116 g; H_2O q.s. 100 ml.

Stock II : $MgCl_2$, $6H_2O$ 2.03 g; H_2O q.s. 100 ml.

Stock III: $CaCl_2$, $6H_2O$ 2.19 g; H_2O q.s. 100 ml.

Mix stock I 5 ml; stock II 1 ml; stock III 2 ml; human sterile albumine 200 g/l (Centre de Transfusion de Strasbourg) 1.75 ml; D(+)-glucose 0.1 g; H_2O q.s. 100 ml. pH is adjusted to 7.3 and osmolarity to 295 mOsm.

c) Prostacyclin (PGI_2). Prostacyclin sodium salt (U-53217 A,

Upjohn Co, Kalamazoo MI, USA) is prepared as a 1 mM stock solution in Tris buffer 0.05 M (Tris HCl 1.23 g; Tris Base 5.13 g; H_2O q.s. 1 l; pH 9.36 at 4°C). It is sterilized by filtration on Millipore filters (0,22 μpore size), distributed sterily in 0.1 ml aliquots and kept at -30°C for at least 6 months.

2. Radioactive products. ^{111}Indium oxinate (Ref. IN-15P) and ^{3}H-5-hydroxytryptamine (Ref. TRK 223) were obtained from Amersham and ^{125}I-albumine (Ref. SARI 125 A_2) from CIS, France.

3. Platelet aggregating agents (6). ADP (Ref. A-0127) and collagen (C-9879 was from Sigma. Bovine thrombin (Ref. 4010) was from Roche.

C. Preparation of ^{111}In-labelled washed human platelets. The method used to prepare washed labelled human platelets for survival studies is a modification of the method developed by Mustard and collaborators (5). To be injected in humans, the platelet suspension has to be prepared in a sterile way, under a laminar flow hood. Apyrase is omitted and replaced prostacyclin (6), a short lasting but powerful inhibitor of platelet functions. Human albumin is included instead of bovine albumin.

Blood is taken from a forearm vein through a transfusion set needle 18/10, the first 2 ml are discarded and the second needle is punched through the sterile cork of the 50 ml Corning conical plastic tube. The blood (42.5 ml) flows directly into the ACD (7.5 ml). It is kept at 37°C in a water bath until it is centrifuged at 37°C, at 175 g (middle of the tube) for 15 min. Platelet-rich plasma (PRP) is removed with a sterile Pastette into a 50 ml tube and centrifuged at 1570 g for 10 to 14 min (for 15 to 35 ml of PRO). The platelet-poor plasma (PPP) is removed carefully and completely to avoid any thrombin generation later on. The platelet pellet is resuspended in the first 10 ml Tyrode-albumin washing solution containing PGI_2 (1 μM). The suspension is kept at 37°C for 5 min and 100 μl of ^{111}Indium-oxine solution is added (final oxine concentration is 0.5 μg/ml). 10 μl of the suspension are removed (aliquot 1). The suspension is incubated at 37°C for 15 min, then centrifuged at 1100 g for 7 min. The supernatant is totally discarded, the pellet resuspended in 10 ml Tyrode-albumin and kept 5 min at 37°C. The suspension is then ready for injection. 10 µl are removed (aliquot 2). 500 µl are removed and used for platelet counting and the remaining is diluted to measure platelet aggregation induced by ADP, collagen and thrombin.

D. In vitro platelet function studies. Platelet aggregation is studied at 37°C using a turbidimetric device (8). For release studies, platelets are prelabelled in the first washing solution with ^{3}H-5-hydroxytryptamine and release into the suspending fluid is measured 3 min after addition of an aggregating agent as described previously (8). Uptake and storage of ^{3}H-5-hydroxytryptamine are studied as described (9).

E. In vivo kinetics and distribution of ^{111}In-labelled platelets. 10 ml of ^{111}In-labelled platelet suspension in Tyrode-albumin (about 100 µCi) are injected, the gamma camera head being in posterior abdominal incidence. A dynamic acquisition of 20 min (40 images of 30 sec duration) is performed. Immediately at the end, 2 static views are obtained in the anterior and posterior abdominal incidence. Each day, for 8 days, the same static views are obtained. 3 regions of interest are selected, corresponding to the projection area of the spleen, the liver and the heart. The computer calculates the time activity curves of the data acquired in these regions during the 20 min after injection of the platelets and also the total radioactive counts in these selected areas.

Every day, following the gamma camera examination, a 5 ml blood-sample is drawn on EDTA. The radioactivity is measured in a well-type γ counter, on a 3 ml sample of whole blood and on 0.5 ml of platelet-poor plasma, obtained after centrifugation in an Eppendorf centrifuge at 9980 g for 3 min. The blood-volume is estimated at the end of the study by measuring the plasma volume with 5 µCi of ^{125}I-albumin, corrected by the hematocrit measured in a capillary tube by centrifugation of venous blood. The radioactivity of each sample is expressed as per cent recovery of the total injected activity, taking into account the measured total blood-volume. To estimate mean survival, the experimental data are subjected to computer analysis. The program was kindly supplied by Dr E.A. Murphy, Johns Hopkins University, Baltimore. 3 mathematical models were used for curve fitting: a linear model, an exponential model, and a maximum likelihood estimate of the integer-ordered gamma function. For each estimate of the survival time, the residual mean square (RMS) was evaluated as a measure of the precision of the curve fitting. These standard methods of curve analysis have been described in detail by Murphy's group (10,11).

F. Subjects studied. 8 healthy male volunteers ranging from 28 to 39 years were studied. No drugs had been taken for the last 10 days and during the study. Half of them were studied with the gamma camera, the other half with the multicrystal external counting system. Among the 8 subjects, 6 received autologous non activated disc-shaped platelets and 2 autologous activated spherocytic platelets. In addition 3 asplenic patients (2 splenectomy, 1 functional asplenia) were studied.

Results

1. Influence of the concentration of oxine on the aggregation of washed human platelets. Fig 1 shows that increasing the concentration of oxine, the carrier of ^{111}In through the platelet membrane, results in inhibition of platelet aggregation induced by ADP, collagen and thrombin. Collagen is the most sensitive and is already completely inhibited by 2 to 5 µg/ml of oxine. In the following platelet survival studies, all the suspensions were labelled at a concentration of oxine not greater than 0.5 µg/ml, a concentration which does not inhibit aggregation by collagen, ADP or thrombin.

2. Labelling of platelets with ^{111}In-oxine. In preliminary studies, the rate of ^{111}In-oxine uptake was studied in the suspensions of washed human platelets. Fig 2 shows, in 2 preparations, that labelling at 37°C is a fast process which is maximum at 10 min. The labelling efficiency at 10 min is about 90%. For further experiments, it was decided to incubate the platelets with ^{111}In-oxine for 10 min at 37°C. ^{111}In labels

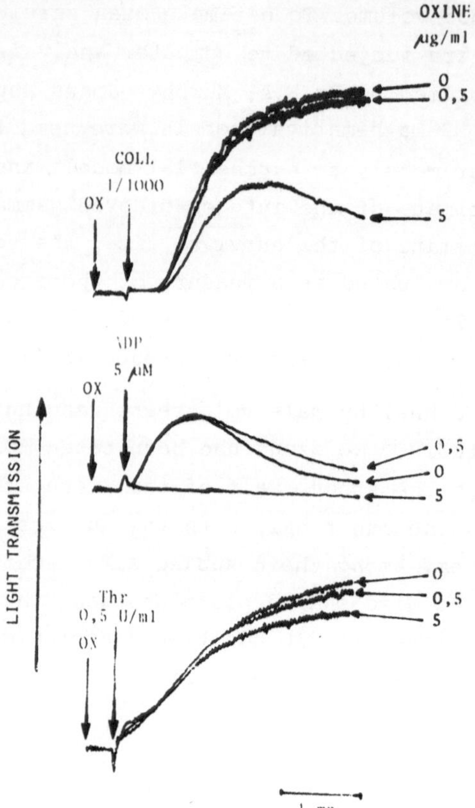

Fig. 1. Effect of oxine on aggregation of washed human platelets induced by collagen, ADP or thrombin.

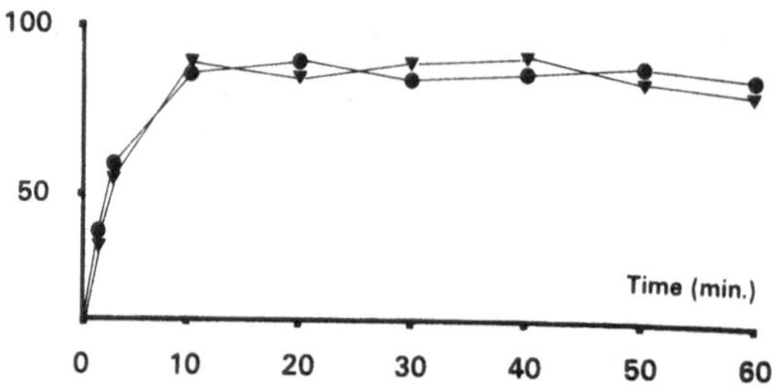

Fig. 2. Kinetics of uptake of the ^{111}In-oxine complex (final oxine concentration is 0.5 g/ml) by washed human platelets in 2 typical experiments.

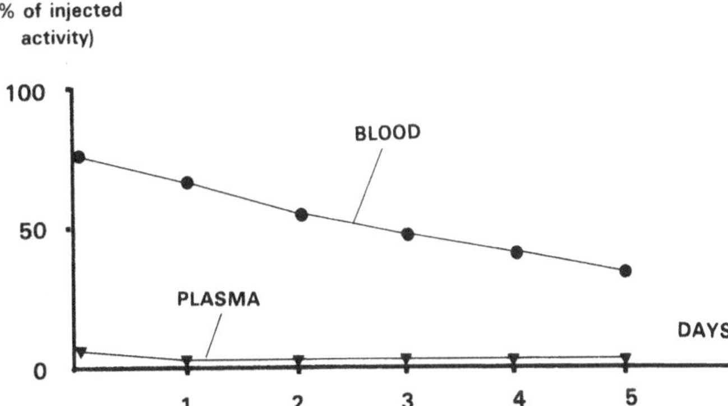

Fig. 3. Typical survival curve of ^{111}In-labelled platelets injected into a normal subject. Blood-radioactivity is measured in the whole blood-sample collected on EDTA. After centrifugation in an Eppendorf centrifuge, the radioactivity is also determined in platelet-poor plasma.

Table 1. In vivo kinetics of autologous ^{111}In-labelled platelets in normal subjects.

	% recovery	Linear Regression		Logarithmic Regression		Gamma Function		Weighted Mean in days
		M.L.S.	R.	M.L.S.	R.	M.L.S.	R.	
1	70.0	8.0	0.019	4.7	10.4	8.0	0.027	8.0
2	61.0	8.9	15.2	4.9	10.5	6.7	1.2	6.6
3	66.3	8.5	18.5	4.4	41.5	7.2	3.7	7.3
4	60.0	8.2	6.1	4.8	18.0	7.3	0.83	7.3
5	67.0	9.4	24.5	4.7	8.4	8.2	7.65	8.4
6	66.7	9.8	4.0	5.9	12.9	9.1	2.5	8.7
Mean	65.2	8.8	-	4.9	-	7.6	-	7.7

M.L.S. = Mean life span in days
R. = Residual sum of squares

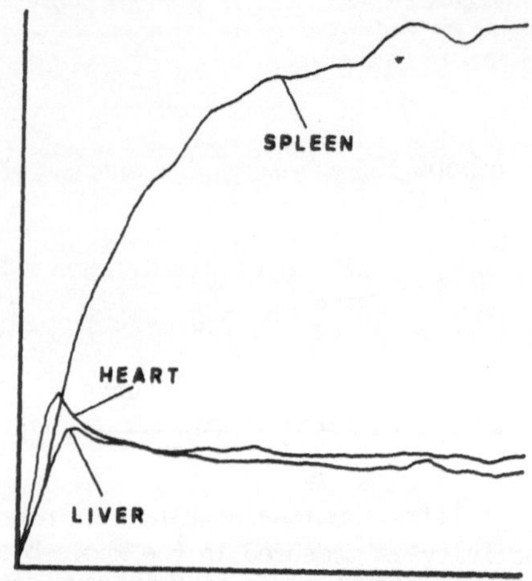

Fig. 4. In vivo distribution of ^{111}In-labelled non activated autologous platelets injected into a normal subject. Typical time activity curves in heart, spleen and liver as acquired by a gamma camera during the first 20 min following platelet injection.

Table 2. In vivo organ uptake in 4 normal subjects (gamma camera data) (a): Percentage of total area activity.

	INITIAL SPLENIC UPTAKE (min^{-1})	activity at 20 min (a)			activity on day 5 (a)		
		HEART	LIVER	SPLEEN	HEART	LIVER	SPLEEN
1	0.173	9.4	11.3	30.6	4.8	11.3	33.9
2	0.22	4.6	6.4	35.6	4.7	8.9	33.2
3	0.20	9.0	9.1	33.6	4.7	10.0	38.7
4	0.173	8.4	7.3	31.4	6.4	8.1	32.6

the platelet cytoplasm and is not released by the effect of high concentrations of thrombin (up to 20 U/ml) on platelets. This is in agreement with previous findings (4,12), which have shown that ^{111}In is not liberated from human platelets by release inducing agents unless release is accompanied by platelet lysis.

3. Shape and function of ^{111}In-oxine platelets. Platelets labelled with ^{111}In at a concentration of oxine not greater than 0.5 μg/ml retain their discoid shape as judged by the "swirling" aspect of the suspension when agitated by gentle rotation. In addition, platelets appear as smooth discoid particles without pseudopod formation when examined with a phase contrast microscope. Initial uptake of ^{3}H-5-hydroxytryptamine (data not shown) is similar to that of control non ^{111}In-labelled platelets. To ascertain that labelled platelets injected for survival studies are functional, it is a routine procedure in our laboratory to test them by performing aggregation studies with ADP (5 μM), collagen (1/1000) and thrombin (0.5 U/ml). In normal subjects, the aggregation pattern of the labelled platelets do not differ in velocity and amplitude of aggregation from that of the normal population of reference of our hemostasis laboratory.

4. In vivo kinetics of ^{111}In-labelled platelets. A typical survival curve of the disappearance of injected ^{111}In-labelled autologous platelets into a normal subject is shown in fig 3. The radioactivity is measured in a sample of whole blood. The bottom curve demonstrates that practically no radioactivity is appearing in the plasma. The data of the platelet survival performed in 6 normal volunteers are presented in table 1. In these subjects, autologous disc-shaped non activated platelets have been injected, their recovery in the circulation at 20 min is 65.2%.

The initial in vivo distribution of ^{111}In-labelled non activated autologous platelets in selected regions is analysed by monitoring the time activity curves obtained by a gamma camera over the spleen, liver and heart. The activity in the liver parallels the activity in the precordial area (fig 4), suggesting that there is no active uptake in the liver. The activity in the spleen increases to reach a maximum in about 15 min.

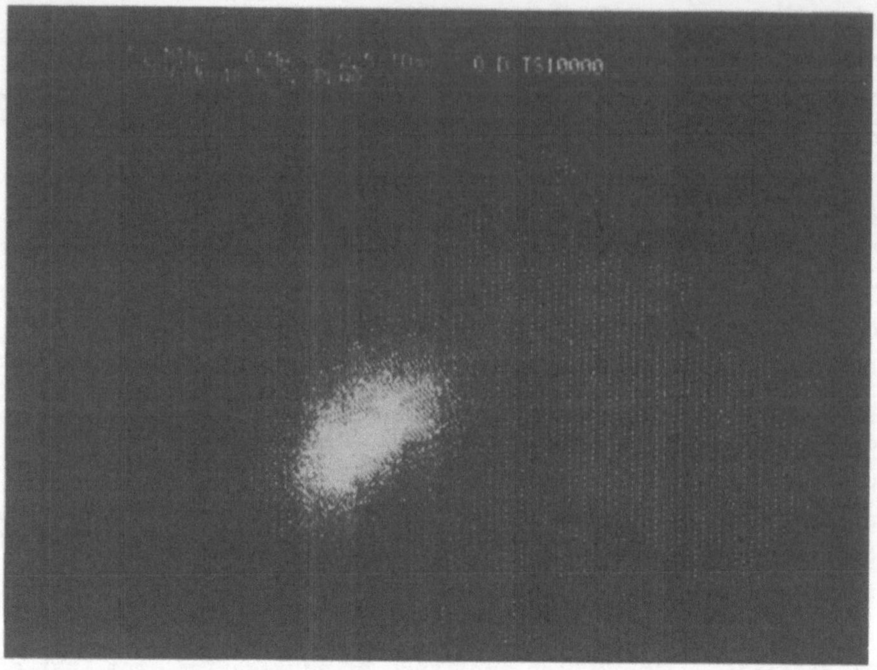

Fig. 5. Scintigraphy of the spleen and the liver 1 day after injection of ^{111}In-labelled autologous non activated platelets into a normal subject.

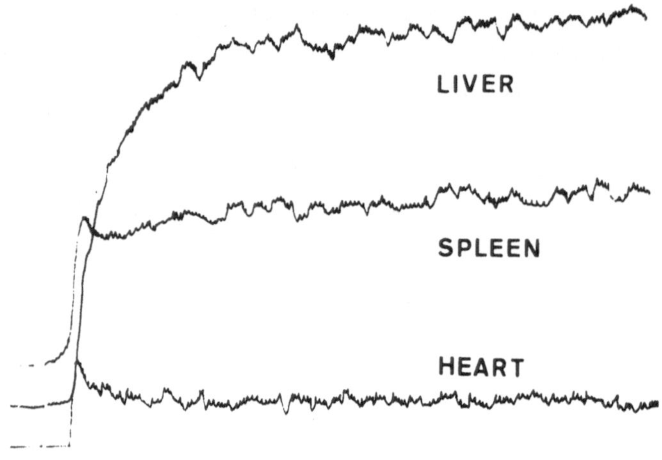

Fig. 6. In vivo distribution of ^{111}In-labelled activated autologous platelets injected into a normal subject. Typical initial time activity curves in heart, spleen and liver obtained with a multicrystal Cardio 4.

Table 3. Comparison of recovery, survival and organ uptake of ^{111}In-labelled autologous activated or non activated platelets in normal subjects.

Platelets	Recovery at 20 min. (%)	Mean life span gamma function (days)	Liver/heart ratio of activity at 20 min.
1 activated	35.0	6.5	2.6
2 activated	30.0	7.0	2.5
non activated (n = 6)	65.2	7.6	1.09

Table 4. Comparison of recovery, survival and organ uptake of ^{111}In-labelled autologous platelets in 3 asplenic patients and in 6 normal subjects.

Patients	Recovery at 20 min. (%)	Mean life span gamma function (days)	Liver/heart ratio of activity at 20 min.
Asplenic 1	95.5	7.3	1.6
Asplenic 2	93.3	6.8	1.4
Asplenic 3	98.0	-	1.3
Normal	65.2	7.6	1.09

The initial rate of uptake by the spleen is calculated by assuming that for a limited period of observation spleen and blood can be assimilated to a closed 2 compartment model (13). Expressed in min^{-1}, the value obtained was 0.188 with a standard deviation of 0.02. The radioactivity of the 3 selected areas, expressed as a percentage of total activity is shown in table 2. The liver activity is not higher than the precordial activity at 20 min. On day 5, the liver activity is very slightly elevated compared to the precordial activity. The scintigraphy (fig 3) demonstrates the very low activity in the liver.

The behaviour of autologous activated, non disc-shaped platelets is different when injected into their recipient. Fig 6, clearly shows that the initial uptake of ^{111}In-labelled platelets in the liver is greater than in the spleen. In addition, the recovery of the labelled platelets in the circulation at 20 min is lower than the recovery of non activated platelets in normal subjects (table 3). Thus, the lower recovery and the increased liver uptake of labelled platelets suggest that loss of discoid shape and activation (in this case by reversible aggregation during the platelet washing procedure) lead to modifications of the platelets which allow recognition and sequestration by the reticuloendothelial system.

To demonstrate that the initial sequestration of about 35% of the injected platelets in the splenic pool is physiologic and not due to a modification of the platelets during their preparation, we examined 3 asplenic patients (table 4). In these patients, the recovery of ^{111}In-labelled platelets at 20 min is close to 100% and no initial uptake is demonstrable.

Discussion

The use of ^{111}In as a label for platelet kinetics and distribution studies has been a major improvement in comparison to ^{51}Cr. In addition to its physical favorable characteristics, the isotopic label is a cytoplasmic marker of human platelets and thus is not secreted when the platelets are activated by release inducing agents, such as collagen or thrombin (14). In contrast, the loss of ^{111}In from platelets indicates that platelet lysis has occured (12).

Because plasma transferrin is a ligand for Chromium and Indium salts, the use of a non plasmatic medium is necessary to label platelets with a high efficiency (2). When platelets are washed in non plasmatic media they may loose their discoid shape and their functional properties. The properties of human platelets washed by the method of Mustard have been extensively studied and are comparable to the properties of platelets in vivo (5). In most of the published reports, the platelets are labelled in acidified (by ACD) saline media, devoided of glucose and protein; this procedure leads to platelet loss of discoid shape and activation (15). Furthermore, high concentrations of oxine are used (15,16), which in our hands is deleterious for platelets. We never use more than 0.5 µg/ml of oxine in order to prevent loss of platelet shape and inhibition of platelet aggregation.

In agreement with Joist (4), who was working with rabbit platelets, we find that labelling of human platelets with ^{111}In-oxine is a rapid process which currently gives at 37°C in less than 15 min an efficiency greater than 85%.

The method of labelling washed human platelets is rapid and can be performed within 1 hour. It needs 42.5 ml of blood, providing the platelet count of the patient is greater than 50 000/mm3.

The in vivo behaviour of ^{111}In-labelled human autologous platelets injected into normal subjects depends on their functional properties and discoid shape. Although activated platelets may survive for a normal period of time (10), a proportion of these injected platelets is rapidly cleared from the circulation and sequestered in the spleen and the liver, resulting in a low percentage of recovery at 20 min. Our data show that there is no measurable initial uptake by the liver when normal subjects are injected with disc-shaped, non activated platelets. In contrast, when the platelets have been activated during the washing and labelling procedure and have lost their shape, they are initially sequestered in the liver and in the spleen, resulting in a low recovery at 20 min in the circulation. In normal subjects, the recovery at 20 min of disc-shaped platelets is 65%, when we use the blood-volume measured by ^{125}I-albumin for the calculation. Most of the authors estimate the blood-volume from published tables. If we used a blood-volume of 70 ml/kg, we would calculate a recovery of injected platelets in the circulation of 70%. In asplenic patients, the recovery of 93 to 98% of the injected labelled platelets provides further evidence that there is no initial hepatic uptake of disc-shaped and functional platelets. In both normal and asplenic subjects, we observed no significant difference between the percentage of recovery at 20 min either measured or extrapolated from the curve.

In conclusion, we suggest that an optimal method for labelling human platelet with ^{111}In-oxine for survival studies should include the following aspects: i) use of a non plasmatic medium to achieve a high labelling efficiency (17); ii) use of a washing medium preventing thrombin generation and containing divalent cations (Ca^{2+} and Mg^{2+}), albumin, glucose and balanced salts. Control the pH, osmolarity, and maintain 37°C during the manipulations. The addition of PGI_2 prevents activation of platelets during preparation and its effects are short-lived; iii) prevent platelet damage and inhibition of function by keeping the concentration of oxine lower than 0.5 μg/ml.

Acknowledgements

The authors wish to thank Mrs. M. Issenhuth for technical assistance and Mrs. C. Schmitt for typing the manuscript.

REFERENCES

1. Mustard JF, Platelet survival, Thrombos. Haemost. 40:154, 1978.
2. Thakur ML, Welch MJ, Joist JH, Coleman RE, Indium-111 labeled platelets. Studies on preparation and evaluation of in vitro and in vivo functions. Thromb. Res. 9:345, 1976.
3. The panel on diagnostic application of radioisotopes in hematology, International Committee for standardization in Hematology: Recommended methods for radioisotope platelet survival studies. Blood 50:1137, 1977.
4. Joist JH, Baker RK, Thakur ML, Welch MJ, Indium-111-labeled human platelets: Uptake and loss of label and in vitro function of labeled platelets. J. Lab. clin. Med. 92:829, 1978.
5. Kinlough-Rathbone RL, Mustard JF, Packham MA, Perry DW, Reimers HJ, Cazenave JP, Properties of washed human platelets. Thrombos. Haemost. 37:291, 1977.
6. Cazenave JP, Hemmendinger S, Beretz A, Sutter-Bay A, Launay J, L'agrégation plaquettaire: outil d'investigation clinique et d'étude pharmacologique. Méthodologie. An. Biol. Clin. (in press).
7. Aster RH, Jandl JH, Platelet sequestration in man. I. Methods. J. clin. Invest. 43:843, 1964.
8. Cazenave JP, Reimers HJ, Kinlough-Rathbone RL, Packham MA, Mustard JF, Effects of sodium periodate on platelet functions. Lab. Invest. 34:471, 1976.
9. Reimers HJ, Allen DJ, Cazenave JP, Feuerstein IA, Mustard JF, Serotonin transport and storage in rabbit blood platelets. The effects of reserpine and imipramine. Biochem. Pharmacol. 26:1645, 1977.
10. Murphy EA, Francis ME, The estimation of blood platelet survival. II. The multiple hit model. Thrombos. Diathos. haemorrh. Stuttg. 25:53, 1971.
11. Scheffel U, McIntyre PA, Evatt B, Dvornicky JA, Natarajan TK, Bolling DR, Murphy EA, Evaluation of Indium-111 as a new high photon yield gamma-emitting "physiological" platelet label. Johns Hopk. Med. J. 140:285, 1977.
12. Joist JH, Baker RK, Loss of ^{111}Indium as indicator of platelet injury. Blood 58:350, 1981.
13. Peters AM, Lavender JP, Factors controlling the intrasplenic transit of platelets. Eur. J. clin. Invest. 12:191, 1982.
14. Baker JRJ, Butler KD, Eakins MN, Pay GF, White AM, Subcellular localization of ^{111}In in human and rabbit platelets. Blood 59:351, 1982.
15. Heyns duP A, Lötter MG, Badenhorst PN, Van Reenen OR, Pieters H, Minnaar PC, Retief FP, Kinetics, distribution and sites of destruction of ^{111}Indium-labelled human platelets. Brit. J. Haemat. 44:269, 1980.
16. Scheffel U, Tasn MF, Mitchell TG, Camargo EE, Braine H, Ezekowitz MD, Nickoloff EL, Hillzobel R, Murphy E, McIntyre PA, Human platelets labeled with In-111 8-hydroxyquinoline. Kinetics, distribution and estimates of radiation dose. J. nucl. Med. 23:149, 1982.
17. Hawker RJ, Hawker LM, Wilkinson AR, Indium (^{111}In)-labelled human platelets: optimal method. Clin. Sci. 58:243, 1980.

4 ^{111}INDIUM LOSS FROM PLATELETS BY IN VITRO AND EX VIVO MANIPULATION

R.J. HAWKER, C.E. HALL, M. GOLDMAN, C.N. McCOLLUM

INTRODUCTION

Since the introduction of lipid soluble chelates of ^{111}In as cell labelling agents (1) there have been a large number of reports on the in vivo and in vitro uses of Indium labelled platelets derived from man and laboratory animals. Such labelled cells have been used for the determination of deep vein thrombosis (2) renal transplant rejection and associated problems (3) and the detection of thrombogenicity in prosthetic arterial graft materials (4). Animal models have been used to evaluate prosthetic materials and medical plastics (5) drug regimes (6) and drug induced normalisation of platelet survival (7). Laboratory assays have been developed to utilize the release of Indium from human platelets and from other cells for the detection and quantification of humoral or cellular antibodies (8,9). The advantages over ^{51}Cr for these tests not only relates to ^{111}In's superior gamma emissions but to the excellent labelling efficiency and very low spontaneous release. The Indium in human platelets is not contained within the storage granules (10) and therefore the granular release initiated upon irreversible aggregation does not cause the loss of Indium. This is not the case with platelets from some other species where Indium is stored in the granules and released upon activation (11). There have been several reports quoting high levels of Indium which are found non-cell bound in samples taken from man and some researchers suggest that Indium may be re-utilized by other blood-cells. Several authors have thus advocated that platelet survival data should be based on the radioactivity associated with separated platelet samples rather than whole blood-samples. This involves a great deal of ex vivo manipulations which introduce their own errors and create artifacts. Reports from a number of centres suggest platelet Indium instability in chronic liver disease and after in vitro experiments involving whole blood (12). Webber et al (13) also concluded that the label in some animal experiments was not associated with platelets and up to 57% of the activity was found in plasma in a 3 hour blood-sample.

These reports are, however, in the minority and it is generally agreed that the Indium is not released during normal physiological platelet function. Joist and Baker (14) have shown that the loss of Indium to the enzyme lactate dehydrogenase (LDH) is much slower than the loss of ^{51}Cr; this may be due to the molecular dimension of the intracellular complexes. They concluded that Indium release was not as good an indicator of sub-lytic or pre-lytic platelet injury as ^{51}Cr. Hudson et al (10) in chromatographic studies showed that Indium derived from labelled platelets was cytosolically bound to a molecule of between 25,000 and 46,000 daltons and DeWanjee et al (15) using human platelets gave an estimate of 52,000 ± 5,000 daltons. The association with lipoproteins, in particular to phosphatidyl-inositol is also documented (16).

The thickness and hence resilence of the layer of surface glycoproteins on the platelet decrease with age, and in vitro removal of surface sialic acid or glycoprotein oxidation reduces in vivo platelet survival proportionally to the chemical alteration (17,18). Such a process of glycoprotein loss occurs ex vivo and spontaneous lysis of platelets may be measured. This is both a combination of aging and of the shear forces to which they are exposed. The amount of spontaneous lysis observed within labelled platelet samples following passing platelets through a microlitre syringe with an orifice of 100 micron diameter was approximately linear with time up to a maximum of 60% loss at 167 hours storage at 4°C (8). This phenomenon was greater in the more fragile platelets of diabetic platelets and may explain Jeysingh's (12) findings in chronic liver disease. Upon repeating these early experiments using larger orifice devices (diameter 500 microns) so as not to exert large shear forces, lysis could be reduced to 20% after 20 days, well beyond the normal in vivo platelet survival, although it should be added that the total releasible Indium also declined, probably as the Indium-lipid chelate became utilized in platelet membranes. It was apparent that lysis and hence Indium release ex vivo was due to handling techniques.

We therefore set out to measure some of the parameters inducing lysis, methods of recuding ex vivo damage, along with a theoretical model to explain the correlation between platelet fragility and the nature and strength of the insult. Thus it would be expected that some drugs which affect platelet metabolism, reactivity or membrane stability would increase their strength and hence ability to survive insults both in vivo and ex vivo. Dewanjee et al (19) have demonstrated that the lysis of platelets induced during cardiopulmonary by-pass surgery in dogs can be reduced by half using either prostacyclin or the cyclo/oxygenase inhibitor Ibuprofen.

Materials and methods

A. Labelling of platelets. Platelets were labelled with ^{111}In-oxine (Amersham International Ltd) by the method of Hawker et al (20). The labelled platelets were resuspended in platelet-poor plasma prior to re-injection and were shown to retain their in vitro function of aggregation to ADP and collagen and of adhesion to glass.

B. Measurement of platelet adhesiveness. Adhesion to glass was carried out using commercially available glass bead columns (Adeplat, Immuno LTD). Non-anticoagulated blood was passed through the columns using an infusion pump. In 3 patients samples were analysed daily for up to 8 days following platelet labelling and in several other patients, samples were investigated on one or more occasions during this period. Using 750 µl volumes of blood pre- and post-passage through the columns, the percentage radioactivity retained was calculated by direct measurement of radioactivity (Searle Automatic Gamma Systems).

Following centrifugation of the same samples (Thrombofuge, Coulter Electronics Ltd) to produce platelet-rich plasma, a platelet count was made (Coulter Model FBI) and the percentage of platelets retained calculated from the numerical data.

C. Measurement of free Indium in ex vivo blood-samples. 5 ml blood-samples were taken in clean venepuncture into standard haematology tubes (Sterilin KE/5) containing potassium EDTA. All samples were processed within 30 min of collection. Quadruplicate 1.0 ml samples of the anticoagulated blood was centrifuged at 1000 xg for 10 min at ambient temperature. The plasma was carefully removed with a siliconised glass pasteur pipette and the cells resuspended in 1.0 ml of 4 mM dipotassium EDTA in phosphate buffered saline (EDTA/PBS) and then further centrifuged at 1000 x g for 10 min. The supernatant was combined with the plasma, and the cells lysed by the addition of 2% Triton x 100 so as to produce a volume of lysed cells equal to the combined plasma/supernatant volume. Both samples were then counted for radioactivity and the amount of activity in the plasma/supernatant expressed as a percentage of the total activity (plasma/supernatant + lysed cells). Blood-samples from patients undergoing treatment with antiplatelet drugs were likewise assayed. Samples were also taken into other anticoagulants or stabilizing agents such as prostaglandins E_1 indomethacin or lignocaine added. Some samples were maintained at +4°C througout in an attempt to stabilize the cell membranes.

D. Artificial circuit (21). The effect of Dazoxiben, a thromboxane synthetase inhibitor, on thromboxane levels, platelet counts and non-cell bound Indium was determined in pre- and post-perfusion samples from an artificial circulation which mimicked the flow in the human femoral artery. To one half of a 600 ml heparinised (2.5 iu/ml) blood donation containing autologous ^{113m}In-labelled platelets, was added Dazoxiben at 33 µg/ml. A comparison was made with the control half of the donation using identical twin circuits made of silastic tubing and containing 15 cm lengths of pre-clotted 6 mm Dacron arterial graft. A pulsatile flow of 140 ml/min at 120/80 mm Hg was maintained at 37°C for 30 min.

E. Measurement of free Indium in in vitro stored platelet samples. Small samples of in vitro aged labelled platelets (stored at +4°C in citrated plasma without agitation and in stoppered plastic tubes) were added to fresh citrated whole blood from the same donor. 1 ml aliquots were then treated exactly as the ex vivo blood-samples collecting the supernatant separately after each centrifugation stage and resuspending the cells in EDTA/PBS. Centrifugation, separation and resuspension were repeated on samples up to 7 times on platelets aged up to 8 days. The amount of radioactivity found in the supernatant was expressed as a percentage of the radioactivity in the samples immediately prior to centrifugation. Samples of platelets dual labelled with ^{113m}In and 14C-5-hydroxytryptamine were treated similarly.

F. Labelling of platelets with 14C-serotonin (5HT) and ^{113m}In. 17 ml of blood was anticoagulated with 3 ml of acid-citrate (71 mM citric acid, 85 mM trisodium citrate) and following mixing, centrifuged at 200 x g for 10 min at room temperature to produce a platelet-rich plasma (PRP). 5 to 10 µl of 14C-5HT (Amersham International) was added to each millilitre of PRP and incubated for 30 min at room temperature. The label incorporation was 60-70%. The PRP was then treated as for Indium labelling being washed and resuspended finally in plasma. ^{113m}In-oxine ($t_{\frac{1}{2}}$: 99 min) prepared as described (22) was used instead of ^{111}In so that following decay of ^{113m}In the 14C-5HT could be measured. If LDH measurements were also made then the platelets were washed and resuspended in buffer.

G. Measurement of lactate dehydrogenase (LDH). LDH was assayed spectrophotometrically by an automated continuous flow technique (23). Briefly using 100 mM lactic acid and 2.6 mM NAD+ dissolved in 100 mM 2-amino-2-methyl-propane-1-01/HCl buffer, pH 9.0, the rate of NADH production was measured at 340 nM using assay conditions which gave a linear release of NADH with time. Samples to be assayed were stored at +4°C and assayed within 24 hours of preparation. All samples were plasma-free and where cell samples were assayed they were lysed using a final concentration of 0.1% Triton-X100.

H. Hypotonic release of ^{111}In and LDH from platelet samples. 100 µl samples of platelets were diluted with phosphate buffered saline (PBS) containing 4 mM EDTA (PBS/EDTA) to give final osmolalities from 5-290 mOs in 10 steps. Following incubation for 30 min at room temperature, the samples were centrifuged at 1000 x g

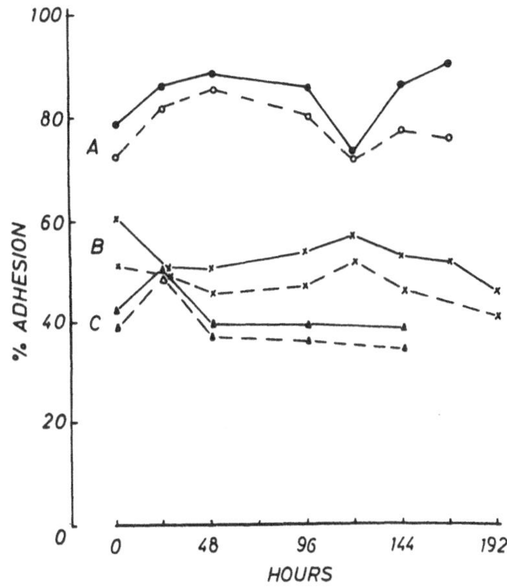

Fig. 1. Adhesion of platelets to glass bead columns (Adeplat T) for 3 individuals. Broken line is the % of radioactivity adherent and the solid line the % of platelets by numerical counts. Platelet survivals of the 3 individuals were linear with survival times of A 228, B 229 and C 220 hours.

Table 1.

Time hours	proportion of labelled plate-lets circulating	% free Indium mean of 4 determinations	% total platelet population*	age (hours prior to death)
1	1.0000	2.37 ± 0.57	3.17	6.63
22	0.9645	2.05 ± 0.66	2.64	5.52
46	0.8645	2.86 ± 0.16	3.29	6.88
70	0.6449	3.47 ± 0.31	2.99	6.26
94	0.5880	3.73 ± 0.06	2.92	6.11
142	0.3432	8.48 ± 0.28	3.88	8.12
166	0.2550	11.49 ± 0.01	3.91	8.17

*assuming max 75% activity can be released

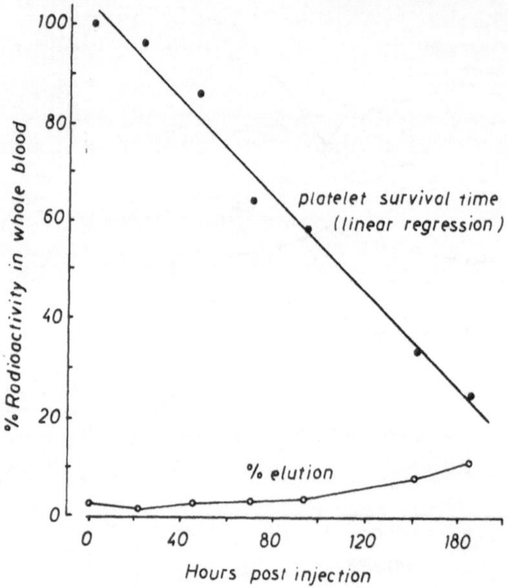

Fig. 2. Plot of platelet survival in a patient using ^{111}In-labelled autologous platelets. The full data is in table 1. Platelet survival time based on 100/slope of the linear regression line of best fit = 209.2 hours. Closed circles represent the % of radioactivity in a 5 ml blood-sample using the initial 1 hour p.i. blood-sample as 100%. The open circle of Indium found in the plasma plus cell washing following centrifugation and washing of the anticoagulated specimen.

for 10 min and the radioactivity or enzymatic activity in the supernatant expressed as a percentage of that released by 0.1% Triton X100.

Results and discussion

1. Ex vivo. Fig 1 shows the close correlation between adhesion measurements using Adeplat-T columns in 3 hospitalized patients both on platelet number and retained radioactivity.

It is apparent that the radioactive platelets retain their adhesive properties for 196 hours which approaches the in vivo platelet life span. The percentage adherence measured by radioactivity was consistently lower than that by numerical platelet count (mean difference 5.32 ± 3.2%. It is unlikely that the difference could be explained by platelet age alone since the

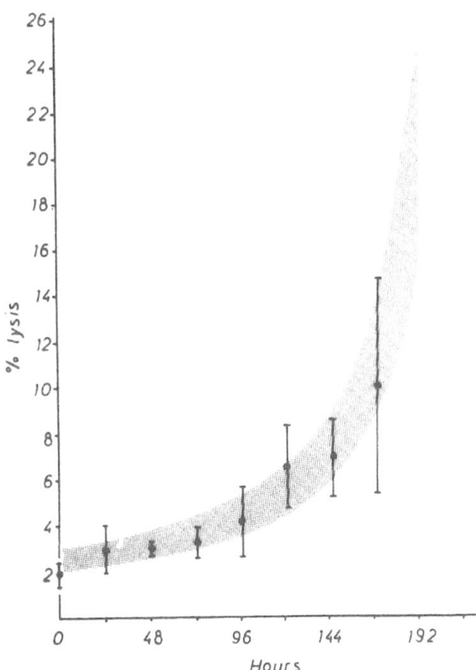

Fig. 3. The amount of Indium found non-cell bound following centrifugation and washing of blood-samples from a group of more than 7 individuals. The vertical bars cover the mean ± 1 SD. The shaded area is a computed plot of the Indium released from platelets which are within 5.8 hours (lower edge) and 8.7 hours (upper edge) of their ultimate calculated in vivo survival (see text).

lines parallel each other and do not diverge with time. The difference can be explained as free radioactivity which does not attach to the glass bead columns as demonstrated by a less than 4% retention following passage of the soluble portion of fragmented labelled platelets. Similarly Indium is released from platelets during the platelet release reaction by agonists such as excess collagen when up to 3% of the Indium may be freed. This of course may only be an expression of the lysis of the older cells. Following passage through the glass bead columns, some Indium will be released by shear forces. This, combined with the use of excess dry EDTA in the collection tube will increase the radioactivity free in the PRP fraction after

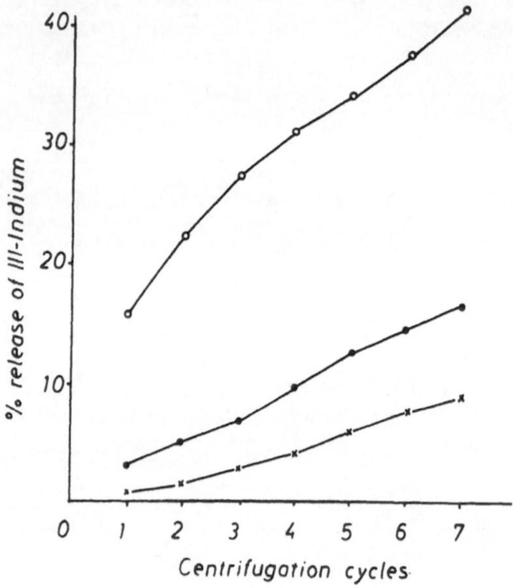

Fig. 4. Repeated centrifugation of labelled platelets. The points are cumulative figures for Indium freed into the washing medium. The lowest line is for freshly labelled platelets. The closed circles are for platelets stored in vitro for 72 hours and the open circles following storage for 7 days.

Table 2. Centrifugal damage of platelets

	% Indium loss		
in vitro age (hours)	first centrifugation	after 7 centrifugation cycles	mean increment per centrifugal insult
1	0.56	9.10	1.42 ± 0.29
72	3.22	16.72	2.25 ± 0.46
168	16.15	42.07	4.32 ± 1.29

centrifugation, and thus decrease the calculated percentage of radioactive platelets adherent on the column.

Table 1 and fig 2 demonstrate the amount of Indium present in the plasma following centrifugation to separate cells and plasma from a single individual. In a group of patients (fig 3) there is a non-linear rise in the Indium found in the plasma starting at 1.42 ± 0.3% (n= 7) immediately following labelling prior to re-injection, and 1.78 ± 0.5% 1 hour following re-injection, this rising to 9.98 ± 4.6% by the 7th day. There was an increase in standard deviation with time (fig 3) which was due to the inter-patient variation of susceptibility of platelets to damage. The errors between replicates was very small with coefficients of variation between 2.1 and 7.2%.

The percentage of Indium in the plasma of blood-samples from patients under treatment with 250 mg b.d. Ticlopidine was consistantly lower than that in the placebo group. The differences in means were maintained with platelet age, but because of individual variations never reached significance.

2. In vitro. In vitro platelets which are repeatedly centrifuged following labelling, can be shown to release Indium in direct relationship to the increasing insult, as shown on fig 4 and table 2. Freshly labelled platelets when repeatedly centrifuged at 1000 x g for 10 min lost an average 1.42 ± 0.3% of the Indium on each occasion, giving a linear loss of from 0.56% following the first centrifugation, to 9.10% after 7 centrifugations. When the labelled platelet suspensions were stored, the platelets became more susceptible to the same insult and by 72 hours the initial release was 3.2% and 2.2 ± 0.5% on each subsequent centrifugation. After 168 hours storage the initial release had risen to 16.0% with a further 5% released by each centrifugation up to 42%. Loss above this became progressively small on each cycle.

Similarly this phenomenon can be induced by exposure to hypotonic solutions as shown in fig 5. Labelled platelets were stored at +4°C and at intervals up to 13 days were titrated against dilutions of phosphate buffered saline in water. After correction for maximum releasible Indium by Triton X100 and for

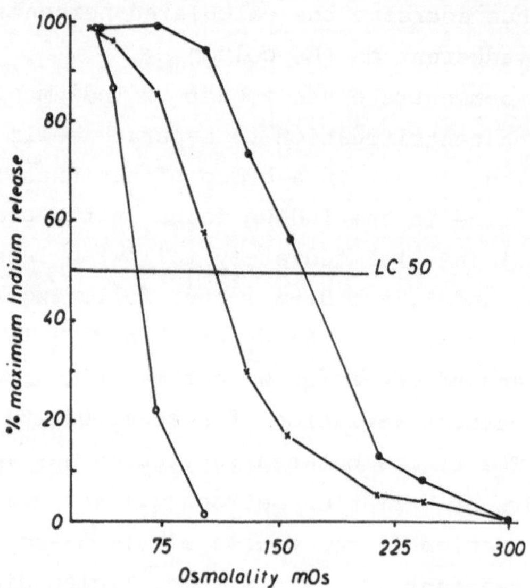

Fig. 5. Titration of platelet lysis measured by ^{111}In release against dilutions of phosphate buffered saline. Osmolality was determined by freezing point depression. Curves (left to right) immediately following labelling, and following 5 and 13 days of in vitro storage at 4°C. Thus 50% lysis concentration (LC 50) is calculated after adjustment for spontaneous lysis in full strength PBS (290 mOs) and for maximum releasible Indium in 2% Triton X100.

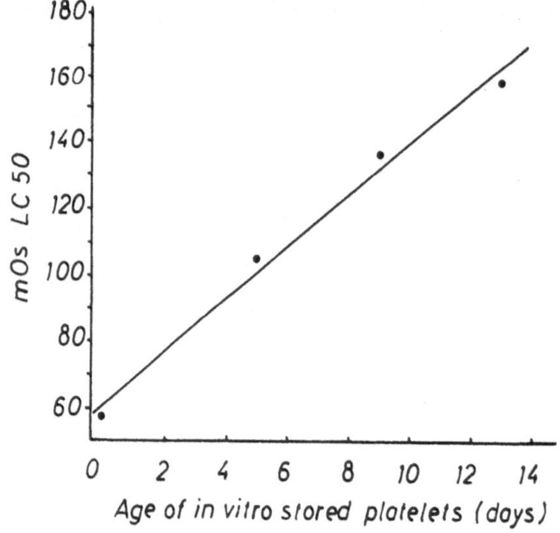

Fig. 6. 50% lytic concentration (mOs) plotted against time of storage. Correlation coefficient r= 0.995.

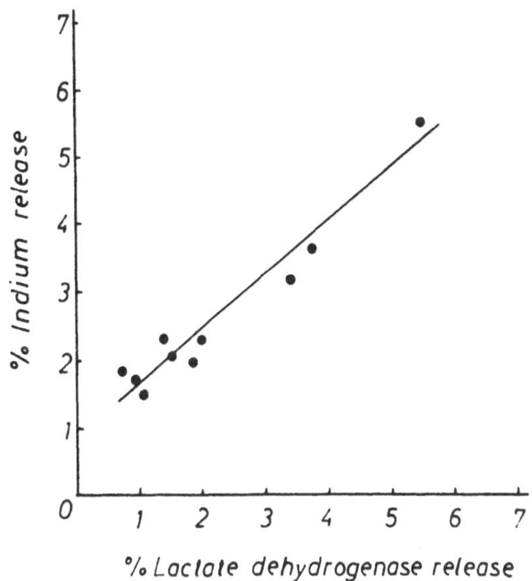

Fig. 7. Correlation of lactate dehydrogenase (LDH) with ^{111}In release using freshly labelled platelets subjected to hypotonic solutions. Correlation coefficient r= 0.972.

spontaneous release in undiluted solutions, the Indium releasible by hypotonic solutions was calculated. Graphs were constructed and the 50% lysis concentration (LC 50) calculated. Fig 5 shows that with increasing length of storage the platelets become more susceptible to hypotonic solution. Fig 6 shows the linearity of LC 50 and time with in vitro aged platelets. The excellent correlation of lactate dehydrogenase release and Indium as shown in fig 7, demonstrates that the latter is measuring lysis and that they appear to be equally good as indicators of injury. This finding supports the results of Joist and Baker (14). The measurement of 14C-5HT release following centrifugation of freshly labelled platelets mimicked the low level loss of both Indium and LDH. Platelets stored in vitro for several days showed a significantly increased release of 14C-5HT compared to Indium. LDH measurement in aged samples proved to be of little value because of enzyme degradation. The difference between 14C-5HT and Indium release would reflect the differing mechanisms involved. Physiological release of platelet 5HT occurs during aggregation induced by centrifugal injury and platelet-platelet interactions. Indium and LDH release are probably caused by lysis of the platelet membrane. Although Indium is not stored in the human platelet granules (11) and released upon aggregation, it is possible that LDH which is stored in some α-granules may be released during processes other than lysis. This may explain why the regression line of Indium versus LDH (fig 7) has a slope $\hat{b}$ of 0.804.

In an attempt to reduce ex vivo damage, stabilizing agents, platelet active drugs and red cell sedimenting agents were added to blood-samples, containing labelled platelets. Following centrifugation at 1000 x g for 10 min at room temperature, unless otherwise stated, the difference between the lysis in the sample containing the added agent and a control was measured by Indium released and expressed as a percentage change.

Both 100 ng/ml prostaglandin E_1 and Indomethacin at final concentration of 0.5 mM significantly reduced the ex vivo damage and hence Indium release by 9.5% and 7.6% respectively. Lignocaine at 0.1 mM and a reduction in temperature to 4°C, both of which alter cell membrane fluidity, only reduced the Indium release by 1.9% and 0.8% respectively. Materials such as excess EDTA (20 mM), Ficoll/Hypaque density gradient and sedimenting agents such as Dextran increased the Indium released by between 3% and 9%.

Table 3 summarizes the results of an experiment using the thromboxane synthetase inhibitor, Dazoxiben added in vitro to blood-samples and then pumped through an artificial circulation (24). The Dazoxiben significantly reduced the plasma thromboxane B_2 level ($p<0.01$) compared to controls but did not maintain the thromboxane B_2 at the pre-circuit level of 70 ± 67 pg/ml. Dazoxiben reduced the loss of circulating platelets ($p<0.05$) either by reducing adhesion or aggregation to the circuit material and/or by preventing lysis caused by the shear forces to which the blood was exposed during circulation. The reduction in the Indium which is found in the plasma of Dazoxiben circuits compared to controls ($p<0.01$) indicates some protection from lysis by the drug.

Table 3. Results of artificial circulation

	Post-circuit plasma TXB_2 pg/ml	% fall in circulating platelet count	% decrease in non-cell bound Indium Dazoxiben/control
Dazoxiben	350 ± 129	6.4 ± 2.4	
			15.8 ± 2.4
Control	2048 ± 799	8.5 ± 3.2	

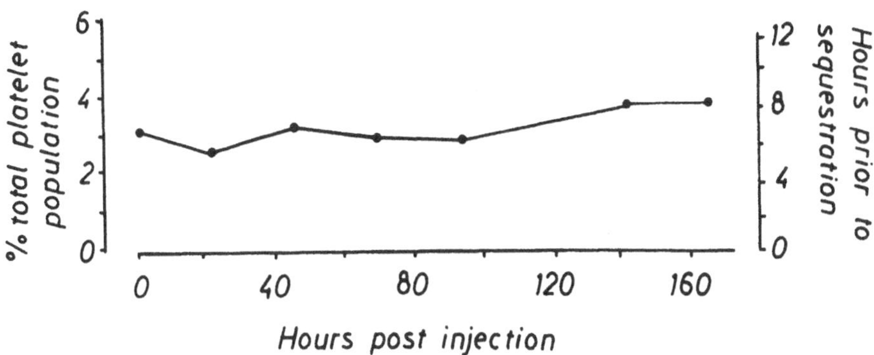

Fig. 8. Calculated percentage of the total platelet population (left hand axis) which have lysed during manipulation plotted against time. The right hand vertical axis is the estimated time prior to sequestration assuming a platelet life span of 209 hours.

Theoretical model to explain plasma-Indium from ex vivo samples. Table 1 shows the results of platelet survival based on the proportion of the original sample for an individual over a period of 166 hours. The survival time based on the slope of the linear regression line of best fit was 209.2 hours. At each sampling time quadruplicate determinations were made of the Indium in plasma and then the percentage of the total platelet population that this lysis represented was calculated.

The data shows that a consistent percentage of the total platelet population is damaged by centrifugation and the manipulations involved in separating cells and plasma. (Table 1, column 4; and fig 8). When related to the calculated platelet survival time and following adjustment for 75% maximum releasable activity probably represents platelets which are within 8 hours of ultimate in vivo sequestration.

The mean percentage value for free Indium over the period of 7 days increases in a non-linear fashion (fig 3). When this data is expressed as the percentage of the platelet population corrected for maximum cytosolic release i.e.

$$\frac{\text{\% free Indium x proportion of labelled platelets circulating}}{0.75}$$

a rather more consistent number of platelets (3.26 ± 0.48) would need to be damaged in order to obtain similar values (fig 8). Thus when 11.49% of the total activity of the whole blood was found in the plasma at 166 hours there was only 0.2550 of the original radioactivity or 3.91% of the total platelets are damaged i.e. possibly those over 201.07 hours.

Fig 3 shows, superimposed on the actual data from a minimum of 7 individuals at each data point, a computed plot of the Indium released by platelets which are within a similar time prior to the calculated in vivo removal from circulation by the reticuloendothelial system. The actual data plotted with standard deviations, fits the computed plot accurately, suggesting that lysis of the older platelets by ex vivo manipulation explains the artifactual plasma levels.

Summary / Conclusion

Indium loss from labelled platelets can be considered as a marker of cell lysis correlating well with lactate dehydrogenase release. Laboratory manipulation of suspensions, including whole blood, containing labelled platelets may cause release of Indium. Simple manipulations such as suspension dispersal, anticoagulation and centrifugation cause lysis. This lysis may be minimized by care and/or the addition of agents such as prostaglandin E_1 or indomethacin. Other materials such as red-cell sedimenting agents may increase lysis. The amount of Indium released by a standard procedure is related to the strength and type of insult (physical, chemical or immunological) and also to the health or age of the platelet. These phenomena can be induced in vitro by repeated centrifugation, hypotonic shock or increased shear stresses and observed during the in vitro ageing of labelled platelets.

Loss of Indium from platelets ex vivo is also related to platelet age and a simple theoretical model based on age fragility has been proposed to explain this phenomenon. This demonstrates that a consistent percentage of the total platelet pool is readily lysed by simple manipulation, such as separation of plasma and cells. These platelets probably represent the oldest platelets within 5 to 8 hours of ultimate sequestration by the reticuloendothelial system.

It is important therefore to use whole blood-samples for radioactive counting and the calculation of platelet survival since the freed Indium is a consequence of ex vivo handling. Other assays such as adhesion measurements based on radioactivity will be inaccurate because of lysis and release of Indium from the platelet cytosol.

Disorders of platelets which affect platelet survival time or fragility or the administration of platelet active drugs will affect the result of manipulative lysis and therefore the comparison of samples either from different individuals or on different occasions from the same individual need be interpreted with caution.

The measurement of platelet lysis by Indium release (following standardized manipulation) may be a useful indicator of cell protection by platelet active compounds or the health of the platelets of an individual.

Acknowledgements

We wish to thank both Pat Cole and Christine Hail for typing the manuscript, skilful drawing and photography of the figures.

REFERENCES

1. Thakur ML, Welch MJ, Joist JH, Coleman RE, Indium-111 labelled platelet: studies on preparation and evaluation of in vitro and in vivo function. Thromb. Res. 9:345, 1976.

2. Fenech A, Nicholls A, Smith FW, Indium (111-In) labelled platelets in the diagnosis of renal transplant rejection: preliminary findings. Brit. J. Radiol. 54:325, 1981.

3. Smith N, Chandler S, Hawker RJ, Hawker LM, Barnes AD, Indium-labelled autologous platelets as diagnostic aid after renal transplantation. Lancet ii:1241, 1979.

4. Goldman M, Norcott HC, Hawker RJ, Hail C, Drolc Z, McCollum CN, Femoro-popliteal bypass grafts- an isotope technique allowing in vivo comparison of thrombogenicity. Brit. J. Surg. 69:380, 1982.

5. Lipton MJ, Doherty PW, Goodwin DA, Bushberg GT, Prager R, Meares CF, Evaluation of catheter thrombogenicity in vivo with Indium labelled platelets. Radiology 135:191, 1980.

6. Zahavi J, Jones NAG, Al-Hassani SFA, Kakkar VV, Prevention of white thrombus formation of Indium-111 labelled platelets in pigs by a thromboxane synthetase inhibitor. Brit. J. Rad. 53:924, 1980.

7. Wilkinson AR, Hawker RJ, Hawker LM, The influence of antiplatelet drugs on platelet survival after aortic damage or implantation of a dacron arterial prosthesis. Thromb. Res. 15:181, 1979.

8. Hawker RJ, Hawker LM, A microcytotoxicity assay using 111-Indium oxine release from platelets. J. Immunol. Methods 33:45, 1980.

9. Frost P, Wiltrout R, Maciorowski Z, Rose NR, An isotope release cytotoxicity assay applicable to human tumours: The use of 111-Indium. Oncology 34:102, 1977.

10. Hudson EM, Ramsey RB, Evatt BL, Subcellular localisation of Indium-111 in Indium-111 labelled platelets. J. Lab. clin. Med. 97-577, 1981.

11. Baker JRJ, Butler KD, Eakins MN, Pay GF, White AM, Subcellular localisation of 111-In in human and rabbit platelets. Blood 59:351, 1982.

12. Jeyasingh K, Barrison IG, Murray-Lyon IM, Jewkes RF, Stability of 111-Indium labelled platelets. Nucl. Med. Commun. 2:119, 1981.

13. Webber MM, Chang B, Buffkin D, Verma R, In-111-labelled platelets or iodinated fibrinogen for the detection of deep vein thrombosis. J. nucl. Med. 20:459, 1979.

14. Joist JH, Baker RK, Loss of 111-Indium as indicator of platelet injury. Blood 58:350, 1981.

15. DeWanjee MK, Roa SA, Didisheim P, Distribution of Indium-111 in labelled human platelets: implications in platelet survival and dosimetry. Thrombos. Haemost. 46:417, 1981.

16. Tsukada T, Effect of solvents on Indium-111 oxine transport in human platelets and on platelet function in vitro. Thrombos. Haemost. 46:416, 1981.

17. Greenberg JP, Packham MA, Guccione MA, Rand ML, Reimers HJ, Mustard JF, Survival of rabbit platelets treated in vitro with chymotrypsin,

18. George JN, Lewis PC, Morgan RK, Studies on platelet plasma membranes. 111. Membrane glycoprotein loss from circulating platelets in rabbits: inhibition by aspirin-dipyridamole and acceleration by thrombrin. J. Lab. clin. Med. 91:301, 1978.

19. DeWanjee MK, Vogel SR, Peterson KA, Kaye MP, Quantitation of platelet lysis, platelet consumption on oxygenator and stabilisation of platelet membrane with prostacyclin and ibuprofen during cardio-pulmonary bypass surgery in dogs. Thrombos. Haemost. 46:263, 1981.

20. Hawker RJ, Hawker LM, Wilkinson AR, Indium (111-In) labelled human platelets: optimal method. Clin. Sci. 58:243, 1980.

21. Hamlin GW, Rajah SM, Crow MJ, Kester RC, Evaluation of the thrombogenic potential of three types of arterial graft studied in an artificial circulation. Brit. J. Surg. 65:272, 1978.

22. Hawker RJ, Hall CE, Aukland A, Goldman M, McCollum CN, The preparation and use of 113m-Indium oxine as a platelet label. Nucl. Med. Biol. 1:910, 1982.

23. Riches DWH, Stanworth DR, Studies on the possible involvement of complement component C3 in the initiation of acid hydrolase secretion by macrophages. 1. Correlation between enzyme-releasing and complement activating capacities of several secretagogues. Immunology 44:29, 1981.

24. Goldman M, Hall C, Hawker RJ, McCollum CN, Dazoxiben examined for platelet inhibitory effect in an artificial circulation. Brit. J. clin. Pharm. 15:61S, 1983.

PLATELETS: KINETIC STUDIES

5 THE MATURATION OF MEGAKARYOCYTES AND THEIR PRECURSORS

J.M. PAULUS

INTRODUCTION

Maturation and amplification of the thrombocytic cells is achieved by a sequence of cells which are termed megakaryocyte progenitors, promegakaryoblasts and megakaryoblasts and finally promegakaryocytes and megakaryocytes. Amplification in these cells follows distinct mechanisms. Cellular multiplication occurs only at the progenitor stage. In promegakaryoblasts and megakaryoblasts a second amplification process does not yield any increase in cell number but rather consists of a series of endoduplications resulting in a polyploid cell whose nuclear and cytoplasmic volume are roughly proportional to ploidy level. Finally arrest of DNA synthesis and endoduplications marks the transition to the megakaryocyte stage. The present paper will briefly review the physiology of these cells.

Megakaryocyte progenitors

Megakaryocytes arise from multipotential stem cells capable of self renewing and no differentiating into the erythrocytic, myelocytic-macrophage and megakaryocyte series. In cultures of mouse bone marrow, megakaryocyte progenitors can form clones (1-3) composed of megakaryocytes (4-9), of megakaryocytes and erythroblasts (2) or of several lineages including megakaryocytes (1,3,10,11). In humans, two culture systems appear to assay distinct progenitor populations (12-14). One of these systems is described in this volume by Breton-Gorius et al.

Whether progenitors of pure megakaryocyte clones belong to a single homogeneous or several distinct populations, possibly descending from each other, is debatable. The possibility exists that distinct populations peak at different culture times. That this is so was recently shown by establishing cumulative doubling distributions in megakaryocyte colonies grown from 3 to 14 days (15). Abrupt shifts of the exponential slopes of these distributions have suggested a model based on three consecutive compartments, each of which is characterized by a given probability for the progenitors to switch to polyploidisation (15). The two late CFU-M compartments appear to parallel the early (day 8 BFU-E) and late (day 3 BFU-E) erythrocytic progenitors also demonstrated in mice (16).

Promegakaryoblast

Staining for acetylcholinesterase in species where this enzyme is specific or quasi specific for the megakaryocyte lineage (17) individualized a class of probably diploid cells which form single megakaryocytes in culture conditions and which support the growth of large colonies from megakaryocyte progenitors (18). Such cells appear to be committed to polyploidisation and may be termed promegakaryoblasts (19). Similar cells were demonstrated in mice using fluorescent antiplatelet sera (17,20) and in man using immunofluorescence (14,21) or the ultrastructural peroxidase reaction which labels the nuclear envelope and endoplasmic reticulum of early and late thrombocytic cells (22).

Megakaryoblast

Polyploidisation takes place exclusively in megakaryoblasts, large cells with a basophilic cytoplasm and a slightly or non indented nucleus (23-26). Microspectrophotometric studies of the nucleus of megakaryoblasts and megakaryocytes have measured in rats, rabbits and guinea pigs cells containing 4, 8, 13, 32 or 64 times the haploid DNA complement (24-27), the number most commonly encountered being 16 N. About the same pattern of ploidy distribution appears to hold for man (28,29). Apparently because of differences in megakaryocyte sampling, a somewhat different distribution was obtained on unseparated, suspended marrow using flow cytophotometry, in which the predominant ploidy class was 8 B (30).

Although appearing immature in Wright-stained smears megakaryoblasts synthetize low amounts of platelet organelles and constituents. The ultrastructure of megakaryoblasts and megakaryocytes has been reviewed (22,31,32). Cells incorporating tritiated thymidine produce low levels of demarcation membranes and specific granules (26,33). Megakaryoblasts also incorporate sulfates in mucopolysaccharides and their Golgi complex concentrates these compounds in the alpha granules (34). Primary lysosomes (35) and catalase granules (36) are also synthesized. In rodents and cats, megakaryoblasts and megakaryocytes synthesize, transport and concentrate acethylcholinesterase for later extracellular secretion (37). By controlling acetylcholine concentration in hematopoietic tissues, the secretion of AchE by megakaryocytes could conceivably modulate the proliferative activity of megakaryocyte progenitors (37,38).

Promegakaryocyte and megakaryocyte

Although synthesis of specialized platelet products is initiated at the promegakaryoblast stage, completion of polyploidisation by massive synthesis of these products. Factor VIII: AGN (21,39) actin (40), fibrinogen, platelet glycoproteins Ib, IIb and IIIa, platelet myosin, fibronectin and platelet factor 4 (21) can be demonstrated in over 85% of megakaryocytes. Dense granules are rarely recognized (35) but serotonin can be incorporated by isolated megakaryocytes and liberated in a typical release reaction (41). Microtubulus and microfilaments are infrequently seen in developing megakaryocytes but their constuent proteins have been identified by a variety of techniques (32,42,43).

Delineation of platelet territories

Demarcation membranes, which individualize future platelet territories, develop through a complex fusion-fission process involving fenestrated tubulus connected to the plasma membrane (44). Demarcation membranes and the enclosed open canalicular system serve as an uptake and extrusion route for products absorbed and secreted by megakaryocytes and platelets (45,46).

In some areas of megakaryocyte cytoplasm, demarcation membranes closely associate with the smooth endoplasmic reticulum or dense tubular system (46,47), determining membrane complexes which resemble the association of transverse tubular system (T system) and sarcoplasmic reticulum in muscle and may have a similar function in the control of calcium fluxes (see fig. 14, in ref. 48).

Determination of platelet size

Several papers, previously reviewed (49,50), have established the approximately lognormal distribution of platelet volumes and dry weights. It has been demonstrated that lognormality may be produced by random variations in the percentage changes in volume or weight undergone by platelet territories during successive steps of megakaryocyte cytoplasmic growth and fragmentation (51). This explanation was shown (49) to account for the correlation between size and platelet functional activity (52), the inverse correlation between size and platelet count (51-55) and the macrothrombocytosis observed in certain clinical conditions (51,53,56). The possibility that platelet size additionally depends on megakaryocyte ploidy (57), particularly in dysthrombocytopoiesis (58), is uncertain. The relationships between platelet aging, size and density have been reviewed (49).

Platelet-releasing megakaryocytes

Platelet liberation by megakaryocytes was discovered in 1910 by Wright who showed that mature megakaryocytes extend filaments of cytoplasm into sinusoidal spaces, where they detach and fragment into individual platelets (59). Later studies, utilizing phase contrast microscopy in tissue culture (60) or electron microscopy (61), have confirmed this view. Most megakaryocytes reside less than 1 μm from a marrow sinus, a distribution which is unlikely to be due to chance (62). Cytoplasmic processes containing longitudinally oriented microtubulus, which probably originate from an organizing centriolar center, extend into sinusoids. There they undergo attenuation and develop constrictions which rupture to release platelets (63). This process indicates that platelet size distribution may depend just as much on the manner the released cytoplasmic processes are fragmented than on the arrangement of megakaryocyte demarcation membranes inside megakaryocyte. Since newborn platelets are already highly heterogenous in size (51), decrease in platelet size with aging may increase or decrease the overall platelet heterogeneity, depending on whether or not it affects platelet fractions uniformly. As an example, computer simultations showed that even a 30% reduction in platelet volume during a normal life span would cause insignificant alterations in the shape of platelet volume distributions and their coefficient of variation of volumes (64).

REFERENCES

1. Metcalf D, Johnson GR, Mandel TE, Colony formation in agar by multipotential hemopoietic cells. J. Cell. Physiol. 98:401, 1979.

2. McLeod DL, Shreeve MM, Axelrad AA, Chromosome marker evidence for the bipotentiality of BFU-E. Blood 56:318, 1980.

3. Hara HV, Noguchi K, Clonal nature of pluripotent hemopoietic precursors in vitro (CFU-mix). Stem Cells 1:53, 1981.

4. Metcalf D, MacDonald HR, Odartchenko N, Sordat B, Growth of mouse megakaryocyte colonies in vitro. Proc. nat. Acad. Sci. USA 72:1744, 1975.

5. Nakeff A, Colony forming unit, megakaryocyte (CFU-M): Its use in elucidating the kinetics and humoral control of the megakaryocytic committed progenitor cell compartment. In: Experimental Hematology Today 1977. Baum SJ, Ledney GD (eds), Springer Verlag, New York, Heidelberg, Berlin, pp 111-123, 1977.

6. Williams N, Jackson H, Sheridan APC, Murphy MJ Jr, Elste A, Moore MAS, Regulation of megakaryocytopoiesis in long-term murine bone marrow cultures. Blood 51:245, 1978.

7. Mizoguchi H, Kubota K, Miura Y, Takaku F, An improved plasma culture system for the production of megakaryocyte colonies in vitro. Exp. Hemat. 7:345, 1979.

8. Burstein SA, Adamson JW, Thorning D, Harker LA, Characteristics of murine megakaryocytic colonies in vitro. Blood 54:169, 1979.

9. Levin J, Levin FC, Penington DG, Metcalf D, Measurement of ploidy distribution in megakaryocyte colonies obtained from cultures: With studies of the effects of thrombocytopenia. Blood 57:287, 1981.

10. Humphries RK, Eaves AC, Eaves CJ, Characterization of a primitive erythropoietic progenitor found in mouse marrow before and after several weeks in culture. Blood 54:746, 1979.

11. Johnson GR, Colony formation in agar by adult bone marrow multipotential hemopoietic cells. J. Cell. Physiol. 103:371, 1980.

12. Vainchenker W, Breton-Gorius J, Introduction of human megakaryocyte colonies in vitro and ultrastructural aspects of the maturation. In: Megakaryocytes in vitro. Evatt BL, Levine RF, Williams N (eds), Elsevier/North-Holland Biomedical Press, Amsterdam, New York, 1981 (in press).

13. Fauser AA, Messner HA, Identification of megakaryocyte, macrophages and eosinophils in colonies of human bone marrow containing neutrophilic granulocytes and erythroblasts. Blood 53:1023, 1979.

14. Mazur ME, Hoffman R, Bruno E, Marchesi S, Chasis J, Identification of two classes of human megakaryocyte progenitor cells. Blood 57:277, 1981.

15. Paulus JM, Prenant M, Deschamps JF, Henry-Amar M, Polyploid megakaryocytes develop randomly from a multicompartimental system of committed progenitors. Proc. nat. Acad. Sci. USA 79:4410, 1982.

16. Gregory CJ, Erythropoietin sensitivity as a differentiation marker in the hemopoietic system: Studies of three erythropoietic colony

responses in culture. J. Cell. Physiol. 89:289, 1976.

17. Jackson CW, Some characteristics of rat megakaryocyte precursors identified using cholinesterase as a marker. In: Platelets: Production, Function, transfusion and storage. Baldini MG, Ebbe S (eds), Grune and Stratton, New York, pp 33-40, 1974.

18. Long MW, Williams N, Relationship of small acethylcholinesterase positive cells to megakaryocytes and clonable megakaryocytic cells. In: Megakaryocytes in vitro. Evat BL, Levine RF, Williams N (eds), Elsevier/North-Holland Biomedical Press, Amsterdam, New York, 1981 (in press).

19. Breton-Gorius J, Megakaryoblastic leukemia. Haematologica 64:517, 1979.

20. Mayer M, Schaefer J, Queisser W, Idenficiation of young megakaryocytes by immunofluorescence and cytophotometry. Blut 37:265, 1978.

21. Rabellino EM, Levene RB, Lawrence LK, Leung LK, Nachman RL, Human megakaryocytes. II. Expression of platelet proteins in early marrow megakaryocytes. J. exp. Med. 154:88, 1981.

22. Breton-Gorius J, Reyer F, Ultrastructure of human bone marrow cell maturation. Int. Rev. Cytol. 46:251,1976.

23. Ebbe S, Stohlman F Jr, Megakaryocytopoiesis in the rat. Blood 26:20, 1965.

24. De Leval M, Contribution à l'étude de la maturation des mégacaryocytes dans la moelle osseuse de cobaye. Arch. Biol. 79:597, 1968.

25. Odell TT Jr, Jackson CW, Polyploidy and maturation of rat megakaryocytes. Blood 32:102, 1968.

26. Paulus JM, DNA metabolism and devlopment of organelles in guinea pig megakaryocytes: A combined ultrastructural, autoradiographic and cytophotometric study. Blood 35:298, 1970.

27. Garcia AM, Feulgen-DNA values in megakaryocytes. J. Cell. Biol. 20:342, 1964.

28. Kinet-Denoël C, Bassleer R, Andrien JM, Paulus JM, Penington DA, Weste SM, Ploidy histograms in ITP. In: Platelet kinetics. Paulus JM (ed), Elsevier/North-Holland Biomedical Press, Amsterdam, New York, pp 280-286, 1971.

29. Queisser U, Queisser W, Spiertz B, Polyploidization in patients with idiopathic thrombocytopenia and with pernicious anemia. Brit. J. Haemat. 20:489, 1971.

30. Levine RF, Bunn PA Jr, Hazzard KC, Schlam ML, Flow cytometric analysis of megakaryocyte ploidy. Comparison with Feulgen microdensitometry and discovery that 8 N is the predominant ploidy class in guinea pig and monkey marrow. Blood 56:210, 1980.

31. Behnke O, Pederson TN, Ultrastructural aspects of megakaryocyte maturation and platelet release. In: Platelet: Production, function, transfusion and storage. Baldini MG, Ebbe S (eds), Grune and Stratton, New York, pp 21-32, 1974.

32. Zucker-Franklin D, Megakaryocytes and platelets. In: Atlas of blood cells, function and pathology. Zucker D, Franklin MF, Greaves MF, Grossi CE, Marmont AM (eds), Vol. 2, Edi Ermes, Milano, Italy and Lea and Febiger, Philadelphia, pp 557-602, 1981.

33. MacPherson GG, Development of megakaryocytes in bone marrow of the rat: An analysis by electron microscopy and high resolution autoradiography. Proc. roy. Soc. B. London, B 177:265, 1971.

34. MacPherson GG, Synthesis and localization of sulfated mucopolysaccharide in megakaryocytes and platelets of the rat: An analysis by electron microscopic autoradiography. J. Cell. Sci. 10:705, 1972.

35. Bentfeld ME, Bainton DF, Cytochemical localization of lysosomal enzymes in rat megakaryocytes and platelets. J. clin. Invest. 56:1635, 1975.

36. Breton-Gorius J, Guichard J, Two different types of granules in megakaryocytes and platelets as revealed by the diaminobenzidine method. J. Microsc. Biol. Cell 23:197, 1975.

37. Paulus JM, Maigne J, Keyhani E, Mouse megakaryocytes secrete acetylcholinesterase. Blood 58:1100, 1981.

38. Burstein SA, Adamson JW, Harker LA, Megakaryocytopoiesis in culture: Modulation by cholinergic mechanisms. J. Cell. Physiol. 103:201, 1980.

39. Nachman R, Levine R, Jaffe EA, Synthesis of factor VIII antigen by cultures guinea-pig megakaryocytes. J. clin. Invest. 60:914, 1977.

40. Nachman R, Levine R, Jaffe EA, Synthesis of actin by cultured guinea-pig megakaryocytes: Complex formation with fibrin. Biochim. biophys. Acta 513:91, 1978.

41. Fedorko ME, The functional capacity of guinea pig megakaryocytes. I. Uptake of 3 H-serotonin by megakaryocytes and their physiologic and morphologic response to stimuli for the platelet release reaction. Lab. Invest. 36:310, 1977.

42. Nachman RL, Marcus AJ, Safier LB, Platelet thrombosthenin: Subcellular localization and function. J. clin. Invest. 46:1380, 1967.

43. Behnke O, Emmersen J, Structural identification of thrombosthenin in rat megakaryocytes. Scand. J. Haemat. 9:130, 1972.

44. Tavasolli M, Fusion-fission reorganization of membrane: A developing membrane model for thrombocytogenesis in megakaryocytes. Blood Cells 5:89, 1979.

45. Behnke O, An electron microscopic study of megakaryocytes of rat bone marrow. I. Development of the demarcation membrane system and platelet surface coat. J. Ultrastruct. Res. 24:412, 1968.

46. White JG, Interaction of membrane systems in blood platelets. Amer. J. Path. 66:295, 1972.

47. Breton-Gorius J, Development of two distinct membrane systems associated in giant complexes in pathological megakaryocytes. Ser. Haemat. 8:49, 1975.

48. Gerrard JM, White JG, Prostaglandins and thromboxanes: Middle-men modulating platelet function in hemostasis and thrombosis. In: Progress in Haemostasis and Thrombosis. Speat TH (ed), Vol. 4, Grune and Stratton, New York, pp 87-125, 1978.

49. Paulus JM, Bury J, Grosdent JC, Control of platelet territory development in megakaryocytes. Blood Cells 5:51, 1979.

50. Dighiero F, Lesty C, Leporrier M, Couty MC, Computer analysis of platelet volumes. Blood Cells 6:365, 1980.

51. Paulus JM, Platelet size in man. Blood 46:321, 1975.

52. Karpatkin S, Heterogeneity of platelet function. Correlation with platelet volume. Amer. J. Med. 64:542, 1978.

53. Von Behrens WE, Mediterranean macrothrombocytopenia. Blood 46:199, 1975.

54. O'Brien JR, Jamieson S, A relationship between platelet volume and platelet number. Thrombos. Diathes. haemorrh. Stuttg. 31:363, 1974.

55. Zeigler Z, Murphy S, Gardner FH, Microscopic platelet size and morphology in various hematologic disorders. Blood 51:479, 1978.

56. Godwin HA, Ginsburg AD, May-Hegglin anomaly: A defect in megakaryocyte fragmentation? Brit. J. Haemat. 26:117, 1974.

57. Penington DG, Streatfield K, Roxburgh AE, Megakaryocytes and the heterogeneity of circulating platelets. Brit. J. Haemat. 34:639, 1976.

58. Paulus JM, Breton-Gorius J, Kinet-Denoël C, Boniver C, Megakaryocyte ultrastructure and ploidy in human macrothrombocytosis. In: Platelets: Production, Function, Transfusion and Storage. Baldini MG, Ebbe S (eds), Grune and Stratton, New York, pp 131-142, 1974.

59. Wright JH, The histogenesis of the blood platelets. J. Morph. 21:203, 1910.

60. Thiery JP, Bessis M, Mécanisme de la plaquettogénèse. Etude in vivo par la microcinématographie. Rev. Hemat. 11:162, 1956.

61. Behnke O, An electron microscopic study of the rat megakaryocyte II. Some aspects of platelet release and microtubules. J. Ultrastruc. Res. 26:111, 1969.

62. Lichtman MA, Chamberlain JK, Simon W, Santillo PA, Parasinusoidal location of megakaryocytes in marrow: A determinant of platelet release. Amer. J. Hemat. 4:303, 1978.

63. Radley JM, Scurfield G, The mechanism of platelet release. Blood 56: 996, 1980.

64. Esch L, Breny K, Paulus JM, A theoretical study of the influence of platelet senescence on platelet size lognormality. Proc. 5th Cong. Eur. Afric. Div. Internat. Soc. Haemat. Hamburg, Vol. 1, p 29, 1979.

6 MEGAKARYOCYTIC PRECURSORS

J. BRETON-GORIUS, W. VAINCHENKER

The recent developments of both culture techniques, determination of differentiation antigens by monoclonal antibodies and cytochemistry has permitted to define several classes of megakaryocytic precursors in murine and human species.

The first megakaryocytic precursor which has been identified is the megakaryoblast. This cell can be recognized by morphological criteriae, particularly by its large size. In the normal bone marrow, nearly only megakaryocytes have a diameter larger than 20 µM (1), and 87-97% of the bone marrow megakaryocytes have a size higher than 14 µm (1). As the size of the megakaryocytes increases with maturation and ploidy level, the first recognizable megakaryocyte precursors have just a larger size than the other marrow cells and corresponds to a ploidy group of 8 N (18 µm diameter) or rarely 4 N (12 µm diameter) (1). This cell has already a bi- or multilobulated nucleus that occupies almost the entire cell volume. At electron microscopic level, this megakaryocytic precursor exhibits some specific cytoplasmic organelles as demarcation membranes and α-granules. This cell has lost its proliferative capacities but retains the capacity of DNA replication and is only able to increase its ploidy level usually to 16 N or 32 N by endomitosis.

It has been demonstrated in rodents and cats, that an enzyme acetylcholinesterase, was nearly specific for the megakaryocytic lineage (2). This enzyme can be easily detected by an optical cytochemical reaction (3). Jackson (4) has demonstrated that a small size (8-18 µM) cell displays this cytochemical marker in the normal bone marrow. These cells have either a round or an indented or lobed nucleus (5). It is the

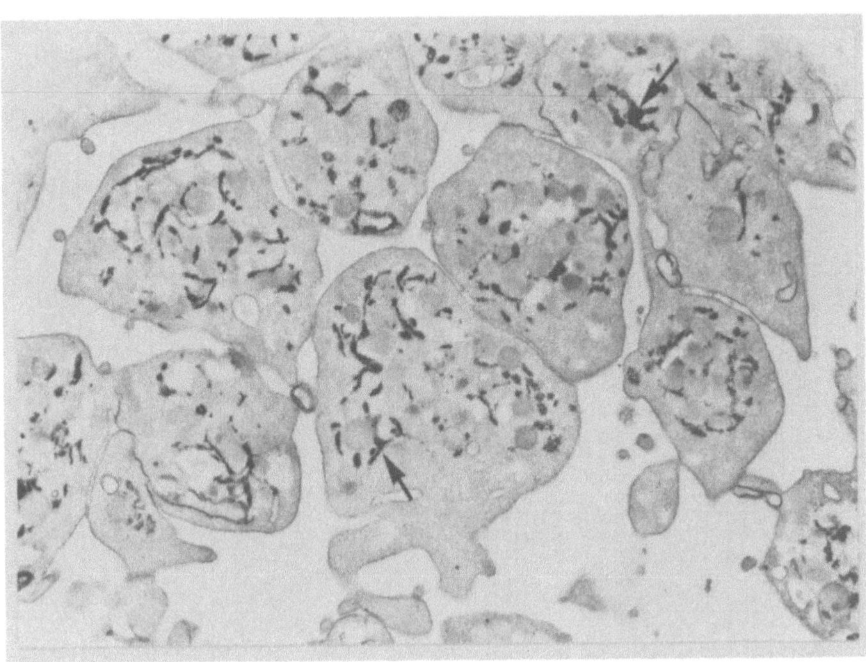

Fig.1: x 17 820. The platelet peroxidase (PPO) is observed in all platelets and marrow megakaryocytes. It is only detected at ultrastructural level, and only is located in the endoplasmic reticulum and the perinuclear space of the megakaryocyte. It is absent from the granules and the Golgi apparatus. Fig 1: x 17 820.

first identifiable cell of the megakaryocytic lineage. Their number (10% of the total number of megakaryocytes) is regulated by the platelet demand (4-7). It is increased or suppressed after induction of thrombocytopenia or thrombocytosis (4,6,7).

Unfortunately, human megakaryocytes are devoid of acetylcholinesterases which are present in the human erythroid serie (2). Breton-Gorius et al have demonstrated that another enzyme, platelet peroxidase (PPO) which is specific of the megakaryocytic lineage can be detected by ultrastructural cytochemistry in platelets (fig 1) megakaryocytes (fig 2). PPO is present in the megakaryocytic serie of all species until now studied (8,9), including human (9). A small diploid cell exhibiting only this enzymatic marker is present in the normal

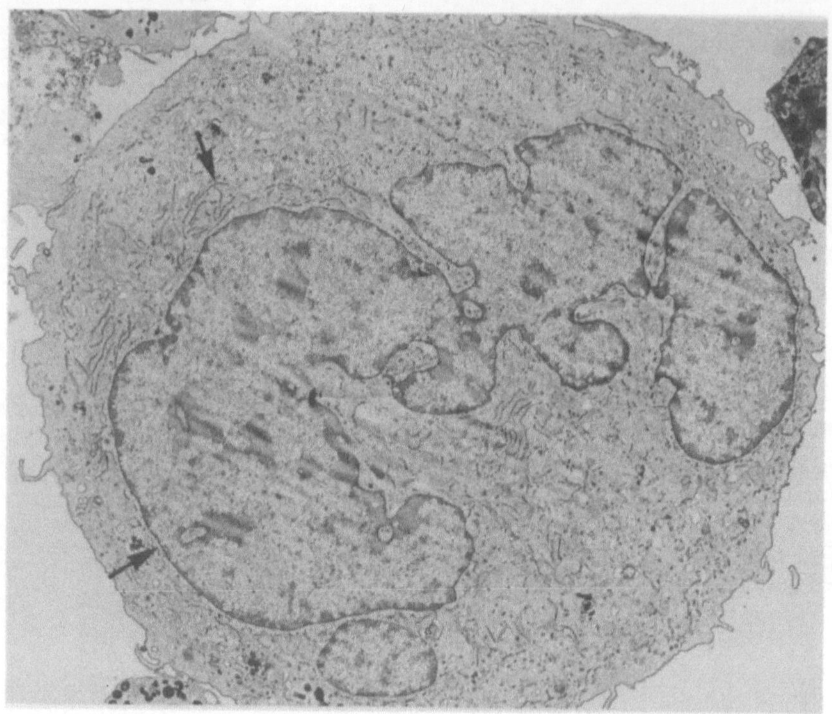

Fig. 2: x 5 200. See legend of fig. 1.

bone marrow (9). This cell does not exhibit any megakaryocytic cytoplasmic organelle (fig 3). This cell has been defined as promegakaryoblast (10). The use of PPO as a specific probe of the megakaryocytic lineage is heavily restricted by its revelation mostly at ultrastructural level (9). The recent development of immunological techniques has permitted to demonstrate that human promegakaryoblasts already synthesize all the platelet specific antigens as platelet glycoproteins (11-13) particularly GpIb (fig 4), GpIs, GpIIIa, GpIIb-IIIa complex, platelet factor IV, fibrinogen, factor VIII (11-16), and are capable of serotonin uptake (17). Therefore, several monoclonal antibodies recognizing platelet glycoproteins as AN 51 (14,16,18), J.15 (14,18,) C 17 (16) are binding to promegakaryoblasts. At EM level, it has been demonstrated that in promegakaryoblastic leukemia, these antibodies bind to "undifferentiated cells"

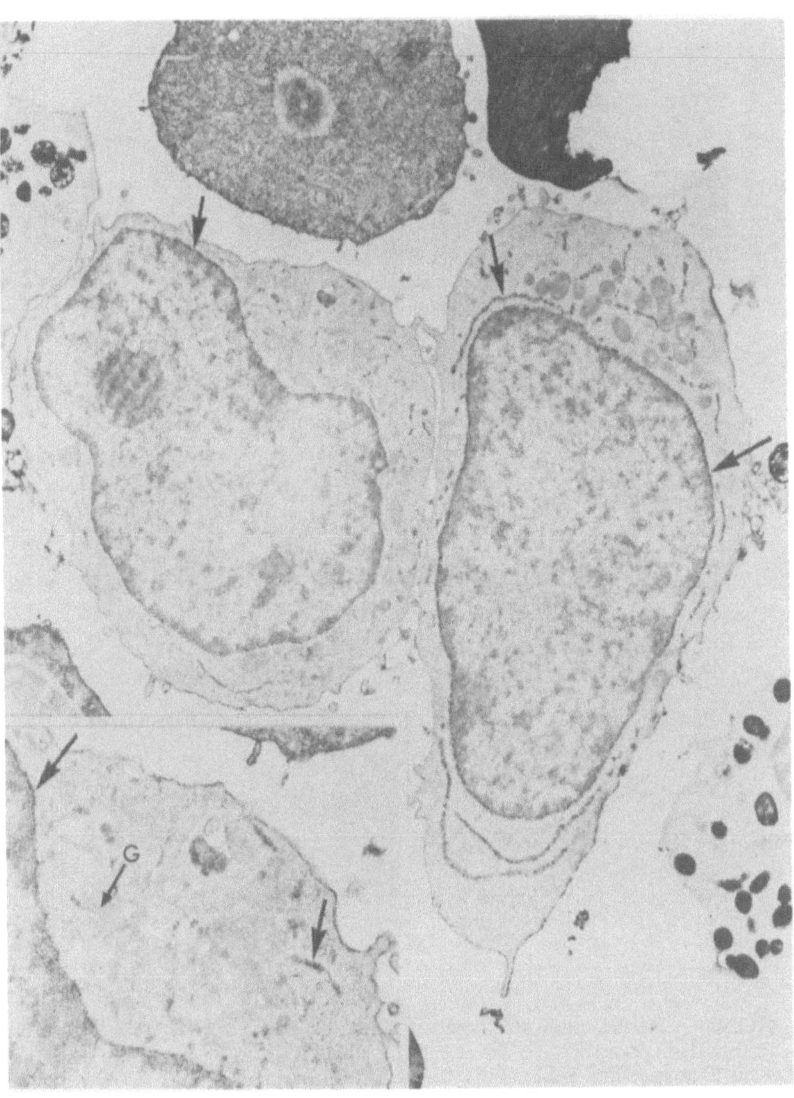

Fig. 3. In a normal bone marrow, rare cells (<0.1%) only exhibiting the PPO marker are present. No specific megakaryocytic organelles as α-granules, or demarcation membranes are present. These cells are called promegakaryoblasts. x 10 100. Inset: An enlargement of fig 3 shows that PPO is present in the perinuclear space, the endoplasmic reticulum but is absent from the Golgi apparatus. x 21 800.

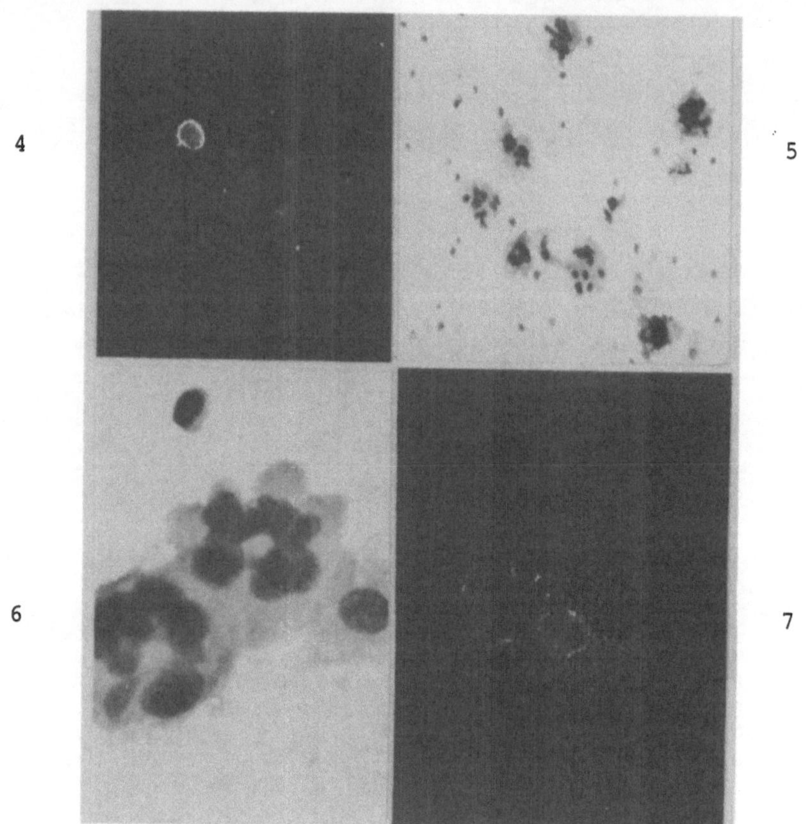

Fig. 4.Using a monoclonal antibody against platelet glycoprotein Ib (AN 51), it is also possible to detect rare small cells ($\simeq$ 8 µm) in the bone marrow by fluorescent labelling. These cells are identical to the promegakaryoblasts described in fig 3.

Fig. 5. A typical megakaryocyte colony is observed at a low magnification. At least, 9 megakaryocytes are loosely aggregated. This type of colony is typical of plasma clot culture. The stimulating factor is PHA-LCM.

Fig. 6. At a higher magnification, the 2 megakaryocytes are easily identifiable by their size, their polylobulated nucleus and cytoplasmic blebs. At the top, a macrophage is present. It has the same large size but exhibits a round nucleus.

Fig. 7. See next page.

Fig. 7. A part of a megakaryocyte colony, 3 cells are stained by the monoclonal antibody AN 51. The use of such fluorescent probe permits a safe identification of the megakaryocyte colonies.

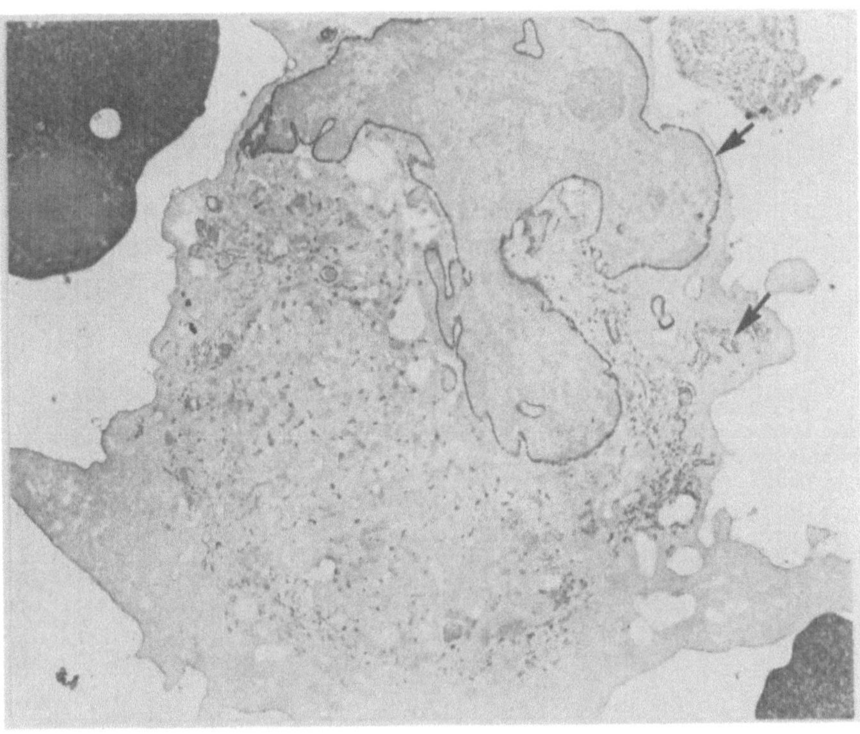

Fig. 8. Ultrastructural studies of a large megakaryocyte grown in culture from adult bone marrow precursors. Platelet peroxidase, α-granules, glycogen, demarcation membranes are present. x 7 920.

exhibiting PPO (18). This result suggests that immunological platelet markers define the same megakaryocytic precursor compartment as PPO or acetylcholinesterase.

It was first considered that the murine promegakaryoblasts were devoid of proliferative capacities and was only capable of endomitosis (5). Recent work demonstrates that promegakaryoblasts are able of at least one mitosis (19). These cells are regulated by the platelet demand,in the mouse as well as in man. Their number can be increased by a factor 100 in idiopathic thrombopenic purpura (14,20). It is suggested that this

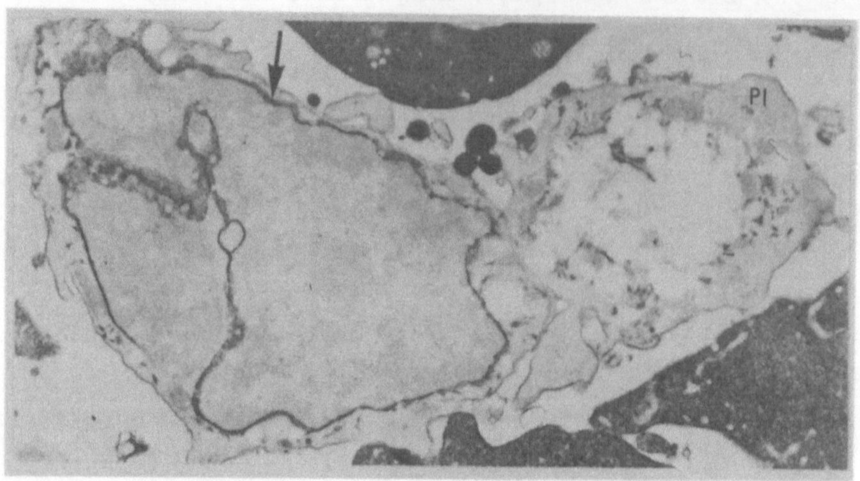

Fig. 9. A mature small megakaryocyte (micromegakaryocyte) has been grown from cord blood precursors. A large number of micromegakaryocytes are present in such cultures. This micromegakaryocyte is shedding a platelet. x 15 000.

cellular compartment (mitosis, endomitosis, cytoplasmic maturation) is regulated by the humoral factor called thrombopoietin (5). The level of thrombopoietin is dependent upon the platelet count.

The development of semi-solid cultures has permitted to define another class of megakaryocytic precursors. These cells called CFU-MK or CFU-M or MK-CFC, are capable to give rise to megakaryocyte colonies in vitro in agar, plasma clot or methylcellulose. Colonies were first obtained from mouse (21,22) and later from man (23) (fig 5,6). Identification of human megakaryocytic colonies has been solved by the use of immunological platelet markers to stain the cultured megakaryocytes (13,14,24) (fig 7). CFU-MK are present in the marrow and bloodcells (22,23) and also in spleen in the mouse (22,25). The maturation of the cultured megakaryocytes can be complete; α-granules, demarcation membranes, glycogen, platelet peroxidase are observed (fig 8). Platelet shedding may be present (fig 9). Addition of a stimulating factor (MK-CSF) is required to obtain growth of colonies. The usual sources of MK-CSF are pokeweed-, or lectin-stimulated spleen cells conditioned medium (22,26,27,28). WEHI-3 conditioned medium (29), Epo preparations (30-33) in the mouse, PHA-leukocyte conditioned medium (24,34,35,36), Epo preparations (37) in man. It has been recently demonstrated that sera from patients exhibiting a thrombocytopenia of marrow origin stimulate human megakaryocyte colony formation (38,39). MK-CSF has been enriched from urine of thrombocytopenic patients (40). Thrombopoietin-enriched preparations are unable by themselves to sustain MK colony formation (13,29,41,42,43,44) but are powerful potentiators (29,41,43,44). Williams et al have suggested that megakaryocyte colony formation was therefore regulated by 2 factors, the first one acting at the early phase of megakaryocyte differentiation, the second one, similar to thrombopoietin at late phase of differentiation (5,19,29,41,43,44). Recent data suggest that there are large differences between human sera and plasma in their capability to sustain megakaryocyte colony formation (24,36). Serum seems to contain a potent inhibitor of megakaryocyte colony formation both on the number and the size of the colonies (35). The size of the MK colonies is extremely variable depending upon culture conditions. Colonies up to a few hundred tight cells have been observed in methylcellulose (24,36) while in plasma clot, they are usualy composed of loose clusters of megakaryocytes (13,23,35,45). There are some differences among the authors in defining the minimum size for a MK colony. Some authors only consider aggregates of 3 or more cells as colonies (13,43,44). However, it has been clearly established that 2 cell clusters have a clonal origin (45); and therefore are truly derived from a single megakaryocytic precursors. In contrast, other authors consider that a single polyploid megakaryocyte may be the equivalent of a colony, i.e. a CFU-E colony may be composed of 8 cells (16 N) 31,33). Indeed, CFU-MK is a multicompartmental system. Some colonies only contain megakaryocytes and therefore are derived from a megakaryocytic committed progenitor, while other colonies are composed of multilineage cells, and are derived from a pluripotent stem cell (23,30,33,34,46,47). Paulus et al have suggested that megakaryocyte progenitors differentiate through 3 successive compartments. The polyploidization of megakaryocytes in culture was dependent upon the compartment of progenitors they derive (33). The regulation of the CFU-MK in vivo is not dependent upon the platelet demand (20,25,42,48). It does not seem that the CFU-MK bear the same antigenic determinants as megakaryocytes or platelets. However, it can not be totally excluded that the compartments of CFU-MKs and promegakaryoblasts are partially intermingled, and that the small size megakaryocyte colonies could arise from a promegakaryoblast (19) i.e. defined by the presence of platelet antigens. Future work using cell sorting and cytotoxicity will permit to more clearly identify the boundaries between these 2 cellular compartments. It has been very recently reported that some antibodies specifically recognize the CFU-MK either by the use of the murine hybridoma technique (49) or in patients exhibiting an amegakaryocytic thrombocytopenic purpura (50).

In the near future, the better identification of the megakaryocyte precursors will permit a better understanding of the megakaryopoiesis and the role of platelets in its regulation.

REFERENCES

1. Levine RF, Hazzard KC, Lamberg JD, The significance of megakaryocyte size. Blood 60:1122, 1982.

2. Zajicek J, Studies on the histogenesis of blood platelets and megakaryocytes. Acta Physiol. scand. 40:138, 1957 (suppl).

3. Karnosvsky MJ, Roots L, A direct coloring thiocholine method for cholinesterases. J. Histochem. Cytochem. 12:219, 1964.

4. Jackson CW, Cholinesterase as a possible marker for early cells of the megakaryocytic series. Blood 42:413, 1973.

5. Long MW, Williams N, Ebbe S, Immature megakaryocytes in the mouse. Physical characteristics, cell cycle status and in vitro responsiveness to thrombopoietic stimulating factor. Blood 59:569, 1982.

6. Long MW, Henry RL, Thrombocytosis induced suppression of small acetylcholinesterase positive cells in bone marrow of rats. Blood 54:1338, 1979.

7. Kalmaz GD, McDonald TP, Effects of antiplatelet serum and thrombopoietin on the percentage of small acetylcholinesterase-positive cells in bone marrow of mice. Exp. Hemat. 9:10002, 1981.

8. Breton-Gorius J, Guichard J, Ultrastructural localization of peroxidase activity in human platelets and megakaryocytes. Amer. J. Path. 66:277, 1972.

9. Breton-Gorius J, Reyes F, Ultrastructure of human bone marrow cell maturation. Int. Rev. Cytol. 46:251, 1976.

10. Breton-Gorius J, Megakaryoblastic leukemia. Hematologica 64:517, 1979.

11. Rabellino EM, Nachman RL, Williams N, Winchester RJ, Ross GD, Human megakaryocytes. I. Characterization of the membranes and cytoplasmic components of isolated marrow megakaryocytes. J. exp. Med. 149:1273, 1979.

12. Rabellino E, Levine RB, Leung LLK, Nachman RL Human megakaryocytes II. Expression of platelet proteins in early marrow megakaryocytes. J. exp. Med. 154:88, 1981.

13. Mazur DM, Hoffman R, Chasis J, Marchesi S, Bruno E, Immunofluorescent identification of human megakaryocyte colonies using an antiplatelet glycoprotein antisera. Blood 57:277, 1981.

14. Vainchenker W, Deschamps JF, Bastin JM, Guichard J, Titeux M, Breton-Gorius J, McMichael AJ, Two monoclonal antiplatelet antibodies as markers of human megakaryocyte maturation. Immunofluorescent staining and platelet peroxidase detection in megakaryocyte colonies and in vivo cells from normal and leukemic patients. Blood 59:514, 1982.

15. Nachman R, Levine R, Jaffe EA, Synthesis of factor VIII antigen by cultured guinea pig megakaryocytes. J. clin. Invest. 60:914, 1977.

16. Vinci G, Tabilio A, Deschamps JF, Henri A, Vainchenker W, Breton-Gorius J, Immunological phenotype of cultured human megakaryocytes. In preparation.

17. Schick PK, Weinstein M, A marker for megakaryocytes: serotonin accumulation in guinea pig megakaryocytes. J. Lab. clin. Med. 98:607, 1981.

18. Breton-Gorius J, Vanhaeke D, Tabilio A, Vainchenker W, Deschamps JF, Xu FS, Glycoprotein I. Identification during normal and pathological megakaryocytic maturation. Blood Cells, 1983 (in press).

19. Long MW, Williams N, McDonald TP, Immature megakaryocytes in the mouse; in vitro relationship to megakaryocyte progenitor cells and mature megakaryocytes. J. Cell. Physiol. 112:339, 1982.

20. Vainchenker W, Tabilio A, Vinci G, Clauvel JP, Breton-Gorius J, Megakaryocyte precursors in ITP: Influence of treatment. In preparation.

21. Nakeff A, Dicke KA, Van Noord MJ, Megakaryocytes in agar cultures of mouse bone marrow. Ser. Haemat. 8:4, 1975.

22. Metcalf D, McDonald HR, Odartchenko N, Sordat B, Growth of mouse megakaryocyte colonies in vitro. Proc. nat. Acad. Sci. USA, 72:1744, 1975.

23. Vainchenker W, Guichard J, Breton-Gorius J, Growth of human megakaryocyte colonies in culture from fetal, neonatal and adult peripheral blood cells. Ultrastructural analysis. Blood Cells, 5:25, 1979.

24. Kantz L, Straub G, Bross KG, Fauser AA, Identification of human megakaryocytes derived from pure megakaryocytic colonies (CFU-M), megakaryocytic/erythroid colonies (CFU/M/E) and mixed hemopoietic colonies (CFU-GEMM) by antibodies against platelet associated antigens. Blut, 45:267, 1982.

25. Levin J, Levin FC, Metcalf D, The effects of acute thrombocytopenia on megakaryocyte-CFC and granulocyte macrophage-CFC in mice. Studies of bone marrow and spleen. Blood 56:274, 1980.

26. Nakeff A, Daniels-McQueen S, In vitro colony assay for a new class of megakaryocyte precursor. Colony forming unit megakaryocyte (CFU-M). Proc. Soc. exp. Biol. Med. 151:587, 1976.

27. Burstein SA, Adamson JW, Thorning D, Harker LA, Characteristics of murine megakaryocytic colonies in vitro. Blood 54:169, 1979.

28. Mizoguchi H, Kubota K, Miura Y, Takaku F, An improved plasma culture system for the production of megakaryocyte colonies in vitro. Exp. Hemat. 7:345, 1979.

29. Williams N, Jackson H, Sheridan APC, Murphy MJ Jr, Elsta A, Moore MAS, Regulation of megakaryopoiesis in longterm murine bone marrow cultures. Blood 51:245, 1978.

30. McLeod DL, Shreeve MM, Axelrad AA, Induction of megakaryocyte colonies with platelet formation in vitro. Nature 261:492, 1976.

31. Dukes PP, Izadi P, Ortega JA, Shore NA, Gomperts E, Inhibitory effects of interferon on mouse megakaryocytic progenitor cells in culture. Exp. Hemat. 8:1048, 1980.

32. Freedman MH, McDonald TP, Saunders EF, Differentiation of murine marrow megakaryocyte progenitors (CFU-M). Humoral control in vitro. Cell Tissue Kinet. 14:53, 1981.

33. Paulus JM, Prenant M, Deschamps JF, Henry-Amar M, Polyploid megakaryocytes develop randomly from a multicompartmental system of committed progenitors. Proc. nat. Acad. Sci. USA, 79:4410, 1982.

34. Fausser AA, Messner HA, Identification of megakaryocytes, macrophages and eosinophils in colonies of human bone marrow containing neutrophilic granulocytic and erythroblasts. Blood 53:1023, 1979.

35. Vainchenker W, Chapman J, Deschamps JF, Vinci G, Bouquet J, Titeux M, Breton-Gorius J, Normal human serum contains a factor(s) capable of inhibiting megakaryocyte colony formation. Exp. Hemat. 10:650, 1982.

36. Messner HA, Jamal N, Izaguirre C, The growth of large megakaryocyte colonies from human bone marrow. J. Cell. Physiol. 45 (suppl. I), 1982.

37. Vainchenker W, Bouquet J, Guichard J, Breton-Gorius J, Megakaryocyte colony formation from human bone marrow precursors. Blood 54:940, 1979.

38. Mazur E, Hoffman R, Bruno E, Regulation of human megakaryocytopoiesis. An in vitro analysis. J. clin. Invest. 68:733, 1981.

39. Hoffman R, Mazur E, Bruno E, Floyd V, Assay of an activity in the serum of patients with disorders of thrombopoiesis that stimulates formation of megakaryocytic colonies. New Engl. J. Med. 305:533, 1981.

40. Enomoto K, Kawakita M, Kishimoto S, Katayama N, Miyake T, Thrombopoiesis and megakaryocyte colony stimulating factor in the urine of patients with aplastic anaemia. Brit. J. Haemat. 45:551, 1980.

41. Williams N, McDonald TP, Rabellino EM, Maturation and regulation of megakaryocytopoiesis. Blood Cells 5:43, 1979.

42. Levin J, Levin FC, Hull III DF, Penington DG, The effects of thrombopoietin on megakaryocyte-CFC, megakaryocytes, and thrombopoiesis with studies of ploidy and platelet size. Blood 60:989, 1982.

43. Williams N, Jackson H, Ralph P, Nakoinz I, Cell interactions influencing murine marrow megakaryopoiesis. Nature of the potentiator cell in bone marrow. Blood 57:157, 1981.

44. Williams N, Eger RR, Jackson HM, Nelson DJ, Two factor requirement for murine megakaryocyte colony formation. J. Cell. Physiol. 110:101, 1982.

45. Vainchenker W, Testa U, Deschamps JF, Henri A, Titeux M, Breton-Gorius J, Rochant H, Lee D, Cartron JP, Clonal expression of the Tn antigen in erythroid and granulocyte colonies and its application to determination of the clonality of the human megakaryocyte colony assay. J. clin. Invest. 69:1081, 1982.

46. Johnson GR, Metcalf D, Pure and mixed erythroid colony formation in vitro stimulated by spleen conditioned medium with no detectable erythropoietin. Proc. nat. Acad. Sci. USA, 74:3879, 1977.

47. Nakahata T, Ogawa M, Clonal origin of murine hemopoietic colonies with apparent restriction to granulocyte-macrophage-megakaryocyte. (GMM) differentiation. J. Cell. Physiol. 111:239, 1982.

48. Burstein SA, Erb SK, Adamson JW, Harker L, Immunologic stimulation of early murine haematopoiesis and its abrogation by cyclosporin. A. Blood 59:851, 1982.

49. Levene RB, Daniel Lamaziere JM, Rabellino EM, Nachman RL, Leung LLK, Phenotypic analysis of human megakaryocyte progenitors. Blood 60:108 (suppl 1), 1982.

50. Hoffman R, Bruno E, Elwell J, Mazur E, Gewirtz AM, Dekker P, Dene AE, Acquired a megakaryocytic thrombocytopenic purpura. A syndrome of diverse etiologies. Blood 60:1173, 1982.

7 METHODS OF QUANTIFICATION OF PLATELET PRODUCTION IN MAN. A CRITICAL ANALYSIS

Y. NAJEAN

INTRODUCTION

In contrast with other myeloid series, and particularly the red cell series, relatively few methods enable to quantify platelet production. So, in clinical practice, only rough (and often questionable) estimation of platelet production can be obtained.

Three methods can be used: - morphological estimation of megakaryocyte density; - indirect calculation of production from direct measure of the destruction; - and direct measurement of production using tracers of the megakaryocytic line.

Morpholocigal study of platelet production

It is well known that megakaryocytic density evaluation is the first, and often sole method used by the physicians to decide if a thrombocytopenia is due to a central or a peripheral mechanism. As all the hematologists and isotopists know, frequent errors of diagnosis are due to the inaccuracy of this method. This is due to the low percentage of megakaryocytes, and to their clustering in some parts of the slide, because of their volume higher than that of the other cells; so the number cannot be given in terms of percentage of the myeloid cells, but only as an empirical estimation (0, +, ++, +++; or using a scale from 0 to 4).

For this reason, some authors tried to quantify the megakaryocytes on bone marrow biopsies. Harker (1) has presented a method, founded on a previous paper of Suit (2), who tried to quantify the number of erythroblasts by using simultaneously the measure of 59 iron uptake into a bone marrow sample and of the number of erythroblasts; knowing the total R B C incorporation of radio-iron (in percentage of the infused radioactivity) and the ratio radioactivity of the sample / infused radioactivity, it is possible to calculate the number of nucleated erythroid cells in the whole body. Harker suggested to count on bone marrow-slides (from B M biopsies) the ratio megakaryocytes / erythroblasts and from this value to measure the total number of megakaryocytes.

Three observations, however, can be made:

1. For erythroblastic quantification, it cannot be quaranteed that the ratio immature / mature erythroblasts in one sample is similar to that of the total erythroid organ; and on another hand the method does not take into account the ^{59}Fe-uptake by reticulocytes of bone marrow (and of the blood obtained with the marrow sample).
2. The ratio megakaryocytes-erythroblasts is not so easy to obtain as expected; due to the large diameter of megakaryocytes, one cell appears 2 or 3 times, at several levels, on consecutive thin slides, in contrast with erythroblasts which are only seen on one slide; a difficult correction is necessary.
3. From a practical point of view, it is worth noting that these methods have never been used in clinical research for immature cell quantification; our own assays have been unsuccessful.

Even if these failures were only methodological, it remains that such a morphological quantification does not have a sense, in many clinical situations. It seems that a large part of the production defects of platelets are due, not to a low number of the nucleated precursors, but to abnormal platelet release from these immature cells. An obvious example is the May-Hegglin abnormality, in which the quantitative platelet defect is due to abnormalities of the demarcation lines appearance into a normal number of megakaryocytes.

A possible progress, at my knowledge not yet explored, could be the cyto-chemical identification of platelet precursors, including the 2n-megakaryocytes not recognized by the present morphological methods; as shown by Breton-Gorius in this volume, fluorescent mono-clonal antibodies risen against specific membrane components, or against constituents of intra-cellular structures (as β-TG or PF-4) could be used after coupling with a fluorescent probe for a convenient quantification of this myeloid series.

Indirect measurement, using the quantification of the platelet renewal

At the present time, the method using the platelet survival time as measured by isotopic methods is the most reliable. The contrast between a normal cell survival and a low platelet count leads to the conclusion of a platelet abnormal production.

Two main criticisms may however be made. The first one is essentially theoretical. For isotopists, a measure of cell survival needs a so-called steady-state; but in fact, this is not important from a practical point of view.

The second one is methodological. When the platelet count is low, the labelling of autologous platelets by ^{51}Cr is difficult, with low yield and infusion of a relatively high percentage of labelled plasma proteins and often labelled red cells. So the curves obtained from the measure of whole blood-samples can be mistaken, if considered as curves of platelet survival; on the other hand, isolation of a reproducible platelet button from blood-samples is technically difficult. In such conditions, it is usual to measure platelet survival of foreign normal platelets infused in the patient, but errors are possible: either if iso-immunization reduces foreign cell survival, or if at the contrary normal survival of foreign cells does not depict a possible abnormal survival of the patients own platelets.

Therefore, in terms of kinetics, the recent introduction of ^{111}In-platelet labelling is a progress. It allows indeed to label autologous platelets even in cases with a low as 30 000 cells per mm^3 with minor plasma contamination. In our experience, the observed cell survival curves are convenient for calculating kinetic parameters (3).

Platelet production (P) is obtained by the following equation:

$$P = \frac{N\ (p)\ \times\ S\ (c)\ \times\ R\ (c)}{N\ (c)\ \times\ S\ (p)\ \times\ R\ (p)}$$

where N (p) and N (c) are the number of circulating platelets in patient (p) and control subjects (c), S (c) and S (p) the survival time,which is the reverse of the renewal rate, and R (p) and R (c) are the values for the platelet recovery after infusion of the labelled material.

This last point is worthy of further discussion. It is obvious indeed that the lower the recovery, the higher the extra-vascular platelet pool, in which in normal persons accounts for 20-30% of the total cell pool. In patients with splenomegaly (but not in all of them) high extra-vascular pool with low recovery is observed (hypersplenism), which could lead to under-estimation of platelet production if only parameters N and S were considered. Recovery is unfortunately a quantitative parameter very sensitive to technical artefacts, and a daily clinical practice of platelet kinetic studies obviously demonstrates the possible errors in its determination. R is calculated from the total infused radioactivity, rapported to the radioactivity measured in the blood-sample at its maximum (15 min in most of the cases; sometimes extrapolation of the survival curve to t_0). In reality, errors are done on the two terms of this ratio: infused radioactivity could not be exclusively platelet-bound (in the case of Indium-labelling, a relatively large part of the radioactivity is bound to the remaining plasma proteins), and similarly circulating radioactivity is also for a part a non-platelet-bound radioactivity. These remarks are particularly true in thrombocytopenic patients, which could explain that some authors considered that in idiopathic thrombocytopenic purpura (ITP), a part of thrombocytopenia could have been due to hypersplenism.

Doubt on the S (p) value may also occur, in these patients in which the "potential" survival is normal, but who demonstrate a curvilinear curve due to random platelet consumption added to normal senescence. In such cases, patients

Table 1. Kinetic data observed in pathological situations in man

	Platelet count (10^9/1)	Platelet survival	Recovery	Production
Severe idiopathic thrombocytopenic purpura (ITP)	<40	very short (homologous)	no valuable value in most of the cases (early destruction)	no valuable calculation
Moderate ITP	40–120	0.5 to 3 days (autologous)	0.4 to 0.7	1 to 3
Hypersplenism (abnormal platelet distribution)	40–120 rarely <40	5 to 9 days (autologous)	0.15 to 0.4	0.5 to 2
Production defect	all values are observed	7 to 10 days (autologous if platelet count >40)	0.5 to 0.8	0 to 0.5
Controls	140 – 440 (2 s.d.)	7 to 10 days	0.6 to 0.8	1 (± 0.5)

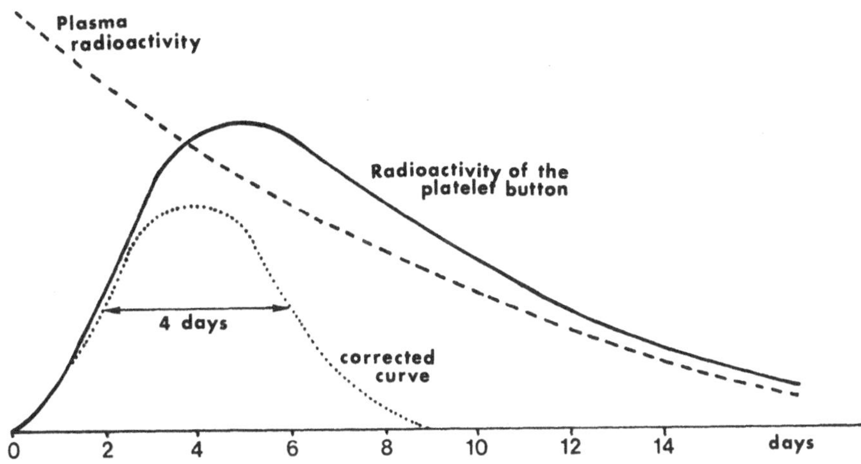

Table 2. ^{75}Se-methionine incorporation into the circulating platelets in humans in several clinical situations

	Maximal incorporation (%) of the injected dose)
Controles	0.18 ± 0.03
Thrombocytosis	1 to 2.2
Aplastic anemia	0.03 to 0.09
I T P (with platelet survival more than 2 days)	0.25 to 0.75

renewal rate could be under-estimated. In spite of these criticisms the method is good, and gives almost accurate values of effective platelet production in a given patient (table 1).

Direct measurement of platelet production, using in vivo uptake of radioisotopes by platelet precursors

From an ideal point of view, the best method for measuring cell production and in vivo kinetics is using a specific tracer incorporated in the proteins of the precursors. Such an ideal has been obtained with ^{59}Fe for the red cell line, since this marker is almost exclusively incorporated into haemoglobin, and this protein exclusively synthetized by red cell precursors.

Due to the relatively high sulphur content of the platelet proteins, animal and human studies using 35 S-sulfate, 35-S methionine and its analogue ^{75}Se-methionine, have been concluded in the last 10 years. 35 S cannot be used in human beings, because of its long physical and biological period, and is also technically difficult to use (low beta energy). ^{75}Se-methionine has been shown to be a physiological analogue of S-methionine, with metabolism and kinetics similar to those of the normal amino-acid.

Methionine is incorporated into megakaryocytes at the late maturation stages, and several papers have shown the typical clock-curve expected from a cohort label (4,5,6,7,8) and fig. 1): latency, then sigmoid increase of circulating radioactivity, due to the maturation delay and progressive release of labelled platelets from the bone marrow, then a peak, and slow decrease due to platelet removal. Theoretically, the height of the peak (radioactivity of platelets from 1 ml of blood multiplied by the blood volume, rapported to the infused radioactivity, is an index of platelet production (table 2).

In fact many problems make this tracer difficult to use and the curves difficult to analyse.

A radiobiological problem first. As methionine is incorporated into the megakaryocytic cell line in a very low percentage (less than 1%), any physiological study obliges to inject relatively high doses (100 µCi and more). On another hand the physical period of ^{75}Se is long (121 days) and methionine is recycled so that its biological period is also long. Irradiation of patients thus makes the use of this tracer difficult in young patients with non-malignant diseases.

Due to the low percentage of methionine incorporated into the platelets, and to the simultaneous incorporation of its into plasma proteins, red cells, and granulocytes, accurate isolation and washing of platelets from large blood-samples are required before counting.

Still more important is the simultaneous labelling of platelets by direct incorporation of the tracer into the proteins at the time of synthesis, and by adsorption of labelled plasma proteins to the platelet membrane. So the observed curve is the sum of a specific labelling ("cohort" curve" and of a permanent non-specific labelling which reflects the plasma protein life span; we can thus explain why the peak is observed later than expected, and why the decreasing part of the curve is excessively slow (6). That is the reason why we have tried, first to substract from the whole radioactivity the plasma contaminants, by using the curve of plasma radioactivity, and hereafter to isolate actin and myosin from the platelet button in order to measure in terms of specific activity the uptake of radiotracer to the constituent platelet proteins (see Cardinaud and Dassin in this volume).

Even if this problem is solved however, mathematical analysis of platelet production from the methionine incorporation at the peak of the curve will be impaired in two pathological conditions. When there is a doubt on the platelet repartition between circulating and non-circulating pools (hypersplenism), the calculated production deduced from incorporation in the only circulating pool could be under-estimated. If platelet survival is short, due to random destruction, a fraction of the labelled material will disappear before than the material labelled in the bone marrow has completely reached the peripheral blood; here again an under-estimation of the platelet production will occur.

So, in spite of a lot of valuable work, it seems that, at least in man in whom pathological situations differ from the well-controlled experimental situations in animal, and in whom the dose has necessarely to be kept as low as possible, the direct measurement of thrombocytopoiesis still remains out of our possibilities in clinical practice.

Hence we can conclude that, at the present time, indirect measurement of platelet production deduced from the life span and distribution of autologous labelled platelets is the best way to obtain approximate, but accurate enough, data in clinical practice.

Table 3. Direct measure of the platelet production using 35 S or ^{75}Se-methionine

Principle
Cohort labelling with intra-venous labelled amino-acid. Measure of the tracer incorporated (% of the dose) - Measure of the mean life span.
Theoretical problems
- Secondary labelling of platelets from labelled proteins of the plasma. - No value of the test when the platelet life span is short. - Necessary correction for the non-circulating platelet pool. - Low radioactivity used for platelet proteins synthesis. - High irradiation of the recipient.

REFERENCES

1. Harker LA, Regulation of thrombocytopoiesis. Amer. J. Physiol. 218: 1376, 1970.

2. Suit HD, A technique for estimating the bone marrow cellularity in vivo using 59 Fe. J. clin. Path. 10:267, 1957.

3. Vigneron N, Dassin E, Najean Y, Double marquage des plaquettes per 51 Cr et 111 In. Nouv. Presse Méd. 9:1835, 1980.

4. Evatt BL, Levin J, Measurement of thrombocytopoiesis in rabbits using 75-seleno-methionine. J. clin. Invest. 48:1615, 1969.

5. MacIntyre PA, Evatt B, Hadkinson BA, Scluffel U, Se-75-Seleno-methionine as label for erythrocytes, leukocytes and platelets. J. Lab. clin. Med. 75:472, 1970.

6. Najean Y, Ardaillou N, The use of 75-Seleno-methionine for the in vivo study of platelet kinetics. Scand. J. Haemat. 6:395, 1969.

7. Odell TT, Use of 35 S-sulfate for labelling megakaryocytes and platelets. In: Platelet kinetics. Paulus JM (ed), Elsevier/North-Holland Biomedical Press, Amsterdam, pp 123-125, 1971.

8. Penington DG, Assessment of platelet production with 75-Se-methionine. Brit. J. Med. 4:782, 1969.

8 PLATELET PRODUCTION RATE DETERMINATION WITH (^{75}Se)-SELENO-METHIONINE

R. CARDINAUD, E. DASSIN

INTRODUCTION

Platelet production rate measurements can be a useful tool for monitoring thrombopoietic factors. Currently available techniques suffer from a number of drawbacks and we have made an attempt to develop a method which is sufficiently direct to avoid cumbersome empirical corrections; its accuracy and reproducibility have been adjusted so as to obtain a final procedure simple enough for routine use. The isotope incorporation technique is a method currently used for production rate measurements. A loading of a suitable precursor is given (usually by injection) and after an appropriate period of time the amount of radioactivity (RA) incorporated is measured. The production rate is often expressed as the percentage ratio between the label incorporated and the injected dose (1,2) as given by relation 1:

$$\frac{\text{RA in the peripheral platelets}}{\text{RA injected}} \times 100 \qquad (1)$$

The total radioactivity (RA_t) on the peripheral platelets is obtained from measurements of the specific radioactivity of the platelets (RA/platelets) and the total number of peripheral platelets [(number of platelets /ml of blood)x (blood-volume in ml)]. Blood-volume in ml is usually determined from the percentage body weight in grams and varies with the animal considered. However, it has been recognized (2) that two different types of radioactivity are carried by washed platelets: a constituent radioactivity incorporated in the megakaryocyte and directly representative of the production rate and an adsorbed radioactivity originating from the circulating plasma proteins and depending on the complex fluctuations of the plasma protein radioactivity. A more rigorous approach to this problem is therefore to take only the constituent radioactivity into account. Actin accounts for up to about 15 - 20% of the total protein in the platelets (3). Its amino acid composition (16 methionine in skeletal rabbit muscle actin (4), 12-15 in platelets) indicates that it is likely to be one of the most labelled proteins. In this report, a description is given of an attempt made to use actin as a probe to determine platelet production rates.

In relation 1, actin RA should be used instead of peripheral platelet RA, the method then requiring a quantitative recovery of the actin from an aliquot part of a platelet suspension. It was evident from the beginning that actin (or acto-myosin) isolation and purification is not easily reproducible and much too cumbersome a procedure to be used as a routine technique. However, if we assume that the total (polymerized and unpolymerized) actin content of the platelets is constant (for example 25% of the total protein), the total actin radioactivity can be obtained from measurements of the total number of peripheral platelets (from which the total actin weight can be determined) and actin specific radioactivity.

Total actin RA = actin specific RA x total actin weight (2)

Unfortunately, it is again rather difficult to isolate and purify actin from a single animal to obtain specific radioactivity; this excludes the routine use of such a procedure.

It was therefore decided that the accuracy and reproducibility of a quantitative electrophoretic technique based on the following principles should be tested. A given number of solubilized platelets P_e) is deposited on a SDS-polyacrylamide gel and electrophoresis carried out under appropriate conditions. The radioactivity of the isolated actin band is measured; the percentage radioactivity incorporated in the actin is given by

$$\frac{\text{RA in actin}}{\text{RA injected}} \times 100 \qquad (3)$$

or

$$\frac{\text{RA in actin band}}{\text{RA injected}} \times \frac{P_c}{P_e} \times 100 \qquad (4)$$

P_c total number of peripheral platelets

P_e number of platelets used for electrophoretic study

Material and methods

All the experiments reported were carried out on male Wistar-rats weighing between 250 and 300 g. (^{75}Se)-selenomethionine (40-60 mCi/mg, CEA Saclay) was injected via the tail vein. The dose administered is reported in the results.

Blood-samples were obtained by cardiac puncture under ether anaesthesia. After centrifugation (300 g) in the presence of anticoagulant (5), the platelet-rich plasma (PRP) was carefully withdrawn and measured exactly. The number of platelets per µl was counted in a Malassez cell to obtain the number of platelets in the PRP sample (P_{PRP}). The platelets were centrifuged at 1500 g, washed twice with 0.164 M NaCl containing 1/10 Aster solution to remove erythrocytes (the hemoglobin constant was always less than 3.3 mg/ml). The platelets were then incubated in a washing solution containing 1% Triton-X-100 (4°, overnight). An equal volume of solution 1.5 M quinidine-HCl, 1 mM ATP, 20 mM Tris-HCl, pH 7.6 was then added and the mixture left to stand 6-8 hours at 4°. The sample was finally dialyzed overnight against 50 mM PO_4, pH 7.2, 0.1% β-mercaptoethanol, 1% SDS. At this stage and before dialysis the total platelet content of the platelet button was usually dispersed in 200 µl of the solution. However, dialysis inevitably causes an uncontrollable change in dilution. To resolve this uncertainty, each sample is quantitatively collected, the dialysis buffer being used to obtain identical final volumes for all the samples in the experiment (e.g. 400 µl). 200 µl of each sample is then mixed with 40 µl of 50% glycerol in water and boiled for 3 min before applying it to the SDS polyacrylamide gel.

<u>"P_e" determination</u> (see relation (4)). "P_e" is the number of platelets deposited on the SDS polyacrylamide gel and is calculated using the relation:

$$P_e = \frac{P_{RPR}}{400} \times \frac{200}{240} \times \text{volume deposited in } \mu l \tag{5}$$

<u>Total peripheral platelet determination</u>: "P_c". Blood obtained by cardiac puncture was collected on heparine; the platelets were counted on a Malassez cell after dilution. The number of platelets per ml of blood was thus obtained. The total blood-volume was estimated using the assumption that it is proportional to body weight (6).

<u>Actin specific radioactivity</u>. This value is arbitrarily given as the number of cpm found in the actin of 10^9 platelets. It is obtained from the formula:

$$\frac{\text{RA in actin band}}{P_e} \times 10^9 \tag{6}$$

In consequence, an exact determination of the actin content is unnecessary.

<u>Electrophoresis and radioactivity measurements</u>. Electrophoresis were carried out in cylindrical gels rather than slabs in order to conveniently recover the actin band. The SDS polyacrylamide gels and electrophoresis conditions are as described in (7).

<u>Electrophoresis under non denaturing conditions</u>. 7.5% or 8.5% gels were prepared in 0.1 M Tris-HCl buffer pH 8.9 with ATP at a final concentration of 0.2 mM. The running buffer was prepared by a ten-fold dilution of a ∿ 0.1 M Tris-glycine stock solution (57.6 g/l of glycine adjusted to pH 8.3 with a 1M Tris solution) with 0.2 mM ATP in the cathode compartment.

The electrophoresis was performed at constant intensity selected so as to have a 250 volts tension at the start.

The radioactivity distribution in the gel is represented as a histogram; it was obtained by measuring counts from 2 mm thick slices using a sodium iodide crystal counter (Intertechnique CG-4000).

Rabbit actin preparation (8) and labelling by reductive methylation (9). All operations are carried out at 4° unless otherwise specified. Actin was extracted from acetone powder (1 g) with 20 ml of G-buffer (β-mercaptoethanol, 2 mM Tris-HCl, 0.2 mM ATP, 0.2 mM $CaCl_2$, pH 8.0) with 30 min stirring. The slurry was filtered off with a sintered glass filter and washed once with 10 ml of G-buffer; the filtrate was then centrifuged for 30 min at 30000 g (collected volume: 12.8 ml). The G-actin solution was adjusted to pH 9.0; 100 μCi of the ^{14}C-formaldehyde was then added; this was followed by the addition of 4-10 μl of a 5 mg/ml potassium borohydride solution within 30 s and 50 μl after 1 min. The ionic strength was raised to 50 mM KCl with a 3 M KCl solution and 2 mM $MgCl_2$ final concentration with a 0.5 M $MgCl_2$ solution; after 2 hours the ionic strength was increased to 0.6 M KCl; the solution was then left to stand for 90 min. After centrifugation (80 000 g, 2 hours) the pellet was dispersed in G-buffer and dialyzed exhaustively against the same buffer for 36 hours to remove all radioactive dialyzable material. A second polymerization-depolymerization cycle was carried out just before the formation of the actin-DNAse-I complex.

Preparation of actin-DNAse-I complex. Labelled actin and DNAse-I were dissolved independently in the same medium: 5 mM Tris-HCl, pH 7.5, 0.1 mM $CaCl_2$, 0.5 mM DTT, 0.8 mM ATP. The concentration of both proteins was adjusted to 0.035 mM. The complex was formed by mixing the two solutions in proportions indicated in Results. Glycerol was added (10% final concentration) before electrophoresis.

Platelet acto-myosin extraction. In this study a crude platelet actomyosin extract was found to be suitable; it was prepared according to a procedure based on existing methods

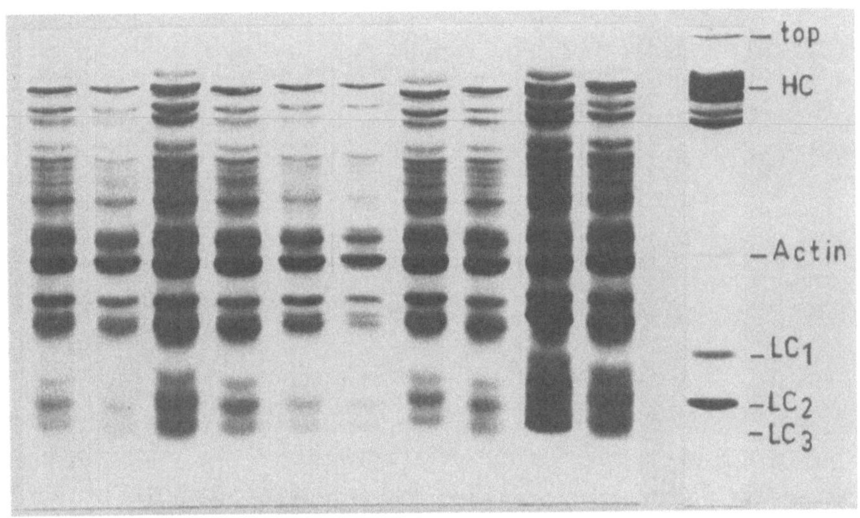

Fig. 1. SDS-polyacrylamide gel electrophoresis of total platelet extracts obtained as indicated in "Material and Methods" from 10 different rats. Note that no material stained by Coomassie Blue remains on top of the gel indicating that all proteins (in particular actin) are completely solubilized. Rabbit skeletal myosin used as a molecular weight marker (last gel).

(10-12) with various modifications. The platelets from 6 to 12 rats were pooled in 40 mM NaCl, 7 mM PO_4, pH 7.0, 5 mM EDTA, 1 mM DTT then ruptured by freezing-thawing at liquid nitrogen temperature. After centrifugation (100000 g, 1 hour) the supernatant (fraction S1) was discarded. The pellet was dispersed in 0.6 m NaCl, 0.04 M $NaHCO_3$, 0.01 M Na_2CO_3, 10 mM DTT, 5mM EDTA (fraction C1) and left to stand 1 hour at room temperature; the solution was gently stirred overnight at 4°. After centrifugation (25000 g, 1 hour) the acto-myosin contained in the supernatant (fraction S2) was precipitated with 3 volumes of mM Mg-acetate adjusted to pH 6.4 with acetic acid and centrifuged (25000 g, 15 min). The supernatant (fraction S3) was discarded. The pellet was dissolved in 0.177 (vol/weight) 3 M NaCl, then diluted with a 0.6 M NaCl, 1 mM DTT, 10 mM Histidine, pH 7.0 solution (fraction C3).

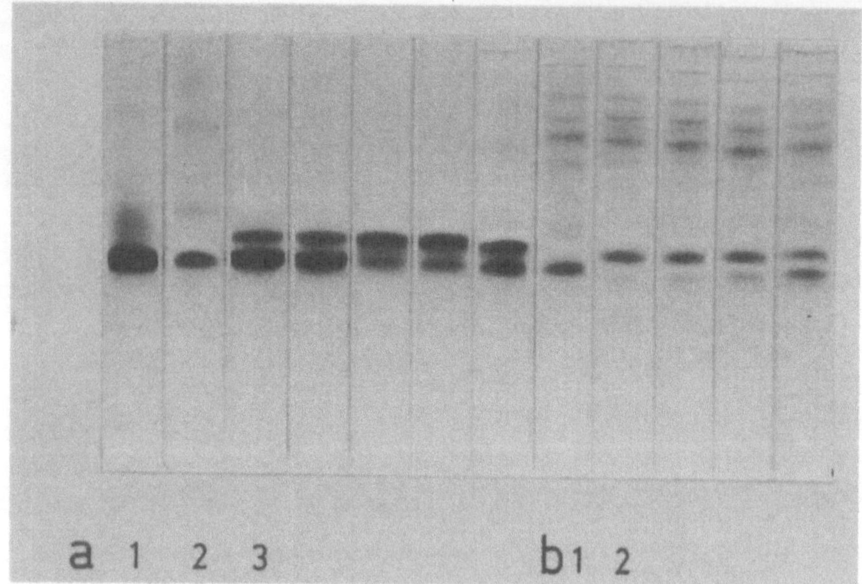

Fig. 2. Polacrylamide gel electrophoresis under non-dissociating conditions (see "Material and Methods") a)-1: actin; 2: DNAse-I; 3: actin-DNAse-I mixture in weight ratio: 1: 0,1; 1: 0,2; 1: 0,5; 1: 1; 1: 2 (conditions suitable to form actin-DNAse-I complex; see "Material and Methods"). b)-1: crude platelet actin; 2: platelet-actin-DNAse-I mixtures in weight ratios: 1:1; 1:1,5; 1:1,75; 1:2.

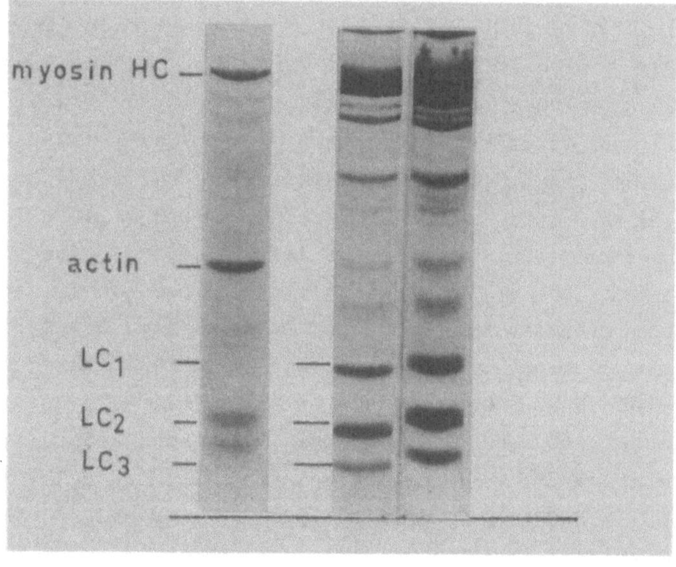

a b

Fig. 3. SDS-polyacrylamide gel electrophoresis of: a) crude platelet actomyosin preparation b) crude rabbit fast skeletal myosin used as a reference with a trace of actin.

Results

Electrophoretic analysis of platelets constituents. Actin identification. The SDS-polyacrylamide gel electrophoresis of total platelet gives a complex pattern. (Fig 1 shows the platelet constituents of 10 individuals. All these samples were prepared as described in "Material and Methods". The reproducibility of the patterns was satisfactory and it could be observed that the procedure enables a complete dissolution of all the constituents since no material could be seen on the top of the gels. Three typical constituents can easily be recognized in the pattern: actin (42500 mol wt), myosin heavy chain (molecular weight of sub-units: 200.000), actin binding protein (ABP, molecular weight of sub-units: 260.000). Tubulin is located just above actin although it was not formally identified. Quantitative densitometry showed our samples to be composed of 15-20% actin, about 7% myosin and 10% ABP. In some electrophoresis the ABP band probably included a 230.000 molecular weight protein as mentioned by Rosenberg et al (13).

In order to assign the actin band, our migration in SDS-PAGE was compared with that of rabbit actin: Rabbit actin labelled by reductive methylation was complexed with DNAse-I (see Material and Methods) and migrated on a non-dissociating electrophoretic system (fig 2). It was observed that: 1) labelling of actin did not alter its migration behaviour and did not hinder the formation of a complex with DNAse-I; 2) the actin-DNAse-I complex was located just above the common actin and DNAse-I position.

This test was also used to show that crude acto-myosin extracts from platelets behave similarly. Crude acto-myosin was obtained in a single precipitation as described in Material and Methods. The SDS-PAGE analysis (fig 3) indicates the state of purity obtained. Increasing proportions of this crude preparation were mixed with DNAse-I under the same conditions as used for rabbit actin. The main platelet component formed the same type of complex with DNAse-I indicating that it was definitely actin (fig 2).

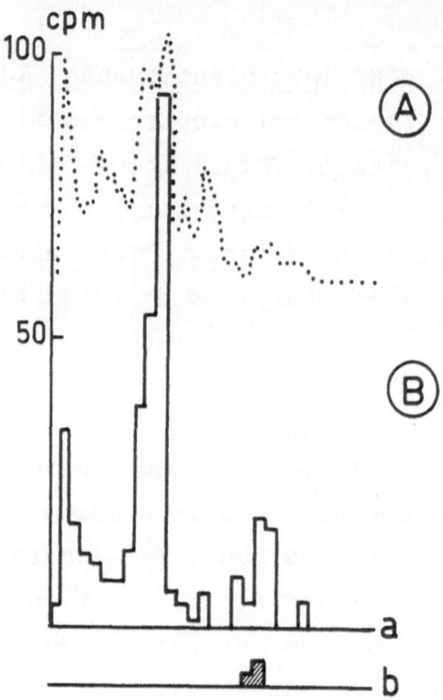

Fig. 4. SBS-polyacrylamide gel electrophoresis of crude acto-myosin extracts from rat platelets. A: densitometric tracing of Coomassie Blue stained gel of a sample from platelets taken 5 days after (^{75}Se)-seleno-methionine injection (arbitrary units); B: histogram of radioactivity (expressed in cpm) of 2 mm thick slices prepared as described in ref. 7. a: Same samples as used for densitometry; b: similar sample taken 10 days after injection.

Radioactivity distribution in total platelet digests. A series of electrophoresis carried out on total digests of platelets obtained 6 days after (^{75}Se)-seleno-methionine injection exhibited typically 2 main radioactivity peaks (fig 4), one corresponding to actin and the other to a faster moving component (apparent mol wt 18-20000). This peak is accompanied by a smaller peak corresponding to an apparent mol wt of 16-17000. These 2 peaks will be refered to as X_M (X major) and X_m(X minor) respectively. Actin is also accompanied by a slightly slower migrating radioactive component - probably tubulin - which must be eliminated if the exact specific radioactivity of actin is to be determined. Actin appears to be a good choice as it is one of the most highly labelled components of platelets. However, the height of the X_M radioactivity peak raises the question whether it is the

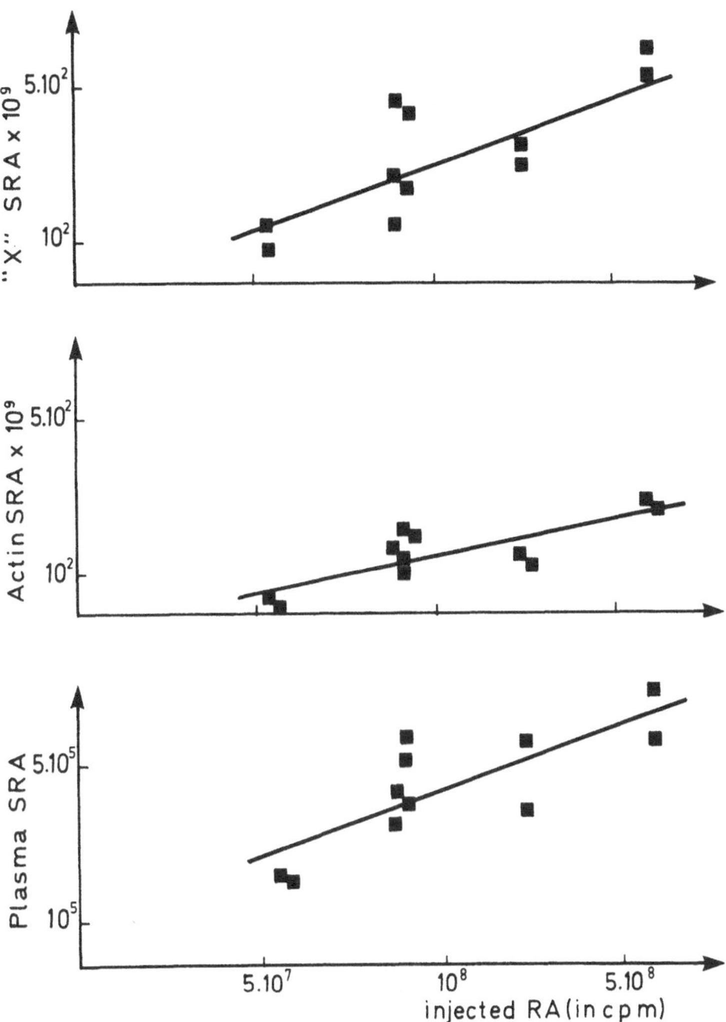

Fig. 5. Specific radioactivity of platelet actin as defined in "Material and Methods". Each point represents the specific radioactivity of a single rat sacrificed 6 days after (^{75}Se)-seleno-methionine injection. "X": $y= 3.61x10^{-6}$ x- 47.32, r= 0.81, $p<0.01$, "actin": $y= 1.93x10^{-6}$ x- 44.16, r= 0.81, $p<0.01$; "plasma": $y= 3.33x10^{-3}$ x + 101308, r= 0.80, $p<0.01$.

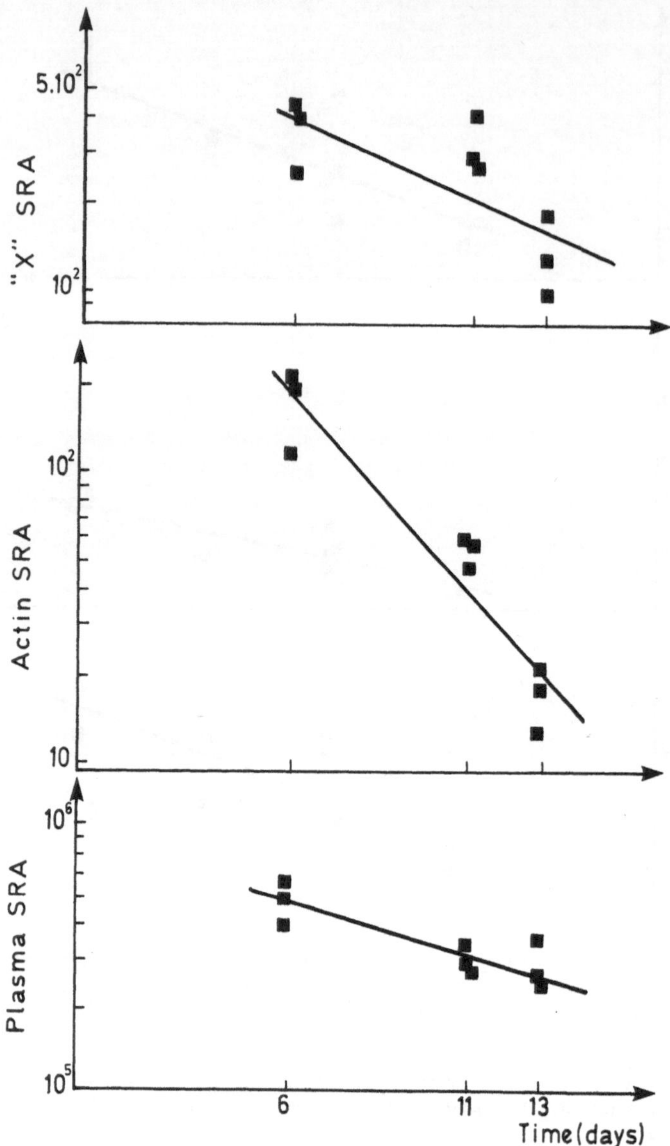

Fig. 6. Plot of specific radioactivity vs time. Specific radioactivity plotted on a logarithmic scale showing a pseudo first order decrease. Each point represents the specific radioactivity of a single rat sacrificed at various times after (^{75}Se)-seleno-methionine injection. "X": $y= 798\ e^{-0.12t}$, $r= 0.69$, $p<0.02$; "actin": $y= 1196,\ e^{-0.31t}$, $r= 0.94$, $p<0.01$; "plasma": $y= 781119\ e^{-0.08t}$, $r= 0.85$, $p<0.01$.

only choice. The radioactivity profile of acto-myosin extracts obtained from animals sacrificed 5 days and 10 days after (^{75}Se)-seleno-methionine injection were measured. The radioactivity of crude acto-myosin was shown to be negligible after 10 days and it was only on the fast migrating component X_M that any radioactivity was found. Earlier kinetic studies have shown that the mean life-span of rat platelets is about 5-6 days; present observations therefore confirm that actin is indeed the best marker for determining platelet production rates; the radioactive low molecular weight component X_M is believed to be a plasma protein adsorbed by the platelets as it has been shown that the plasma radioactivity is still quite high after 10 days. This point will be discussed further on in the text.

In order to investigate the validity of this probe test studies were carried out on populations of normal animals.

Effect of injected dose. This is an important practical problem which must be solved if a useful routine experimental procedure is to be defined. Sufficient quantities of radioactivity must be injected to ensure the required level of accuracy (total incorporation into platelets is currently of the order 0.01 - 0.05%). However, the dose must not produce any pertubation in the platelet production rate. A study of the specific radioactivity of actin, X_M and plasma showed a satisfactory linear dependence for injected radioactivities of up to 1 mCi/kg animal (fig 5). This linear relationship indicates that: a) the amount of seleno-methionine injected does not significantly modify the methionine pool; b) the radioactivity introduced has no apparent irradiation effect as this would have resulted in a lower production rate and a greater dilution of the radioactive platelets by the subsequently produced platelets. In both cases, a lower

$$\frac{\text{SRA actin}}{\text{injected Se-Met}}$$

ratio would have been observed.

Change in specific radioactivity with time (fig 6). A semi-log plot of SRA vs time for actin, X_M and plasma exhibited a pseudo first order decrease in radioactivity. It was observed that the "rate constants" for X_M and plasma were quite close to each other but significantly different from that of actin. This suggests that X_M may well be an adsorbed plasma protein in equilibrium with the plasma. Moreover the "rate constants" for plasma and X_M were not expected to be strictly identical since a comparison is being made between the SRA decrease in one (major) radioactive protein (X_M) and the sum of the decreases in all the radioactive constituents of the plasma. The hypothesis will have to be carefully checked because one of its consequences is that X_M should be rejected as a probe for production rate determination.

Conclusion

Our experimental results indicate that actin is a reasonable choice as a probe for platelet production rate measurements. Procedures involving the quantitative extraction of actin are not realistic since it is commonly observed that actin easily denatures, and is found for one part under a monomeric form no longer able to polymerize and for another part under an irreversible polymeric form. Purification is a lengthy procedure and would be quite impractical with a single extract; consequently specific radioactivity can not be established in this way. Electrophoretic separation of total digests was however shown to be a rapid and easy procedure to obtain specific radioactivity and percentage incorporation. A relevant remark about the accuracy likely to be obtained with the method is that at the optimum injection level the actin band will contain about 300 cpm and the main uncertainty will probably arise from the electrophoretic procedure: in particular the deposited volume and the selection of the actin zone. It is observed that with a single rat extract it is possible to carry out at least 6 identical electrophoreses and therefore to improve considerably the determination accuracy. It is hoped that this method and other complementary methods will lead to a better and easier way of monitoring platelet production rates.

REFERENCES

1. McDonald TP, Proc. Soc. exp. Biol. Med. 144:1006, 1973.
2. Dassin E, Ardailloux N, Eberlin A, Bourebia J, Najean Y, Biochem. biophys. Res. Commun. 81:329, 1978.
3. Crawford N, In: Platelets in biology and pathology Gordon (ed), Elsevier/North-Holland Biomedical Press, Amsterdam, pp 121-157, 1976.
4. Collins JH, Elzinga M, J. biol. Chem. 250:5915, 1975.
5. Levy-Toledano S, Bredoux R, Rendu F, Jeanneau J, Savariau E, Dassin E, Nouv. Rev. franc. Hémat. 16:367, 1976.
6. Everett NB, Simmons B, Lasher EP, Circulat. Res. 4:419, 1956.
7. Cardinaud R, Biochimie (paris) 61:807, 1979.
8. Spudich JA, Watt S, J. biol. Chem. 246:4866, 1971.
9. Means GE, Feeney RE, Biochemistry 7:2192, 1968.
10. Bettex-Galland M, Lüscher EF, Advanc. Protein Chem. 20:134, 1965.
11. Cohen I, Kaminski E, De Vries A, FEBS Lett. 34:315, 1973.
12. Landon F, Huc C, Thomé F, Oriol C, Olomucki A, Eur. J. Biochem. 81:571, 1977.
13. Rosenberg S, Stracher A, Lucas RC, J. Cell. Biol. 91:201, 1981.

9 PLATELET KINETICS: THE STATE OF THE ART

A. duP HEYNS

INTRODUCTION

In this paper an overview of the "state of the art" of platelet kinetics 1982, will be presented.

Six main subjects will be considered. Firstly, a review of some problems involving the procedures whereby platelets are isolated from whole blood; thereafter a discussion of the advantages and disadvantages of some of the many radionuclide platelet labels; focussing briefly on the mathematical models employed for analysis of platelets survival; introducing the concept of analysis of the shape of the platelet survival curve as a parameter for assessing platelet behaviour in the circulation; demonstrate some platelet kinetic studies with measurement of in vivo distribution and lastly a brief introduction of a promising new technique that may prove to be of value in the future.

Isolation of platelets from whole blood

In the methods commonly used, platelets are isolated from whole blood by single step differential centrifugation. The main disadvantage of this method is that only 50-60% of platelets are recovered in the platelet-rich plasma (1). This non-representative platelet subpopulation is mainly a less dense and smaller platelet fraction. It has been suggested that the larger sized subpopulation, excluded by this procedure, may be younger and thus physiologically and functionally more effective (2). This has of course several important implications, the main one being that current studies may not be appropriate or even clinically relevant.

Several techniques have been employed to harvest a fully representative platelet-population: Ficol-Hypaque was used by

Imandt et al (3) as a "cushion" preventing damage to platelets during centrifugation. Corash et al (4) used red cells for a similar purpose in a procedure where platelets are removed by multiple washings. We have modified the Corash-technique slightly and have harvested 88 ± 8% of whole blood platelets. Platelet size and density was fully representative of that of whole blood platelets. The usual single step differential centrifugation technique yielded a population with a mean platelet survival time of 200 ± 29 hours, and with the multiple wash technique platelet survival was 223 ± 16 hours. Although this increase in survival is statistically not significant, it indicates that the younger platelets may be more efficiently harvested. Recently however, there have been reports suggesting that the less buoyant platelets are not necessarily the younger platelets (5,6). This question awaits final clarification.

Platelet labels

Several isotopes have been employed as platelet labels and a non-isotopic method for measuring platelet life span has also been described:

1. ^{32}P-diisopropylfluorophosphate
2. ^{75}Se-selenomethionine
3. ^{32}P-phosphate
4. ^{35}S-sulphate
5. Malondialdehyde (MDA) formation
6. ^{51}Cr-sodium chromate
7. ^{111}In-oxinate and other ^{111}In-complexes
8. Others: ^{14}C-Serotonin; Tc^{99m}; ^{68}Ga; Rubidium.

It is not appropriate to discuss all these labels in this presentation and I would like to limit my remarks to selected aspects.

The MDA formation technique, although simple and not associated with radiation exposure, has several disadvantages: Firstly, it is necessary to give aspirin to patients and this may be inadvisable in certain clinical situations. Relatively large blood samples are required for the assay of MDA and platelet survival may be affected by aspirin administration. It has also suggested that MDA production may vary from platelet to platelet and that this may be dependent on the age of the platelets (7).

<u>^{51}Cr-sodium chromate</u> has been the platelet label of choice for many years, recommended as such by the International Committee for Standardization in Hematology in 1977 (8). Chromium has several disadvantages as platelet label, one of which is a low labelling efficiency. The placing of external probes as is commonly used for detection of in vivo ^{51}Cr-distribution is subject to variation, making this a relatively insensitive technique.

<u>An ^{111}In-chelate</u> has become the platelet label of choice (9). The most widely used chelate is oxinate, but acetone acetate (10) tropolonate (11) and the recently introduced chelate, MERC (Thakur, personal communication) have their adherents.

^{111}In is a cyclotron-produced isotope with a 2.8 day half-life. Its very efficient gamma emission permits visualization and quantification of <u>in vivo</u> distribution of labelled platelets (12). The label does not elute significantly, is not re-utilized, and the radiation dose is acceptable for human studies (13). It should however be noted that contamination of ^{111}In with ^{114}In may significantly increase the radiation dose. The high labelling efficiency of about 90% allows labelling of a small number of platelets. Kinetic studies with autologous platelets are possible even in the presence of severe thrombocytopenia with a blood platelet count of less than $10x10^9$/l (14) and for kinetic studies in subjects with normal platelet counts enough platelets may be harvested from 50 ml blood.

^{111}In-oxinate is not an ideal label. One of the major problems is that labelling efficiency is low if not carried out in a plasma free medium (9). It is said that the chelate MERC permits platelet labelling in plasma, but results have not yet been published (Thakur, personal communication).

To prevent <u>in vitro</u> aggregation, prostaglandins such as PGE_1 and PGI_2 have been added to the labelling medium (15,16). This is unnecessary and only complicates an already unphysiol-

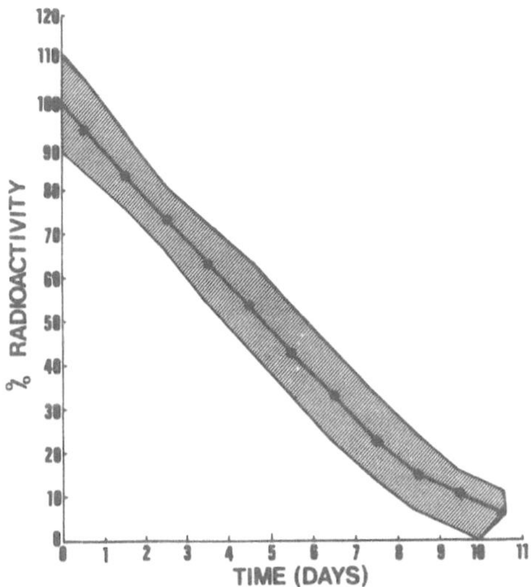

Fig. 1. Survival of ^{111}In-labelled platelets in normal humans. The boundary lines indicate the spread of values around the mean.

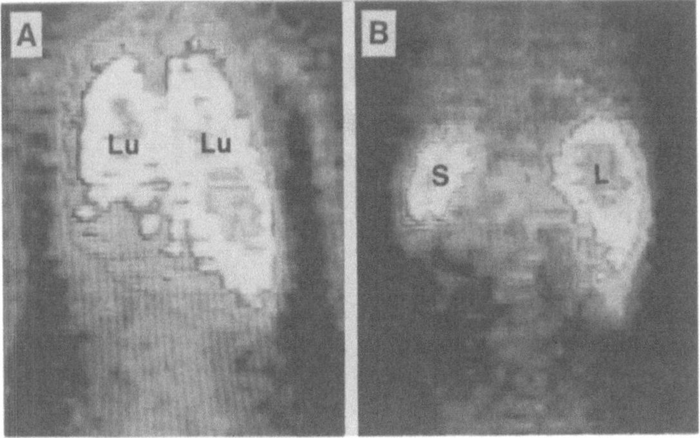

Fig. 2. Transient sequestration of ^{111}In-labelled platelets in the lung of a patient with lupus erythematosus. Fig. 2A is a scintigraph done 15 min after reinjection of labelled platelets, whereas fig. 2B illustrates that the platelets were not present in the lung 24 hours later. (Lu= Lungs; S= Spleen; L= Liver).

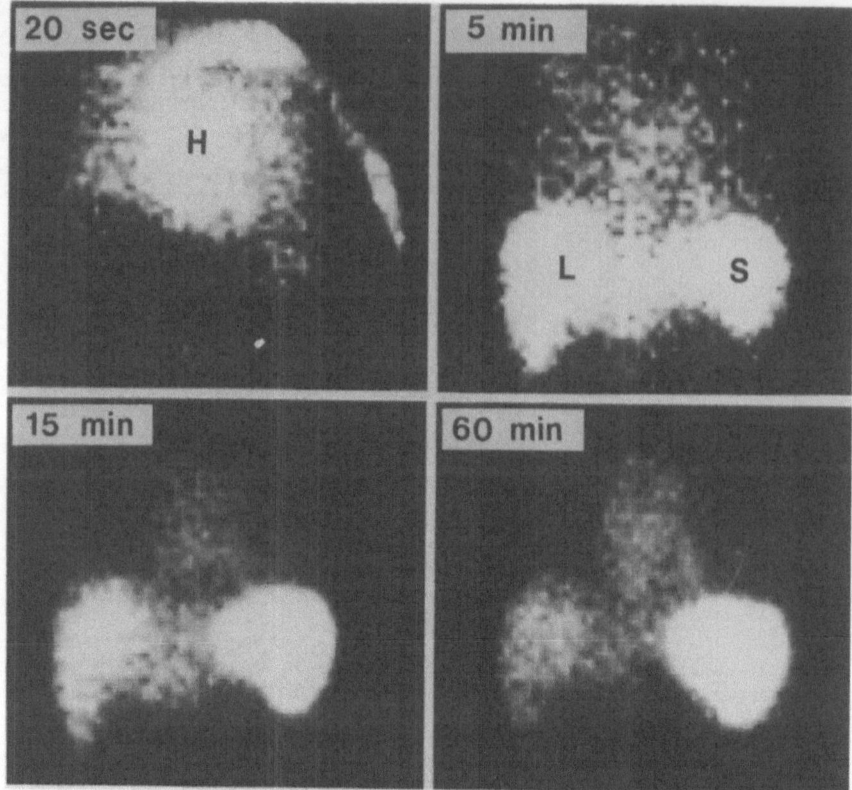

Fig. 3. Serial scintillation camera images taken 20 sec, 5 min, and 60 min after reinjection of ^{111}In-labelled platelets. The splenic pool (s) and the transient accumulation of platelets in the liver (L) is evident. The heart (H) is clearly visible.

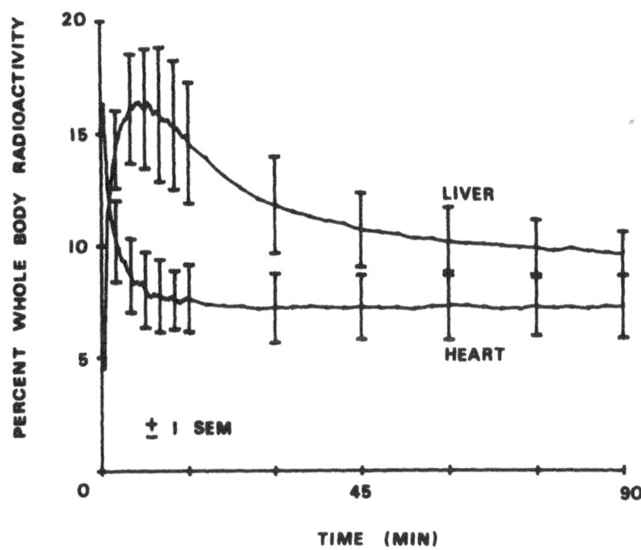

Fig. 4. Time-activity curves of organ radioactivity generated by a scintillation camera and computer assisted imaging system. The splenic pool, and the transient hepatic sequestration due to "Collection injury" is evident.

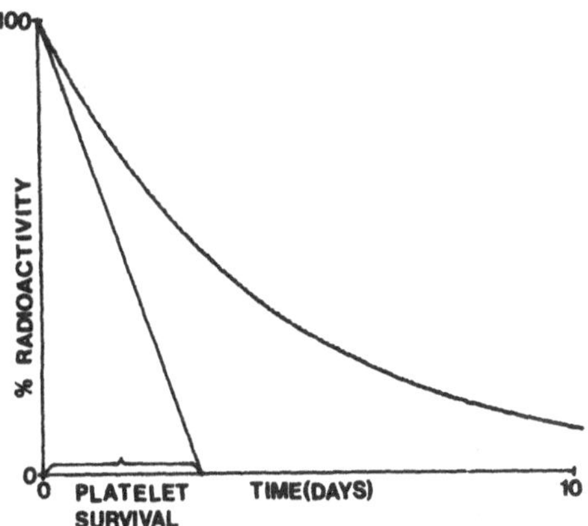

Fig. 5. The analysis of platelet survival curves: platelet survival is calculated as the ratio of the y-intercept and the initial slope of the regression curve.

ogical procedure further.

Analysis of platelet survival curves

In normal subjects, the platelet survival curve may be divided into 3 phases (fig 1). Initially, platelet activity in the blood may reach a plateau, but on the first day after re-injection of labelled platelets radionuclide levels in the blood remain unstable and variable. Thereafter, blood radioactivity decreases as a linear function for about 8 days. "Tailing" of the curve, produced by about 5% of the radioactivity present on day 8, then becomes evident.

The early, unstable, phase may be ascribed to the "collection injury" which may vary considerably from subject to subject. In fig 2 a rather rare, unexplained phenomenon is illustrated. A patient with systemic lupus erythematosus was studied with autologous ^{111}In-oxinate labelled platelets. Marked accumulation of platelets in the lungs was evident. This was transient, and the following day platelets had been mobilized. Platelet survival however did not differ from that of a similar study repeated a week later. We can only interpret this as a variant of a severe "collection injury", inducing transient platelet segregation in the lungs, without affecting platelet survival.

The more common, and almost inevitable, "collection injury" variant is illustrated in figs 3 and 4. Shortly after reinjection of labelled platelets, one observes a transient accumulation of platelets in the liver, attaining a maximum after about 15 min. Hepatic radioactivity then decreases, to reach equilibrium 60-90 min after reinjection. This collection injury clearly must influence calculation of platelet recovery in the circulation markedly if this is based on the radioactivity of a 5 min specimen. Determination of platelet survival, which includes analysis of the data points collected during the initial 60 min, must also be affected.

It should always be kept in mind that the analysis of the platelet survival in all instances is dependent of the ratio of the y-intercept and the initial slope of the regression curve (fig 5). The analysis of the platelet survival simply by expressing results either as a linear, or patterns of an exponential function has proved unsatisfactory, since many patterns of survival are a mixture of these 2 components. Mathematical models have been evolved to facilitate the calculation of platelet survival by fitting the data points of the survival curve more accurately and with less bias.

Mathematical models for analysis of platelet survival

1. Linear function (8): This is appropriate in the calculation of platelet survival in normal subjects and reflects an age dependent destruction of platelets in the circulation.
2. Exponential function(8): This is appropriate when platelets are removed from the circulation in a random fashion, independent of platelet age.
3. Weighted mean of linear and exponential function (8): Since many instances of platelet survival fit neither a linear or an exponential function adequately, it has been suggested that this could be overcome by a simple calculation of the weighted mean of these 2 survival times. It has the advantage of simplicity.
4. Multiple hit (gamma function) model (17): The model is based on physiological assumptions, some of which may not be valid. The mean platelet survival is calculated as a computed number of "hits" multiplied by the waiting time between these "hits". A "hit" is an insult imposed on the platelet by its environment, and may vary in intensity. The number of hits may give some indication of the shape of the curve: a single hit is found in an exponential curve, whereas a linear survival is reflected by an infinite number of "hits".
5. Dornhorst model (18): It is assumed that platelets have a determined life span and that they are exposed to destruction by external mechanisms. Platelet survival is calculated from these parameters. The model may be extended to give the mean age of circulating platelets, and the production rate may be calculated.
6. Alpha Order model (19): This model has been employed in pharmacokinetc studies. It also evaluates survival time varying from linear to exponential. The formula is derived from a

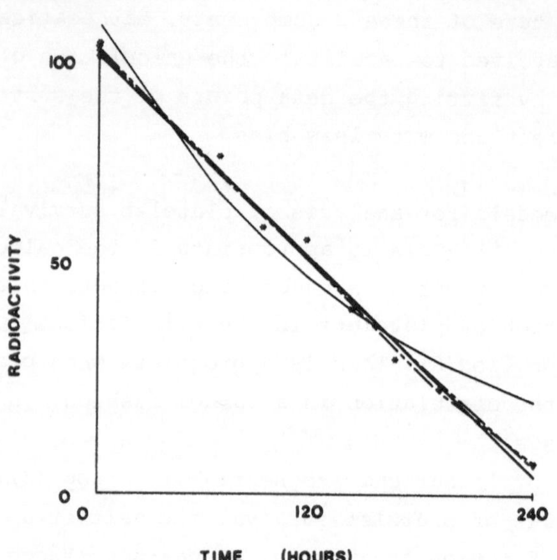

Fig. 6. An example of fitting data points of platelet survival with different mathematical models. In this normal subject, all models except the exponential function, fit data equally well.

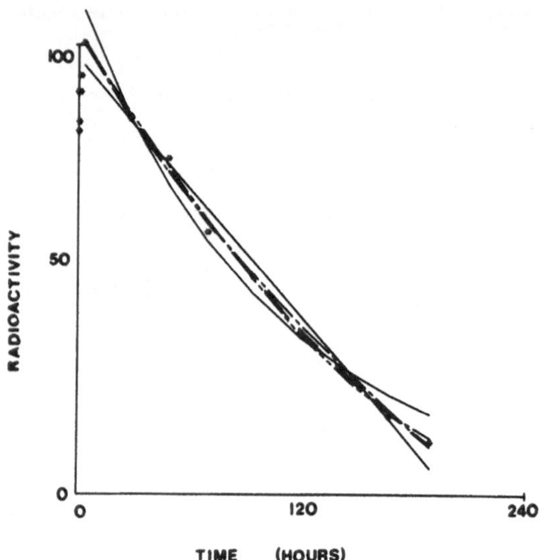

Fig. 7. An example of fitting data points of platelet survival with different mathematical models. In this patient with a linear-exponential survival curve, the linear and exponential functions do not fit the data well, but the other models are equal and satisfactory.

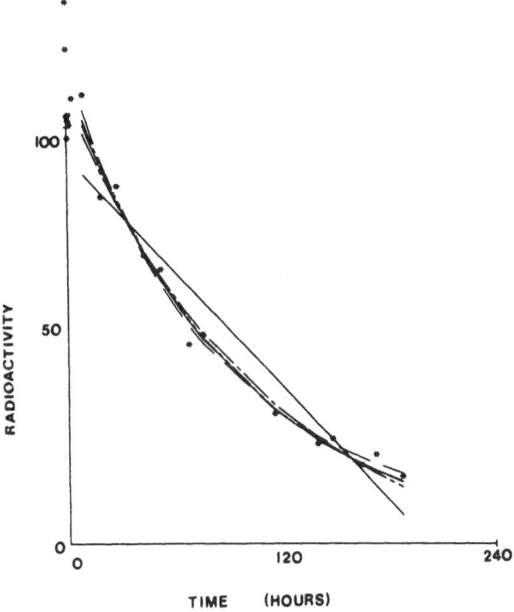

Fig. 8. An example of fitting data points of platelet survival with different mathematical models. In this patient with a random clearance of platelets from the circulation, all models except the linear function, fit data equally well.

general compartment, non-linear differential model:

$$dC/dt = kC\,\alpha$$

where C = concentration

t = time

k = rate parameter ($k < 0$)

α = order parameter ($\alpha \geqslant 0$)

The shape of the survival curve may be evaluated by calculating alpha in the above equation, since zero-order (α=0) and first-order (α=1) kinetics are particular cases.

7. Other models: Several other models have been employed for calculating platelet survival. The polynomial model was widely investigated by Paulus (20) and Meuleman in 1980 proposed another model (21). We have no experience with these models, but there is little doubt that the results obtained with these mathematical manipulations will closely correspond to those studied in

in our series.

Comparison of mathematical models

The results of comparative studies are discussed elsewhere in this issue (22). These findings may be briefly illustrated. We investigated 3 groups of patients: those with a linear platelet survival (fig 6); those with a survival that may be described as linear-exponential (fig 7); and those patients with a complete exponential survival (fig 8). As is evident from inspection of these graphs, the gamma function, Dornhost, Alpha Order, and weighted mean models all fitted the data points well and gave similar platelet survival times. In those patients with a linear platelet survival, the exponential model was inappropriate; and conversely in those with an exponential clearance of platelets from the circulation, the linear function fitted the data poorly. Not one of any of these mathematical models was superior in the calculation of platelet survival time.

We conclude that these models are equally suitable. These are simply manipulations of the data and the preference for a specific model is a matter of choice or experience. It would however be wise in clinical practice to compare data from a patient to another directly only if the same mathematical model is employed.

Problems of interpretation of platelet survival curves

Interpretation of platelet survival time is not as simple as it may seem. A major difficulty arises from the observation that platelet deposition at a site of sequestration, such as a thrombus, may not be permanent. We have evidence that platelets may partake in a thrombotic lesion, but that the final site of platelet sequestration may not differ from that seen in normal subjects (23). This is illustrated in figs 9 and 10, taken from a quantitative kinetic study performed in patients with abdominal aortic aneurysms. It is evident from fig 9 that there is a gradual deposition of ^{111}In-platelets in the aneurysm wall, but this reaches a plateau with time. Quantification of the final sites of sequestration showed that platelets were deposited in the liver, spleen and reticuloendpthelial system (RES),

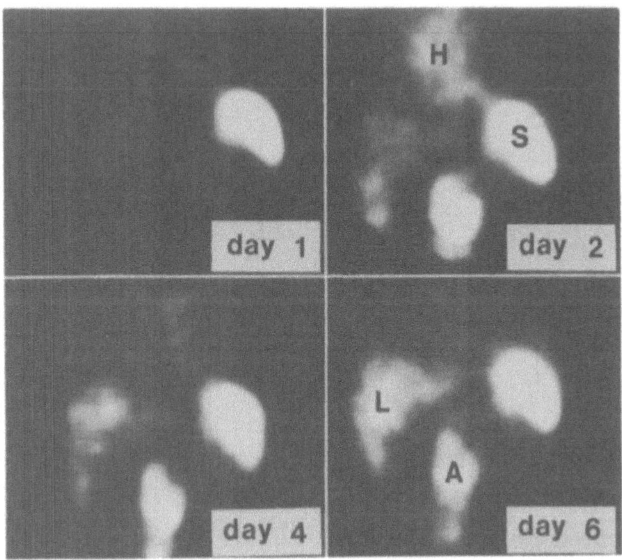

Fig. 9. Scintigrams of a patient with an abdominal aortic aneurysm. Imaging was done on the first, second, fourth and sixth day: the accumulation of ^{111}In-labelled platelets in the aneurysm is clearly visible. (A=aneurysm; S=spleen; L=liver and H=heart).

not significantly different from that of normal subjects (23). This finding implies that the platelets deposited in the superficial layers of the thrombus are eventually released, are in equilibrium with circulating platelets, and are finally deposited in the RES. Since we do not know how long the released platelets remain in the circulation, interpretation of the platelet survival curve and platelet survival time becomes very difficult. Obviously, a similar state of affairs may be operative in other diseases with increased platelet consumption.

Platelet survival and shape of the survival curve

Since there are so many difficulties associated with analysis of platelet survival curves, we have also approached the problem differently. Platelet survival is to some extent dependent on the shape of the clearance curve. It thus seems appropriate to

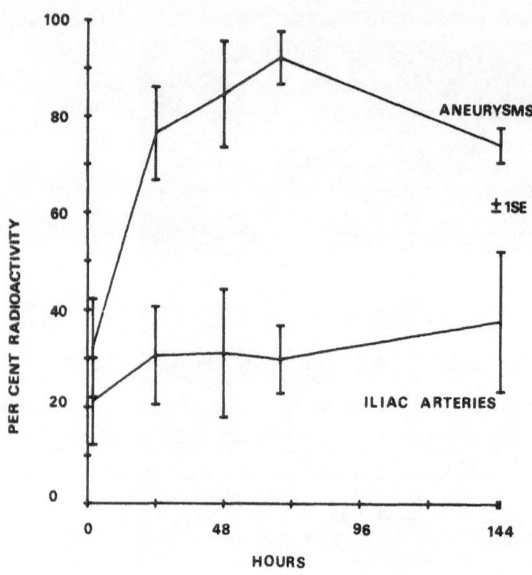

Fig. 10. Time-activity curves of ^{111}In-labelled platelet deposition in patients with abdominal aortic aneurysms. Radioactivity in the aneurysm increases rapidly but reaches a plateau suggesting that circulating and deposited platelets are in equilibrium.

analyse the shape of the curve. This approach is fully discussed by Lötter et al elsewhere in this volume (22). This is a different, and promising method of analysis of platelet clearance from the circulation. Further experience with analysis of these shape factors is necessary before a final verdict on the application will be possible.

Illustrative applications of quantitative platelet kinetic measurements

Physiology of normal platelet kinetics. ^{111}In-oxinate labelled platelets allows quantitative measurement of in vivo distribution of platelets (12). This is illustrated in fig 11: the platelet splenic pool is evident, and the final sequestration of senescent platelets in the spleen, liver and bone marrow may be seen. Quantification shows that the liver and spleen are major sites of sequestration (fig 12). Animal studies have shown that the

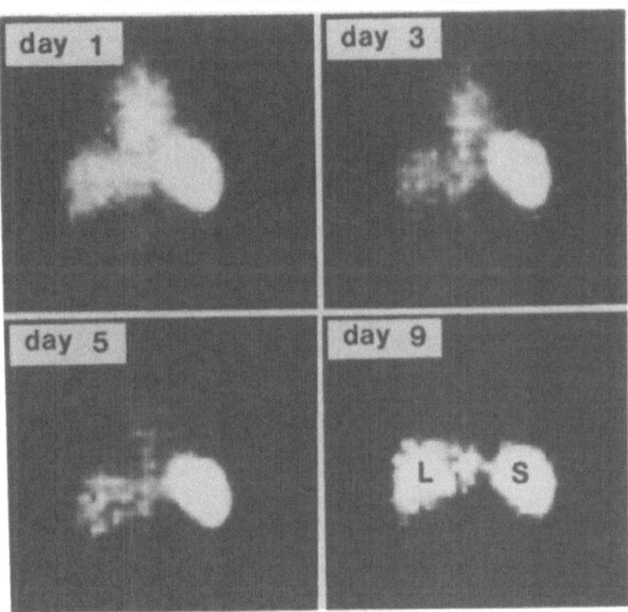

Fig. 11. Scintigrams of in vivo platelet distribution in a normal subject. The splenic pool and hepatic (L) and spleen (S) sequestration of senescent ^{111}In-labelled platelets is clear.

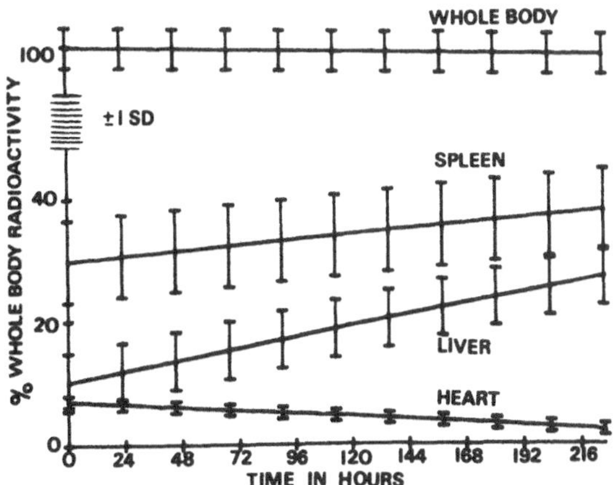

Fig. 12. Time-activity curves of whole body and organ radioactivity after reinjection of autologous In-labelled platelets to normal subjects.

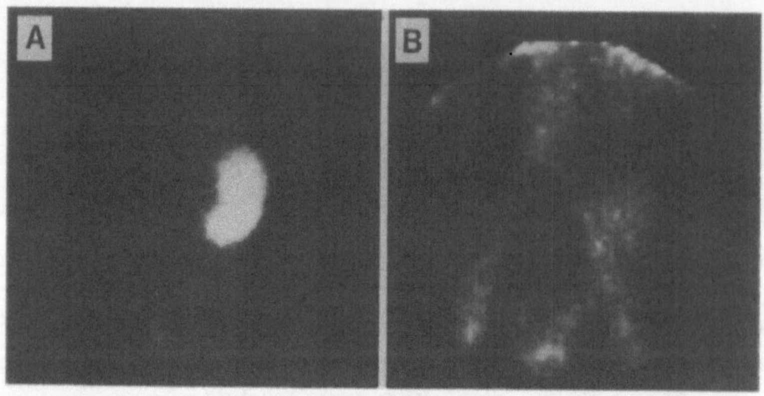

Fig. 13. Accumulation of ^{111}In-labelled platelets in a transplanted kidney during an acute rejection periode (A).

remainder of the platelets are sequestrated in the bone marrow (24). We have not been able to demonstrate significant deposition of platelets in the vasculature of normal subjects, (12) but this is evident in patients with severe atherosclerosis (23). Whole body radioactivity does not decrease significantly with time, indicating that there is no significant loss of radionuclide during the time of platelet survival studies.

Immune thrombocytopenic purpura (ITP)

Three patterns of sequestration of platelets in ITP are evident, as illustrated in fig 13: mainly splenic; hepatic; and diffusely in the RES, with a major component in the bone marrow. Quantitative data have been published (14). This approach to ITP will lead to a better understanding of the role of the components of the RES, the importance of platelet surface antibody levels and the influence of these on therapy. It should also be noted that ^{111}In makes it possible to investigate ITP with autologous labelled platelets. This has raised new problems. Autologous platelet survival is significantly longer than results obtained with ^{51}Cr labelled isologous platelets. These results suggest that in ITP platelet production by megakaryocytes may

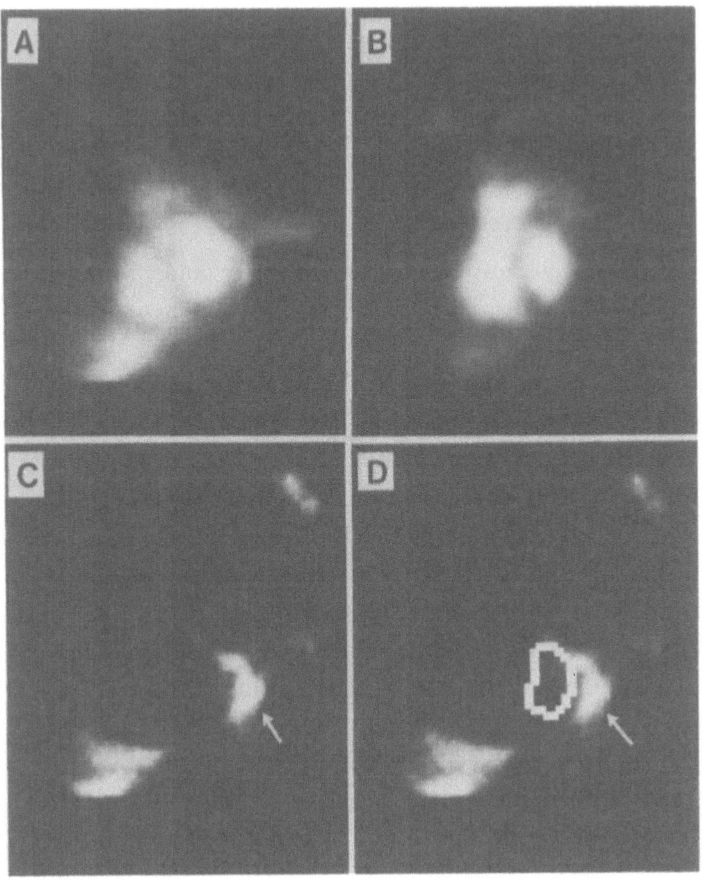

Fig. 14. After subtraction of circulating ^{111}In-platelet radioactivity deposition of platelets in a myocardial infarct becomes evident (D). Image A is Tc^{99m}-red cell activity; this is the sum of circulating activity and activity accumulating in the left ventricle.
Images C and D demonstrate deposition of platelets in the infarct (arrow); the left ventricular blood-pool is outlined in image D.

not always be normal as has previously been assumed (25).

Renal transplant rejection

^{111}In-labelled platelets provide an elegant, simple and accurate method of demonstrating acute renal transplant rejection (26,27). It is evident (fig 13) that platelets accumulate in the rejected kidney and that this is reversible by successful immunosuppression. In chronic transplant rejection, or in acute renal tubular necrosis there is no significant deposition of platelets in the kidney. This makes this technique a valuable adjunct to the diagnosis of the cause of oligo uria in the post-transplantation period.

Further applications

One of the most promising techniques, and one that will certainly be applied more frequently in the near future, is the subtraction of the radioactivity of circulating platelets in order to facilitate detection of platelet radioactivity deposited in an organ or vessel. This is illustrated (fig 14) in a patient with myocardial infarction. Circulating platelet radioactivity was quantified by measurement of blood-flow with Tc^{99m}-labelled red cells. ^{111}In-radioactivity due to circulating platelets is subtracted with the help of a computer. As is evident it then becomes possible to demonstrate deposition of ^{111}In-platelets in the wall of the left ventricle. Without this technique, background radioactivity of circulating platelets obscures the lesion completely.

Conclusions

1. It is necessary to isolate and label a representative platelet population for kinetic studies. This platelet population must be viable, and uniformly labelled. An ^{111}In-chelate is the prefered radiolabel.
2. The analysis of platelet survival curves is dependent on the precision of the data points. It is essential to analyse all data points obtained throughout the platelet survival time period. The "Collection injury" jeopardises overdependence on analysis of only the early part of the survival curve.
3. In normal subjects the survival curves are predominantly linear, but there is usually an exponential element. This exponential element becomes more evident in patients with increased

peripheral platelet consumption. In these cases mathematical models must be employed to decrease bias in assessment of minor differences. Results obtained with the various models are comparable, and there is no evidence that any one of these is superior.

4. There may be some merit in analysing the shape of the survival curve as a further parameter of assessing the clearance of platelets from the circulation.

5. ^{111}In-labelled platelets permits exploitation of the technology of the scintillation camera interfaced with a computer. Quantitative in vivo platelet kinetic studies are now possible. Elegant studies delineating the role of platelets in disease and the influence of antiplatelet drugs, may be performed.

Acknowledgements

This project was supported by The South African Medical Research Council, The South African Atomic Energy Board, and The University of the Orange Free State.

The contributions of my co-workers P.N. Badenhorst, M.G. Lötter, H. Pieters, P. Wessels, H.F. Kotzè, P.C. Minnaar and L.J. Duyvenè de Wit, are gratefully acknowledged.

REFERENCES

1. Reiss RF, Katz AJ, Optimizing recovery of platelets in platelet-rich plasma by the simplex strategy. Transfusion 16:307, 1976.
2. Karpatkin S, Heterogeneity of human platelets. VI. Correlation of platelet function with platelet volume. Blood 51:307, 1978.
3. Imandt L, Genders T, Wessels H, Haanen C, An improved method for preparing platelet-rich plasma. Thromb. Res. 11:429, 1977.
4. Corash L, Shafer B, Perlow M, Heterogeneity of human whole blood platelet subpopulations. II. Use of a subhuman primate model to analyse the relationship between density and platelet age. Blood 52: 726, 1978.
5. Mezzano D, Hwang K, Aster RH, Characteristics of total platelet populations and of platelets isolated in platelet-rich plasma. Transfusion 22:197, 1982.
6. Schmidt et al, Comparative kinetic studies of dense and light platelets. Symposium "Methodology of platelet labelling and analysis of platelet kinetics", Paris 1982.
7. Stuart MJ, Murphy S, Oski FA, A simple nonradioisotope technic for the determination of platelet life span. New Engl. J. Med. 292:1310, 1975.
8. The Panel on Diagnostic Application of Radioisotope in Hematology, ICSH, Recommended methods for radioisotope platelet survival studies. Blood 50:1137, 1977.
9. Thakur ML, Welch MJ, Joist JH et al, Indium-111 labeled platelets: Studies on preparation and evaluation of in vitro and in vivo functions. Thromb. Res. 9:345, 1976.
10. Sinn H, Silvester DJ, Simplified cell labelling with Indium-111 acetylacetone. Brit. J. Rad. 52:758, 1979.
11. Dewanjee MK, Rao SA, Didisheim P, Indium-111 tropolone, a new high-affinity platelet label: Preparation and evaluation of labeling parameters. J. nucl. Med. 22:981, 1981.
12. Heyns duP A, Lötter MG, Badenhorst PN et al, Kinetics, distribution and sites of destruction of ^{111}Indium labelled human platelets. Brit. J. Haemat. 44:269, 1980.
13. Van Reenen OR, Lötter MG, Minnaar PC et al, Radiation dose from human platelets labelled with Indium-111. Brit. J. Radiol. 53:790, 1980.
14. Heyns duP A, Lötter MG, Badenhorst PN et al, Kinetics and sites of destruction of ^{111}Indium-labeled platelets in idiopathic thrombocytopenic purpura: A quantitative study. Amer. J. Hemat. 12:167, 1982.
15. Hawker RJ, Hawker LM, Wilkinson AR, Indium (^{111}In)-labelled human platelets: Optimal method. Clin. Sci. 58,243, 1980.
16. Sinzinger H, Angelberger P, Höfer R, Platelet labeling with In-111-oxine: Benefit of prostacyclin (PGI_2) addition for preparation and injection. J. nucl. Med. 22:292, 1981.
17. Murphy EA, Mustard JR, Studies of platelet economy. In: Platelet Kinetics, Paulus JM (ed), Elsevier/North-Holland Biomedical Press, Amsterdam, p 24, 1971.

18. Dornhorst AC, The interpretation of red cell survival curves. Blood 6:1284, 1951.

19. Simon TL, Hyers TM, Gaston JP, Harker LA, Heparin pharmacokinetics: Increased requirements in pulmonary embolism. Brit. J. Haemat. 39:111, 1978.

20. Paulus JM, Measuring mean life span, mean age, and variance of longevity in platelets. In: Platelet Kinetics, Paulus JM (ed), Elsevier/North-Holland Biomedical Press, Amsterdam, p 60, 1971.

21. Meuleman DC, Vogel GMT, Stulemeyer SM, Moelker HCT, Analysis of platelet survival curves in an arterial thrombosis model in rats. Thromb. Res. 20:31, 1980.

22. Lötter MG, Herbst C, Badenhorst PN et al, Evaluation of models to determine platelet life span and survival curve shape. Symposium "Methodology of platelet labelling and analysis of platelet kinetics", Paris 1982.

23. Heyns duP A, Lötter MG, Badenhorst PN et al, Kinetics and fate of ^{111}Indium-oxine labelled platelets in patients with aortic aneurysms. Arch. Surg. 117:1170, 1982.

24. Heyns duP A, Lötter MG, Kotze HF et al, Quantification of in vivo distribution of Indium-111-oxine labeled platelets. J. nucl. Med. (in press) 1982.

25. Harker LA, Thrombokinetics in idiopathic thrombocytopenic purpura. Brit. J. Haemat. 19:95, 1970.

26. Kolbe H, Sinzinger H, Angelberger P, Leithner Ch. Früherkennung von Abstoszungsreaktionen mit ^{111}Indium-oxin markierten Thrombozyten. Radiol. Diagn. 21:821, 1980.

27. Heyns duP A, Lötter MG, Pieters H et al, A quantitative study of Indium-111-oxine platelet kinetics in acute and chronic renal transplant rejection. Clinical Nephrol.(in press) 1982.

10 PLATELET KINETICS

A.M. PETERS

The subject of platelet kinetics can conveniently be subdivided into three areas:

1. Platelet distribution.
2. Platelet life span.
3. Sites of platelet destruction.

Distribution

Following intravenous injection, a substantial fraction of radiolabelled platelets is taken up by the spleen (1-3). These splenic platelets are in dynamic equilibrium with extrasplenic, circulating platelets, and have a transit time through the spleen such that at any time, about one third of the total platelet population is "pooled" in the spleen. The so-called recovery of radiolabelled platelets following re-injection is very nearly equal to the difference between the dose and the splenic uptake. Why a platelet spends a third of its life span in the spleen is unknown, as, also, are the mechanisms controlling its transit through the spleen. This transit time is about 10 min in the normal subject (4), as can be shown by dynamic imaging over the spleen and cardiac blood-pool following bolus intravenous injection of platelets labelled with a gamma emitting isotope such as ^{111}In or ^{113m}In (fig. 1). Transit time does not appear to correlate with splenic blood-flow (SBF), which can be measured at the same time, but does show a significant inverse correlation with splenic perfusion (i.e. SBF per unit volume of spleen) (4) (fig. 2). It might be expected to increase in splenomegaly, as SBF does, but in fact remains essentially the same as in normal sized spleens (4). The pooling capacity of the spleen tends, therefore, to be dependant on SBF rather than on platelet transit time, and the in-

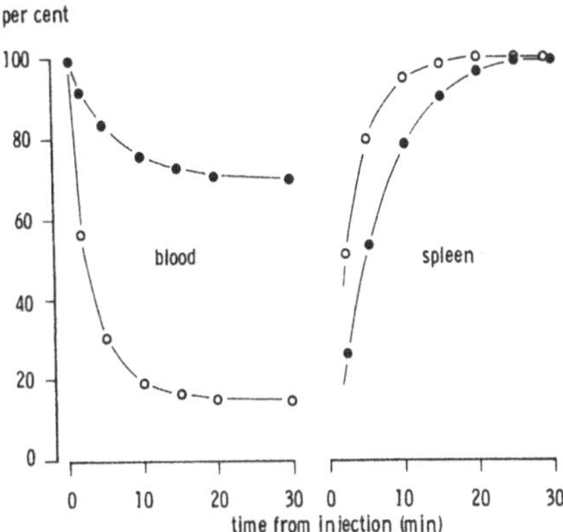

Fig. 1. Simultaneous time activity curves recorded over the cardiac blood-pool and spleen following bolus i.v. injection of ^{111}In-labelled platelets in a patient with a normal sized spleen (closed circles) and a patient with massive splenomegaly (open circles) (ordinate: percent of maximum).

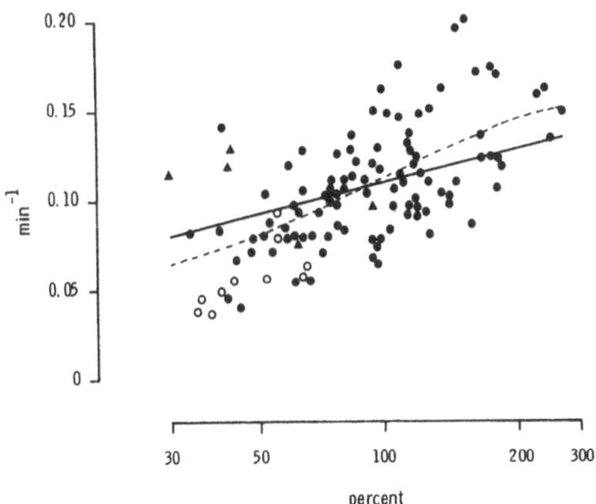

Fig. 2. Relationship between intrasplenic platelet transit time (shown as the reciprocal-ordinate) and splenic perfusion. Patients have been placed into 5 groups, according to spleen size, and the mean SBF calculated for each group. Each patient's SBF has then been expressed as a percentage of the mean for his spleen size group (abscissa). The continuous line is the regression slope for $y = a + b \log x$ (r=0.62) and the dotted line for $y = A(1 - e^{-kx})$ (r=0.57). In the latter relationship, A, represents the minimum transit time (6.3 min). Triangles - primary polycythaemia; open circles-secondary polycythaemia. Closed circles: others.

creased pooling capacity in the abnormally enlarged spleen (fig. 1) is explained by the direct relationship between SBF and spleen size (4).

It is possible that platelets also pool normally in the liver, as has been suggested by non-isotopic approaches to platelet kinetic studies (5). Following re-injection of ^{111}In-labelled platelets about 10-15% of the dose is rapidly taken up by the liver (2,6-8) but, because the liver also removes nonviable cells, the interpretation of this early activity is uncertain. Furthermore, although the liver activity subsequently falls, it does not strictly parallel blood-activity which it should if it represented platelet pooling within the liver (2-4). Platelets maintained in plasma during isolation and labelling with ^{111}In-tropolone display almost no liver uptake (S.H. Saverymuttu, F. Malik, unpublished), suggesting that liver activity, when seen, is "artefactual". This is strongly reminiscent of the pulmonary granulocyte sequestration which is seen following exposure of cells to plasma-free media during labelling with ^{111}In-oxine but is greatly reduced if the cells are maintained in plasma and labelled with ^{111}In-tropolone (9).

The lung has also been put forward as a platelet pooling region on the basis of both non-isotopic (10) and isotopic studies utilizing ^{51}Cr as the platelet label (11). Absolute quantitation of ^{111}In-distribution, shortly after the injection of ^{111}In-labelled platelets, has, however, consistently shown that the entire dose can be accounted for in spleen, liver and circulating blood (2,6-8

Life span

The normal platelet survival is almost linear when determined using ^{111}In-labelled platelets, with a life span of 9-10 days. With ^{51}Cr it has been found by some to be linear whereas by others to be curvilinear or truly exponential. For linear survivals life span is usually expressed as the time at which the plot cuts the time axis. It should be realized that this time is the platelet life span from the time of the platelet's release from bone marrow to the time of its destruction, not the time from its re-injection. For non-linear survivals, a variety of analytical approaches are possible.

The most versatile is the use of the gamma function (12) which is based on the so-called multiple-hit model and which for any shaped survival curve indicates the mean number of hits required for the platelet to be removed from the circulation; one hit yields an exponential survival, whereas an infinite number is required for a truly linear survival. Another approach, based on the equally plausible model of random destruction superimposed on age dependant destruction, is the Mills-Dornhorst equation which quantitates the relative magnitude of random destruction (13). Other techniques are less rigorous but do not require computer facilities; they include the initial slope and weighted harmonic mean (14). Very short survivals are satisfactorily fitted with an exponential function. For accurate survival curve data it is necessary to subtract plasma isotope levels (15). With ^{111}In for instance, with its slow biological turnover, plasma isotope is probably in equilibrium with reticuloendothelial isotope rather than circulating platelet activity and therefore tends to remain constant over the duration of the survival study. It, therefore, progressively rises as a percentage of total blood activity.

Platelet survival is a poor indicator of intravascular platelet consumption as can be inferred from theoretical considerations (16). Abnormal ^{111}In-labelled platelet uptake in diseased (17) or artificial vessels (18), identifiable with the gamma camera, has been observed to have no impact on platelet life span, and, conversely, in conditions in which reduced platelet life span is thought to be the result of intravascular consumption, no abnormal activity has been identified on imaging even though reduced life span has been confirmed (16). Reduced life span in these circumstances is more likely the result of premature platelet senility. Thus a relationship between splenic destruction and life span was recently demonstrated in diabetic patients (19), whereas the reverse would have been expected if reduced life span resulted from intravascular consumption. However, in other circumstances, reduced life span has been found to be associated with scintigraphic evidence of peripheral (i.e. non-reticuloendothelial) platelet uptake, such as in the rejecting transplanted kidney (20). We have recently looked for a relationship between platelet life

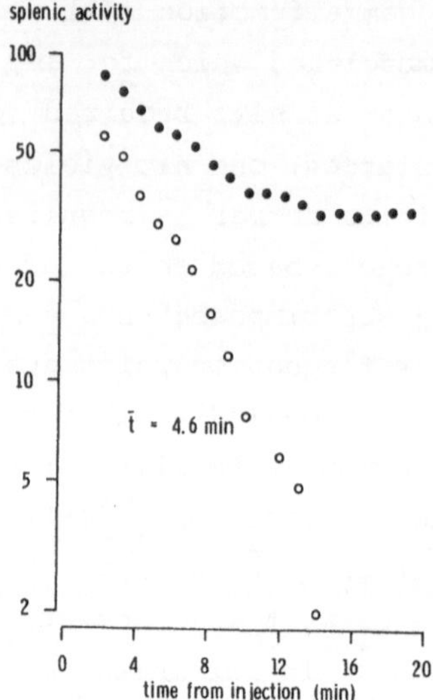

Fig. 3. Splenic platelet "wash-out" curve (closed circles) predicted by deconvolution analysis in a patient with ITP who had a platelet count of $20x10^9/1$ and a mean platelet life span of 1.1 hour. Subtraction of the asymptote yielded the open circles which represents "wash-out" of un-extracted platelets and which resembles the predicted "wash-out" curve seen in normals. t- intrasplenic platelet transit time.

span and intrasplenic transit time, based on the possibility that platelets, like erythrocytes, become susceptible to increased splenic trapping when damaged or senescent. However, the use of deconvolution analysis (21), (fig. 3) in addition to compartimenta analysis (3), for the measurement of transit time, has shown that even very short lived platelets have essentially normal transit time through the spleen, suggesting that pooling is not related to destruction in the spleen (A.M. Peters et al, unpublished).

Sites of destruction

Based on ^{51}Cr-labelled platelet studies it has long been held that the main sites of destruction are the liver and spleen. Because of its superior gamma emission, the availability of ^{111}In as a platelet label provides the opportunity to study sites of platelet destruction more accurately. Soon after ^{111}In-platelet injection the sum of activities in liver, spleen and blood is

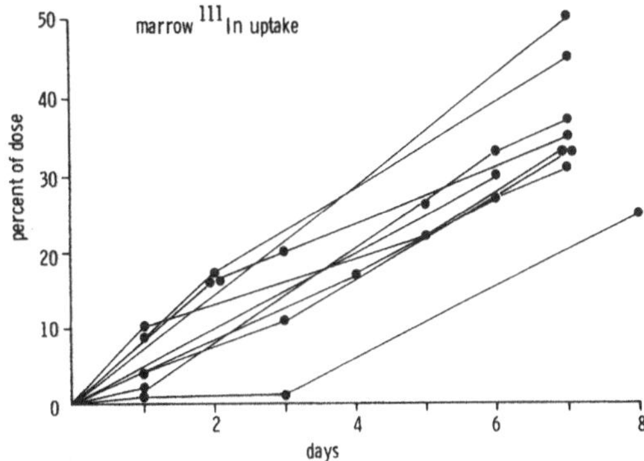

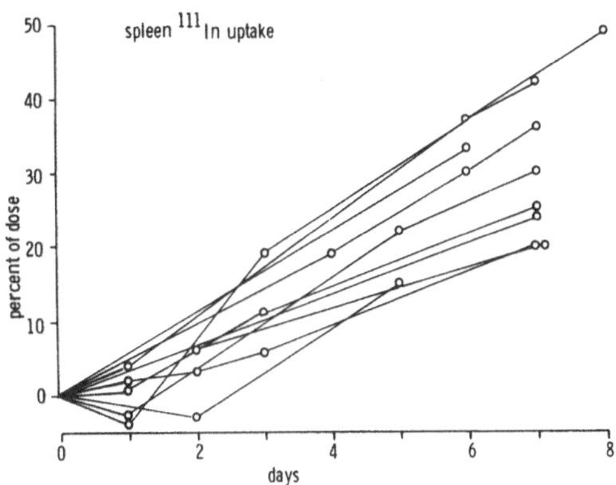

Fig.4.Uptake of ^{111}In by bone marrow and spleen following injection of ^{111}In-platelets in normal subjects. The splenic activity has been corrected for activity present in platelets pooled in the spleen. Marrow activity has been estimated by subtraction of the sum of activities in liver, spleen and circulating blood from 100%.

equal to 100% of the dose (2,6-8). This sum falls progressively throughout the life span of the radiolabelled platelets, and, because i) there are essentially no losses of ^{111}In via urine (22) or faeces (23) and ii) a bone marrow image becomes increasingly visible, it is likely that the rising ^{111}In "deficit" is present in bone marrow (7). Since ^{111}In is relatively stable in the spleen and liver, the increasing bone marrow activity probably represents uptake of platelets rather than of "free" ^{111}In (24).

Based on this approach, it has been concluded that approximately as many platelets are destroyed in the bone marrow as in the spleen, about 40% to 50% (fig. 4). The remainder, about 15% appear to be destroyed in the liver, but, because a significant fraction of this may represent immediate uptake of platelets damaged from the labelling procedure, it must be concluded that the liver is not normally an important site for platelet destruction.

Because the radioactivity signal from the spleen remains almos constant between 1 hour after reinjection of ^{51}Cr (1) or ^{111}In, (2,6-8) labelled platelets and completion of life span, the fracti of the total platelet population pooling in the spleen is essentia ly equal to the fraction destroyed there. This constancy holds in splenomegaly and reduced platelet life span (25), except in idiopathic thrombocytopenic purpura (ITP) (A.M. Peters et al, unpublis ed). In ITP, the destruction: pooling ratio may be elevated,incriminating the spleen as a site of abnormal, or inappropriate, destruction, or it may be reduced, suggesting the liver as an abnormal destruction site. In the latter instance, the platelet life span is generally greatly reduced, and liver destruction can often be identified as a rising signal on dynamic gamma camera imaging (A.M. Peters et al, unpublished).

Acknowledgements

The author was supported by the Cancer Research Campaign. The secretarial assistance of Miss C. Debnam is gratefully acknowledged.

REFERENCES

1. Aster RH, Studies of the fate of platelets in rats and man. Blood 34: 117, 1969.

2. Heyns A du P, Lötter MG, Badenhorst PN et al, Kinetics, distribution and sites of destruction of ^{111}Indium labelled human platelets. Brit. J. Haemat. 44:269, 1980.

3. Peters AM, Klonizakis I, Lavender JP et al, Use of ^{111}In-labelled platelets to measure spleen function. Brit. J. Haemat. 46:587, 1980.

4. Peters AM, Lavender JP, Factors controlling the intrasplenic transit of platelets. Eur. J. Clin. Invest. 12:191, 1982.

5. Freedman M, Altszuler N, Karpatkin S, Presence of nonsplenic platelet pool. Blood 50:419, 1977.

6. Robertson JS, Dewanjee MK, Brown ML et al, Distribution and dosimetry of ^{111}In-labelled platelets. Radiology 140:169, 1981.

7. Klonizakis I, Peters AM, Fitzpatrick ML, Radionuclide distribution following injection ^{111}Indium labelled platelets. Brit. J. Haemat. 46:595, 1980.

8. Scheffel U, Tsan MF, Mitchell TG et al, Human platelets labelled with In-111-8-hydroxyquinoline, kinetics, distribution and estimates of radiation dose. J. nucl. Med. 23:149, 1982.

9. Saverymuttu SH, Peters AM, Danpure HJ et al, Lung transit of ^{111}Indium labelled granulocytes. Relationship to labelling techniques. Scan. J. Haemat. 30:151, 1983.

10. Bierman HR, Kelly KH, Cordes FL et al, The release of leukocytes and platelets from the pulmonary circulation by epinephrine. Blood 7:683, 1952.

11. Martin BA, Dahlby R, Nicholls I et al, Platelet sequestration in the lung with haemorrhagic shock and re-infusion in dogs. J. appl. Physiol. 50:1306, 1981.

12. Murphy EA, Francis ME, The estimation of blood platelet survival II. The multiple hit model. Thrombos. Diathes. haemorrh. (Stuttg) 25:53, 1971.

13. Dassin E, Najean Y, Poirer O et al, In-vivo platelet kinetics in 31 diabetic patients. Correlation with the degree of vascular impairment. Thromb. Haemost. 40:83, 1978.

14. ICSH, Recommended methods for radioisotope platelet survival studies. Blood 50:1137, 1977.

15. Heaton WA, Davis HH, Welch MJ et al, Indium-111: a new radionuclide label for studying human platelet kinetics. Brit. J. Haemat. 46:613, 1979.

16. Peters AM, Rozkovec A, Bell RN et al, Platelet kinetics in congenital heart disease. Cardiovasc. Res. 16:391, 1982.

17. Davis HH, Siegel BA, Sherman LA et al, Scintigraphic detection of carotid atherosclerosis with Indium-111-labelled autologous platelets. Circulation 16:982, 1980.

18. Goldman M, Norcott HC, Hawker RJ et al, Platelet accumulation on mature Dacron grafts in man. Brit. J. Surg. 69:538, 1982 (suppl).

19. Porta M, Peters AM, Cousins SA et al, A study of platelet relevant parameters in patients with diabetic microangiopathy. Diabetologia 1983 (in press).

20. Leithner C, Sinzinger H, Schwartz M, Treatment of chronic kidney transplant rejection with prostacyclin-reduction of platelet deposition in the transplant, prolongation of platelet survival and improvement of transplant function. Prostaglandins 22:783, 1981.

21. Williams DL, Improvement in quantitative data analysis by numerical deconvolution techniques. J. nucl. Med. 20:568, 1979.

22. Goodwin DA, Bushberg JT, Doherty PW et al, Indium-111-labelled autologous platelets for location of vascular thrombi in humans. J. nucl. Med. 19:626, 1979.

23. Saverymuttu SH, Peters AM, Hodgson HJ et al, Assessment of disease activity in ulcerative colitis using ^{111}In-labelled leucocyte faecal excretion. Scand. J. Gastroenterol. 1983 (in press).

24. Peters AM, Klonizakis I, Lavender JP et al, Elution of ^{111}Indium from reticuloendothelial cells. J. clin. Path. 35:507, 1982.

25. Ries CA, Price DC, ^{51}Cr platelet kinetics in thrombocytopenia: correlation between splenic sequestration of platelets and response to splenectomy. Ann. Intern. Med. 80:702, 1974.

11 EVALUATION OF MODELS TO DETERMINE PLATELET LIFE SPAN AND SURVIVAL CURVE SHAPE

M.G. LÖTTER, C.P. HERBST, P.N. BADENHORST, A. duP HEYNS, P. WESSELS, P.C. MINNAAR

INTRODUCTION

The value of radionuclide platelet survival studies to delineate the mechanisms of thrombocytopenia and factors contributing to it has been proven (1), and the effect of various diseases and therapies on platelet survival may be evaluated by the same technique. The recent introduction of ^{111}In-oxine as a cellular label allowing in vivo imaging of platelet distribution, has renewed interest in platelet kinetic studies (2,3).

Platelet kinetics may be assessed by the mean platelet survival time in the circulation (PS) and the shape of the survival curve (CS). These parameters are best estimated by the fitting of a mathematical model to the blood radioactivity data, thus eliminating human bias. The mathematical models are either empirical, or the parameters may have a physiological basis. All models have a similar theory: If the survival of platelets is strictly age-dependent, or, platelets have a finite life-span, a linear survival curve will result. On the other hand, if platelet destruction is fully random, the platelet survival curve will be exponential. It is also generally accepted that platelet survival curves of a platelet population consisting of platelets of different random ages, are in general neither strictly linear nor exponential.

Different mathematical models to evaluate platelet kinetics have been proposed (ICSH 1977),but it is not clear which is the most appropriate.

The aim of this study was to assess and compare results obtained with several different mathematical models for analysis of PS and CS found in different clinical situations. ^{111}In-oxine

Table 1. Patient population divided into 3 groups of linear, linear-exponential and exponential survival

Patients	Number	Platelet survival curve
Normal	19	Linear function; normal life span (180-240 h)
Vascular diseases	3	Linear-exponential function; intermediate life span (120-180 h)
Renal transplantation	8	
Cardiac valve disease	2	
Immune thrombocytopenia	9	Exponential function; short life span (less than 120 h)
Vascular diseases	3	
Renal transplantation	9	
Cardiac valve disease	2	
Total:	55	

was the platelet label in all instances. We propose a new curve shape factor, the variance shape factor (VS), which is independent of the mathematical model used.

Models

Patient selection. 55 patients gave informed written consent for an investigation that was approved by the Ethical Committee of the Province and the University of the Orange Free State. These patients were divided into 3 groups according to PS (table 1).

The first group consisted of 19 normal volunteers with multiple hit PS between 180 and 240 hours.

The PS of the second group of 13 patients ranged between 120 and 180 hours. This group consisted of 3 patients with vascular disease. 8 patients had had transplantation and 2 patients had cardiac valvular disease.

The PS of the third group was less than 120 hours. It consisted of 9 patients who had immune thrombocytopenia, 3 with vascular disease, 9 who had renal transplantation and 2 patients had cardiac valvular disease.

Reagents and labelling of platelets. ^{111}In-oxine (Radiochemical Centre, Amersham, UK) was supplied as a 1 ml isotonic solution of 0.75% NaCl containing 37 MBq (1 mCi) of ^{111}In complexed with 50 µg 8-hydroxyquinoline, 6 mg HEPES buffer, and 100 µg Polysorbate 80.

Labelling of platelets was performed with a method based on that previously described (3). Briefly, 84 ml of blood was collected in a polystyrene syringe containing 16 ml ACD NIH formula A as anticoagulant. Platelet-rich plasma (PRP) was obtained by centrifugation at 180 g for 15 min and the PRP was transferred to polystyrene tubes. Platelets trapped with the red cells were recovered by repeating resuspension and centrifugation at 750 g for 3 min of red cells 4 times. After acidifying to pH 6.2 - 6.5 with ACD, platelets were sedimented by centrifuging at 800 g for 30 min, resuspended in physiological saline, incubated for 30 min with ^{111}In-oxine, washed once with platelet-poor autologous plasma (PPP) and finally resuspended in PPP.

A dose not exeeding 18.5 MBq (500 µCi) of ^{111}In was adminstered to patients. Labelled platelets were used for in vivo studies only if aggregation with collagen in vitro was satisfactory.

Calculation of mean platelet survival time. Whole blood-samples of 3 ml were directly collected in the counting vials, the mass determined and water added to a constant final volume of 4 ml. The samples were counted in a well scintillation counter with the pulse height analyzer set to include the 172, 247 keV and sum peak of ^{111}In. Count rate was corrected for background and normalized to unit mass.

In all mathematical models, PS was calculated by the ratio of the y-intercept and the initial slope of the curve, i.e. the intersection of the x-intercept by the tangent (fig 1).

Platelet survival was calculated for each of the following 6 mathematical models.

1. Linear function (4)

$N = N_o (1-kt)$

N = circulating platelet activity at time t

N_o = y-intercept

k = rate of platelet removal

L = 1/k This is referred to as Linear PS

2. Exponential function (4)

$N_e = N_o \exp(-ft)$

f = fractional rate of random platelet removal

E = 1/f This is referred to as exponential PS

3. Weighted mean function

A weighted mean function has been proposed to allow goodness of fit evaluation with this approach:

$$N_w = \frac{N_e S_p + N_p S_e}{S_p + S_e}$$

S_p and S = Sum of squares of deviations of the data points for fitted linear and exponential functions

$$W = \frac{L S_e + E S_p}{S_e + S_p}$$

4. Multiple hit function (4)

$$N = \frac{No}{n} \sum_{i=o}^{n-1} \frac{(n-i)}{i!} e^{-at} (at)^i$$

a = the reciprocal of the mean waiting time between hits

n = number of hits that result in platelet destruction

M = n/a This is referred to as the multiple hit PS

5. Dornhorst function (4)

$$N = \frac{No\ (\exp(-ft) - \exp(-fT))}{(1 - \exp(-fT))}$$

T = Senescent PS if random removal is absent

D = $-(1-(\exp-fT))/f$ This is referred to as the Dornhost PS

6. Alpha-order function (5)

$N = 1+(\alpha-1)(k_o-kt))^{1/(1-\alpha)}$

α = order of function

k_o = normalization constant

A = $(1+(\alpha-1)k_o)/k$ This is referred to a alpha-order PS

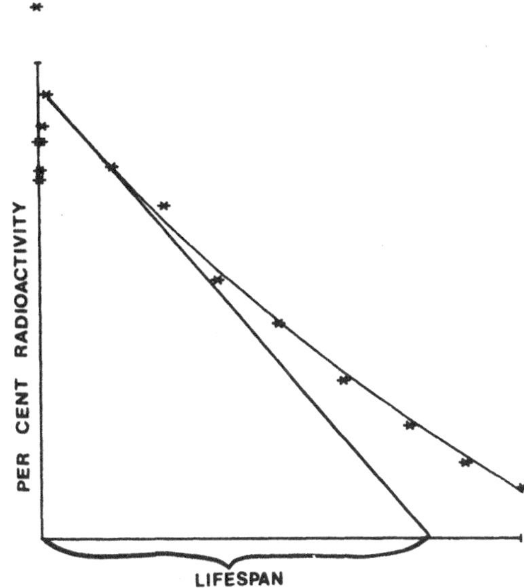

Fig. 1. The mean platelet life span (PS) is calculated by the ratio of the y-intercept and initial slope of the regression curve fitted to the survival data; that is the time to the X-intercept by the tangent.

Table 2. Goodness of fit for each model was expressed as the standard deviation of data points around the fitted lines. All models except the LN and EXP function fit data well

Standard deviation (SD) of data points around the fitted line (n=55)

MODEL	Linear	Exponential	Weighted mean	Multiple hit	Dornhorst	Alpha-order
MEAN SD	6.0	4.3	3.6	3.1	3.7	3.4
VARIANCE ANALYSIS	S	S	NS	NS	NS	NS

S = significant NS = not significant

The mathematical models were fitted to the survival curve data by a least squares non-linear Newton iteration method. Iteration was terminated when fractional changes in regression constants were less than 0,0001. A computer program to perform the calculations were written for a Medical Data System A^2 imaging system. Curve data was entered by keyboard and the curve was displayed on a graphical terminal for selection of the curve fitting range. Curve fitting was started when splenic pooling was completed and platelets, temporarily damaged during labelling, released from the liver. Curve fitting was stopped when sample activity was less than 10 percent of the maximum curve value. Measured and fitted curves were stored according to a patient directory on magnetic disc and graphs could be obtained in colour with a graphics plotter. Other results such as the PS, CS and goodness of fit for each model were tabulated using a line printer.

The goodness of fit of the different models to the data was evaluated by calculating the standard deviation of the data points around the fitted line as a percentage of the regression curve y-intercept. One-way variance analysis was performed to determine if the differences between the goodness of fit and survival times for each of the models investigated were statistically significant.

Analysis of curve shape. CS was evaluated by the number of "hits" in the multiple hit model. Platelet removal by a single hit represents random exponential destruction. As platelet removal becomes age-dependant and linear the number of hits increases to infinity.

The alpha value (α) of the alpha-order model also represents curve shape. For α = o a linear and for α = 1 an exponential survival curve is obtained.

A variance curve shape factor (VS) which is independent of the mathematical model used is proposed.

$$VS = \frac{S_p - S_r}{(S_p - S_r) + (S_e - S_r)}$$

Sr = sum of squares of deviations of the data points for a

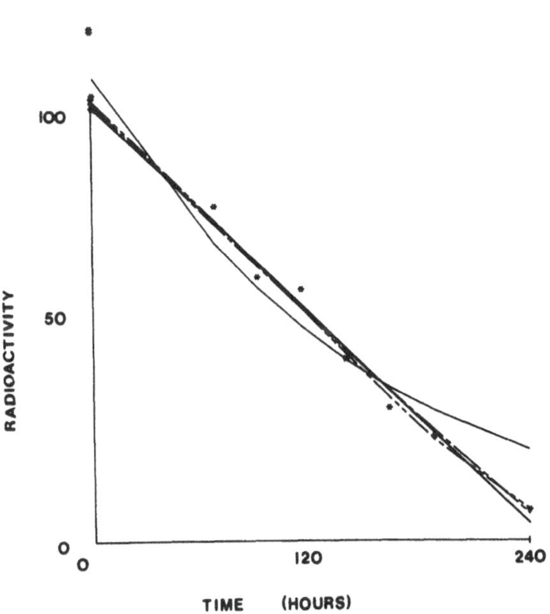

Fig. 2. When mathematical models were fit to normal patients (PS longer than 180 h) all models except the EXP function fit data well. Models are indicated by:

LN, EXP, WM,
MH, DH, AO.

Table 3. Survival times and variance curve shape values for patient platelet survival curves in figs 2 to 4

Typical survival times and variance curve shape factors for each patient group

	Linear		Linear-Exponential		Exponential	
Mathematical Model	PS hours	VS	PS hours	VS hours	PS hours	VS
Linear	250		200		208	
Exponential	148		102		99	
Weighted Mean	237	0,00	161	0,37	122	1,09
Multiple Hit	243	0,06	171	0,38	97	0,99
Dornhorst	232	0,02	144	0,38	97	0,99
Alpha Order	234	0,02	153	0,38	95	0,99

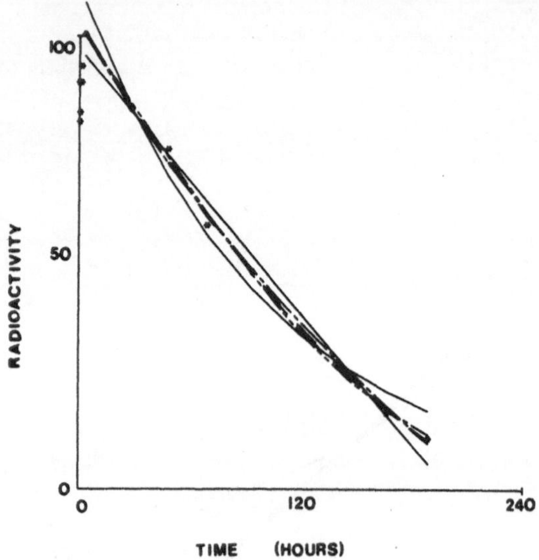

Fig. 3. In a renal transplant patient with linear exponential survival (PS between 120 and 180 h), data were fitted well by all models except the LN and EXP functions, indicated by solid lines. Other models are represented by similar broken lines as explained in fig 2.

fitted regression curve.

The value of VS varies between = 0 for fully linear, and VS = 1.0 for exponential platelet survival.

Statistical differences between the VS for each model were tested by one way analysis of variance. The VS was also correlated with the number of "hits", alpha value and platelet survival.

Results

Evaluation of models. The goodness of fit of models investigated was evaluated by calculating standard deviation (SD) of data points around the fitted line, expressed as a percentage of the y-intercept. The results for 55 studies representing the full spectrum of platelet survival times are presented in table 2. One way analysis of variance demonstrated no significant differences in the goodness of fit of the weighted mean, multiple hit, Dornhorst and alpha-order functions.

Fig 2 demonstrates the measured and fitted survival curves

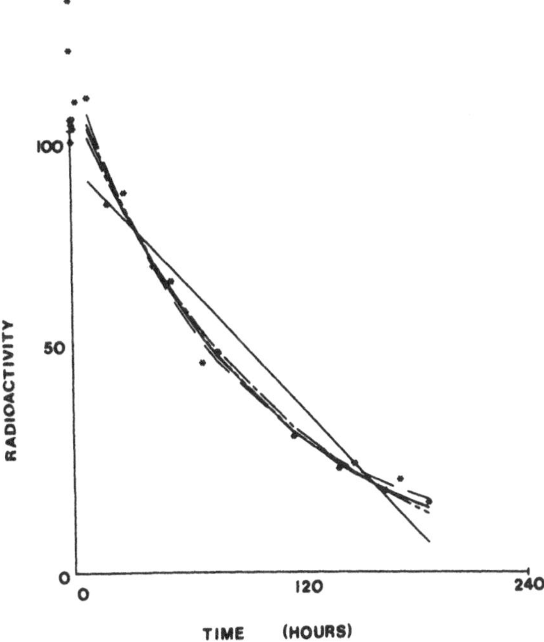

Fig. 4. The LN function (solid line) did not fit data well for a patient with immune thrombocytopenic purpura and exponential survival (PS less than 120 h). Other models are represented by similar broken lines as explained in fig 2.

Table 4. The mean platelet survival average values and standard deviations for the reference patient group (n=19) and all patient groups combined (n=55) are presented in this table

Estimated platelet survival (hours ± 1SD)

MODEL	Linear	Exponential	Weighted mean	Multiple hit	Dornhorst	Alpha-order
Reference group	234 ± 21	130 ± 25	216 ± 19	223 ± 16	211 ± 27	220 ± 26
Variance analysis	S	S	NS	NS	NS	NS
All patients	191 ± 55	104 ± 36	150 ± 59	155 ± 67	147 ± 67	142 ± 70
Variance analysis	S	S	NS	NS	NS	NS

S = significant NS = not significant

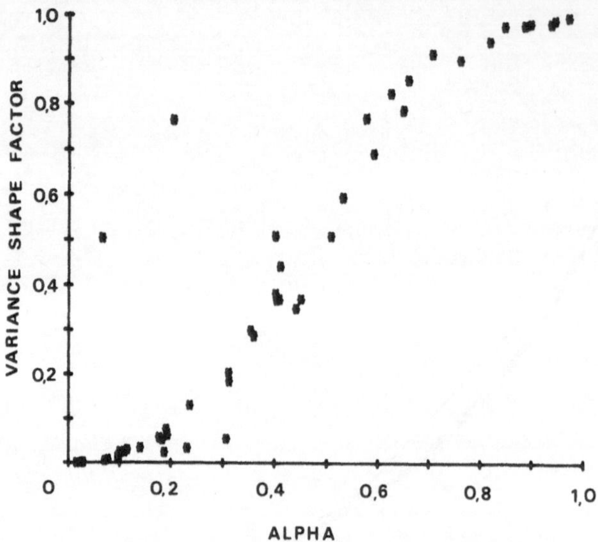

Fig. 5. The variance shape factor (all models) and the α value (alpha order function) correlated well in the range 0,2 to 0,8.

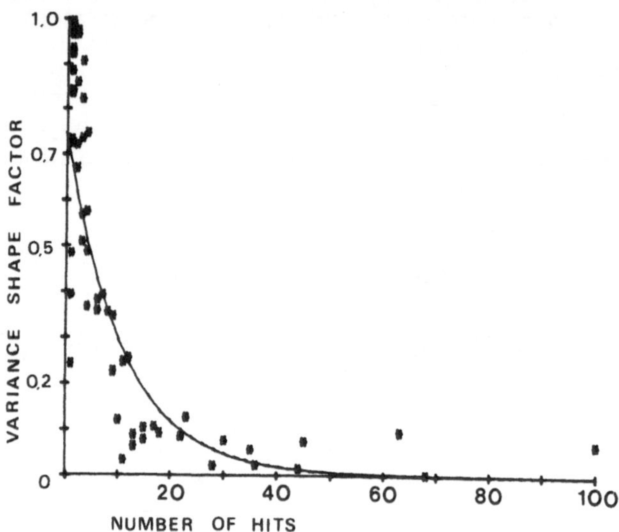

Fig. 6. A non-linear correlation was obtained between the variance shape factor (all models) and number of "hits" (Multiple hit function).

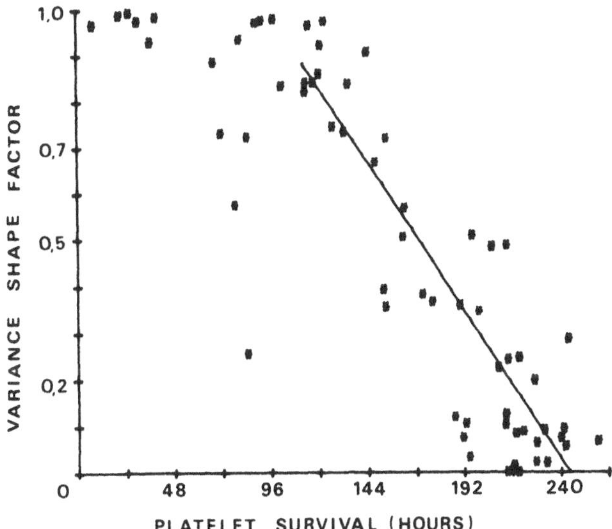

Fig. 7. A good correlation between variance shape factor (all models) and PS was obtained for the interval 96 to 240 h. For survival periods less than 96 h, survival curves were exponential with CS close to one.

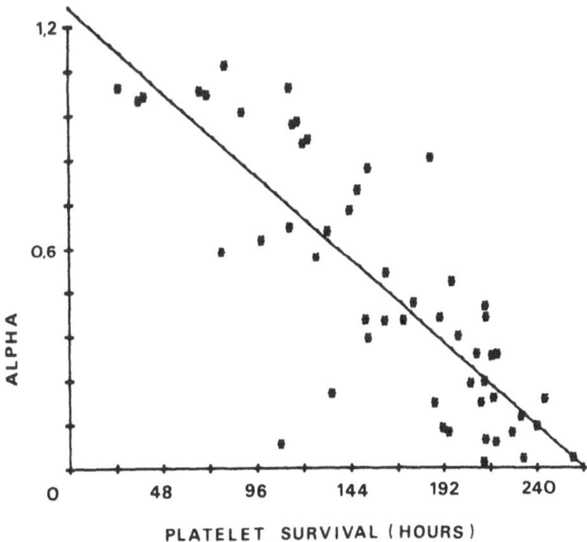

Fig. 8. A good correlation between the shape factor alpha (alpha order model) and PS was obtained for the PS range 96 to 240 h was found.

for a single patient in the linear survival group. In this group all functions fit measured data well, except the exponential function. This is also demonstrated by the calculated PS and CS (table 3). In the linear-exponential survival group, neither the exponential nor the linear fitted the data well (fig 3 and table 3). In the patient group with an exponential platelet survival, the data were not fitted well by the linear curve, but adequately by the other mathematical models (fig 4 and table 3).

Estimate of mean platelet survival. Mean platelet survival was calculated for each mathematical function evaluated for the 3 patient groups. Table 5 presents the PS for the reference normal group (n=19). One way analysis of variance did not demonstrate a significant difference for the estimated PS between the weighted mean, multiple hit, Dornhorst and alpha-order models. A significant difference could also not be demonstrated when all patients were grouped.

Estimate of the shape of the platelet survival curve. The VS was compared with the number of "hits", the alpha value and the PS.

Fig 5 illustrates the correlation between alpha and the VS: There was good agreement in the middle zone. The VS and number of "hits" were not linearly related (fig 6).

There was a negative linear correlation (r= -0,8317) between the PS and VS in the range of platelet survival of 120 to 260 hours. Survival times shorter than 120 hours were almost always associated with an exponential curve shape (fig 7).

The correlation coefficient of the alpha value and PS was r = -0,8207 (fig 8).

Conclusions

The weighted mean, multiple hit, Dornhorst and alpha-order models were all equally satisfactory for the analysis of platelet survival data. There was not a statistical significant difference in PS as calculated with these models. Since the models were evaluated over a wide spectrum of platelet survival times, the results suggested that any of these models would be appropriate for the analysis of platelet survival curve data.

It must be emphasized that since the survival time is calculated by the ratio of the y-intercept and initial slope of the regression curve, frequent and accurate measurements must be obtained during the initial part of the study. However, only sample counts obtained after the splenic and liver pool has reached a steady state, should be included for curve fitting. This certainly complicates analysis of PS in patients with rapid clearance of platelets from the circulation, e.g. immune thrombocytopenic purpura.

Because of the inaccuracies associated with estimation of platelet survival, the CS was also investigated as a means of evaluating platelet kinetics. This approach is based on the assumption that the survival curve of normal platelets is nearly linear, and that it becomes more curved with increasing random platelet destruction.

The VS correlated well with the alpha value and the results indicated that as shape factors, they reflect the shape of the survival curve. The VS has the advantage that it may be employed independent of the mathematical model used for fitting the data of the survival curve.

The VS and PS correlated well in the range of between 120 and 260 hours. For PS of less than 120 hours, survival curves were all exponential and this resulted in a VS close to one. There was poor agreement in the 4 patients with a PS of around 70 hours. These studies were performed in patients after acute renal transplant rejection episodes when platelet kinetics were almost certainly not in a steady state. As a steady state is a theoretical prerequisite for these analyses, it would explain the discrepancy.

These results indicated that the variance curve shape warrants further investigation in clinical situations and may be applied to the assessment of the therapeutic efficacy of antiplatelet drugs.

REFERENCES

1. Davey MG, In: The survival and destruction of human platelets. Karger S (ed), Basel, pp 85-117, 1966.

2. Thakur ML, Welch MJ, Joist H, Coleman RE, Indium-111-labelled platelets: Studies on preparation and evaluation of in vitro and in vivo functions. Thromb. Res. 9:345, 1976.

3. Heyns duP A, Lötter MG, Badenhorst PN, Van Reenen OR, Pieters H, Minnaar PC, Retief FP, Kinetics, distribution and sites of destruction of Indium-111-labelled human platelets. Brit. J. Haemat. 44:269, 1980.

4. The panel on diagnostic application of radioisotopes in hematology, International Committee for standardization in Hematology: Recommended methods for radioisotope platelet survival studies. Blood 50:1137, 1977.

5. Simon TL, Heyers TM, Gasron JP, Harker LH, Heparin pharmacokinetics: Increased requirements in pulmonary embolism. Brit. J. Haemat. 39:111, 1978.

12 COMPARISON OF THREE METHODS EVALUATING PLATELET SURVIVAL TIME IN PATIENTS WITH PROSTHETIC HEART VALVE

J. SCHBATH, D. VILLE, B. MATHY, B. SANCHINI, E. BENVENISTE, J. BELLEVILLE, M. DECHAVANNE, J.P. BOISSEL, J. GILLET

INTRODUCTION

In determining the mean life span in ^{51}Cr platelet survival studies, the survival parameters could be estimated by visual fitting (graphical method). In addition, 3 methods have been recommended for computing the mean survival time (1): the weighted mean of linear estimate or logarithmic estimate, the truncated exponential model and the gamma model. In our study these 2 later models and graphical method were used for evaluating platelet survival time (PST). The study was a randomized controlled clinical trial (2) carried out with patients with aortic or mitral valve replacement, operated by the surgeons of Hôpital Cardiologique, Lyon, France.

Data concerning treatment groups and strata (valves) have been published elsewhere. The purpose of this presentation is to provide with the main data of the comparison between different means of calculating PST and to evaluate correlation between PST and other variables (3).

Materials and methods

1. The population sample consisted of 40 males and 15 females ages 40-70 years (average 53 years); 32 received Bjork-Shilley in aortic position, 22 underwent mitral valve replacement: 3 with Cooley-Cutter, 11 with Lillehei Kaster 500 and 9 with Starr-Edwards 6120 prostheses.
2. Trial medication was either dipyridamole 375 mg a day, or RA 233 (another pyrimido-pyrimidine derivative) 1,5g a day, or matched placebo. All patients received oral anticoagulants concomitantly. The study began 2 to 3 weeks after surgery and lasted 2½ months, i.e. an average of 3 months after valve

replacement. Compliance to trial medication has been assessed by pills counting and patients questioning. Compliance to oral anticoagulants was checked by prothrombin time at the start and at the end of the follow-up and used to titrate the dosage in between (range 25-35%). Extended haematological investigations were performed at the beginning and at the end. 1 week before the end of the treatment, platelet survival time was determined.

Investigation on platelet survival. The method for PST determination was derived from that of Aster and Jandl (4) by 2 of us (D. Ville and M. Dechavanne). A platelet-rich fraction was obtained from a series of 3 centrifugations at constant temperature (37°C) with citric acid as anticoagulant (4). Each time the supernatant or platelet-poor fraction was saved. It is refered below as PPP. The final platelet button was then resuspended and incubated for 30 min with 400 to 500 µCi of ^{51}Cr (Na_2CrO^4). The labelled platelets were washed with the patient's PPP, centrifugated and finally injected to the patient using a disposable plastic syringe after a homogenous aliquot has been removed for determination of platelet bound radioactivity (PBR). Samples of blood were obtained at 30 min and 4 hours after injection, and thereafter twice a day on days 1,2,3 and once a day, in the morning, on days 4, 5,6 and 7. 12½ ml of blood were drawn without stasis into a glass tube containing 0.5 ml 5% EDTA. 2 centrifugations were performed at 280 g for 10 min. The supernatant was harvested and 4 ml of isotonic saline was added to the sediment, which was centrifugated again. The pooled PPP isotonic extracts were then centrifuged at 2400 rpm for 10 min and the radioactivity of the platelet button measured with a Packard counter.

PBR was calculated as follows:

PBR = (radioactivity of aliquot) x (weight of injected suspension) x (weight of aliquot)$^{-1}$.

Platelet recovery (PR) was obtained from:

PR : (platelet radioactivity per ml of blood) x (total blood-volume) x $(PBR)^{-1}$

The total blood-volume was determined from the body surface value.

Calculation of mean survival time. Mean survival time was calculated by the following 3 methods:

The graphical method (GM). The tangent to the curve at zero time is fitted visualy and cuts the x-axis at time equal to the mean life span.

The linear exponential model (LEM) is based on an equation originally described by Dornhorst (5) (issued from a model developed from red cell survival study) and used by Dassin (6) and Najean (7). The population curve is shown as:

$$N(t) = \frac{No \; (e^{-bt} - e^{bT})}{1 - e^{-bt}}$$

where N_o is the radioactivity at the origin, b is the constant instantaneous rate of random destruction, and T is the maximum platelet survival time. Those values of N_o (the y intercept), b and T that minimize the residual sum of squares S, are obtained by the method of least square:

$$S = \sum_{i-1}^{n} (Ni - Nt)^2$$

where N_i is the observed radioactivity and N_t is the theoretical activity at time t.

The mean survival time (L) is calculated as:

$$L = - \frac{1 - e^{-bT}}{b}$$

The multiple hit model (MHM) leads to a gamma function:

$$N_i = \frac{N_o}{n} \quad \Sigma_{i=0}^{n-1} \left[\frac{n-i}{i!} e^{-at} \cdot (at)^i \right]$$

Those values of N_o, a and n that minimize the residual sum of squares of the n data points (see above) are obtained by iteration on a digital computer. N_i is the observed radioactivity at time t_i; a is the reciprocal of the mean waiting time between hits, n is the number of hits before destroyed and No is estimated by y intercept. The mean survival time is calculated by n/a. This model was performed by Murphy and Francis (8) and assessed by Tsukada and Tango (9) as the best method for calculating the mean survival time of platelets from observed decrease of radioactivity of ^{51}Cr labelled platelets. They based their choice on the values of residual mean squares. The computer program, which is available from the International Committee for Standardization in Hematology (1) has been adapted by one of us.

Statistical methods. Possible confounding factors of PST were accounted for through a mathematical relation. The easiest estimate was obtained by assuming a linear relationship: PST, called the dependant variable, is assumed to be a linear combination of other variables, called explicative variables. This linear model has been fitted with the following explicative variables: Starr valve, Lillehei-Kaster valve, Bjork valve, dipyridamole, RA 233, placebo, sex, age, body surface, follow-up duration, mean number of pills a day, number of concomitant treatments, leucocyte count, platelet count, platelet adhesiveness, plasmatic antithrombin 3, alpha-2 macroglobulin, haptoglobulin, compliance to treatment, cardiac rhythm. During the analysis, significance of coefficient of each variable was tested. This process has been performed again after elimination of some explicative variables whose coefficients appeared to be negligible. The remaining variables were supposed to be important. The multiple linear regression was performed for 42 patients for whom all data were available.

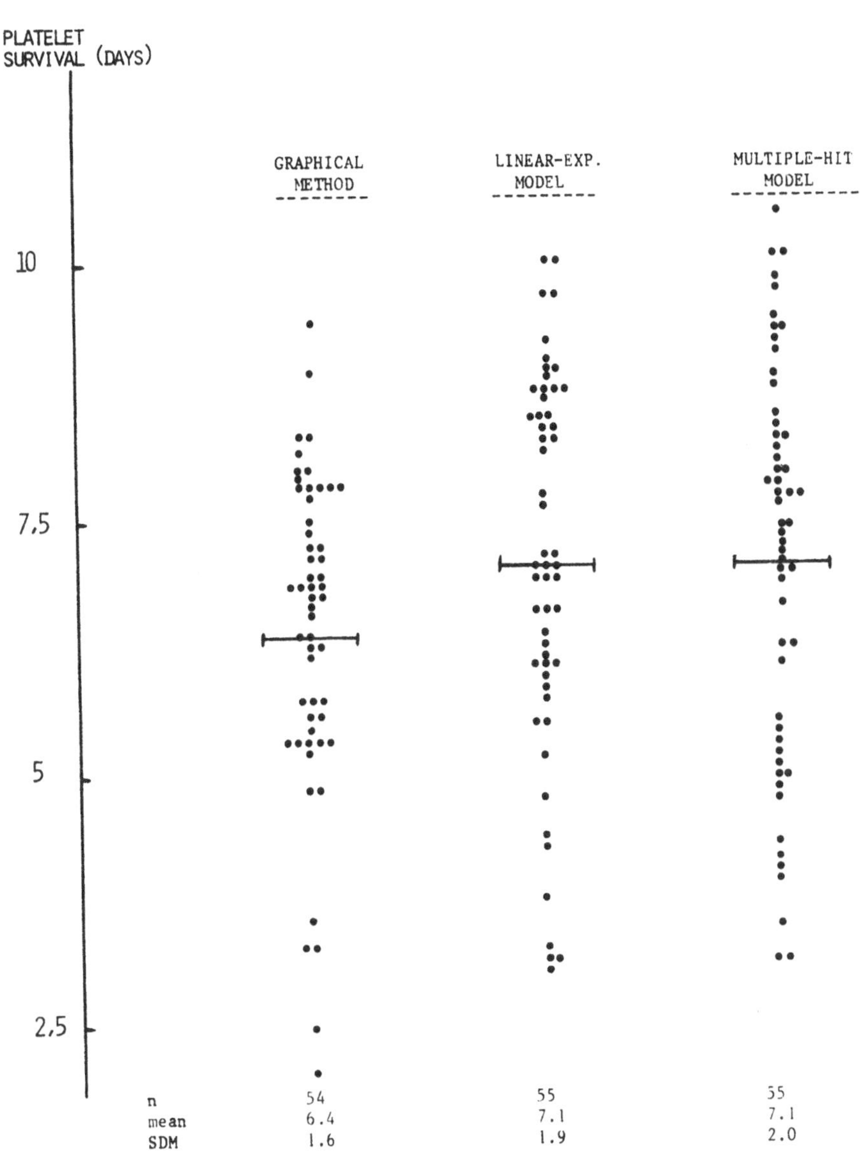

Fig. 1. Platelet survival time (days) in 55 patients by using 3 different models for calculation.

Table 1. Correlations between the 3 methods of calculation

methods	a graphical	c multi-hit
a graphical		R = 0,86345
b. linear-exponential	R = 0,92559	R = 0,92021

Results

The platelet mean life span, in days, computed from the same set of experimental data are given in fig 1. The individual differences between the values for platelet mean life span, given as by graphical method, or linear exponential or multiple hit model are very small.

The averages of platelet mean life spans were respectively 6.4 days, calculated by the graphical method, 7.1 days, calculated by the linear exponential method and 7.1 days, calculated by the multiple hit model.

Whatever the method, PST's were in average "normal". Linear correlation coefficients were calculated between GM and LEM, between GM and MHM, between LEM and MHM as shown in table 1. All coefficients were greater than 0.80 ($p \ll 0,001$).

Since the gamma model was the recommended method (see above), it has been used as the dependant variable in multiple linear regression. Explicative variables, remaining in this regression were: type of valve, type of treatment (although not significant), body surface, platelet number (3rd month) and leucocyte count (3rd month).

The percentage of accounted variance was 36%; the model was significant ($F_{34}^{7} = 2.74$, $p = 0.05$).

The t-test was significant for leucocyte counts ($t = 2.07$, $p = 0.05$), for body surface ($t = 2.63$, $p = 0.01$), for platelet count ($t = 3.64$, $p = 0.001$).

Conclusion

This study showed that PST's, calculated either with graphical method, or linear exponential model or gamma model, in patients with modern (non thrombotic) cardiac valves were similar. These 3 models used to estimate PST gave results in close agreement. The multiple linear approach showed that several factors do correlate with PST. Thus any study comparing PST from different patients samples should give account for these variables.

REFERENCES

1. The panel on Diagnostic Application of Radioisotopes in Haematology. International Committee for Standardization in Haematology. Recommended methods for radioisotope platelet survival studies. Blood 50:1137, 1977.

2. Schbath J, Boissel JP, Mathy B, Ville D, Benveniste E, Sanchini B, Leizorovicz A, Dechavanne M, Maitre P, Gillet J, Bentamar A, Drugs effect on platelet survival time: comparison of two pyrimido-pyridimine derivatives in patients with aortic or mitral replacement. Submitted for publication, 1983.

3. Kutti J, Weinfeld A, Platelet survival in man. Scand. J. Haemat. 8:336, 1971.

4. Aster RH, Jandl JH, Platelet sequestration in man: I. Methods. J. clin. Invest. 43:843, 1964.

5. Dornhorst AC, The interpretation of red cell survival curves. Blood 6:1284, 1951.

6. Dassin E, Balitrand N, Najean Y, An analysis of the effect of random and ageing mechanisms on the survival of platelets. Biomedicine 25:23, 1976.

7. Najean Y, Dassin E, Renner C, Wacquet M, Cinétique plaquettaire au cours des maladies artérielles. Nouv. Presse Med. 8:3813, 1979.

8. Murphy EA, Francis ME, The estimation of blood platelet survival: II. The multiple hit model. Thrombos. Diathes. haemorrh. Stuttg. 25:53, 1978.

9. Tsukada T, Tango T, On the methods calculating mean survival time in ^{51}Cr-platelet survival study. Amer. J. Haemat. 8:281, 1980.

13 IN VIVO KINETICS OF SIMULTANEOUSLY INJECTED ^{111}IN- AND ^{51}CR-LABELLED HUMAN PLATELETS: ON THE SIGNIFICANCE OF THE PLATELET ISOLATION YIELD FROM BLOOD PRIOR TO LABELLING

K.G. SCHMIDT, J.W. RASMUSSEN, A.D. RASMUSSEN, H. ARENDRUP, M. LORENTZEN

INTRODUCTION

Platelets, which have been isolated from the blood and labelled with a radioactive isotope, most frequently ^{51}Cr or ^{111}In, are normally used for in vivo platelet kinetic studies and it is essential that the labelled platelets represent a cross-section of the blood's platelets. This means that during isolation of the platelets from the blood, platelets having another age composition than those later injected into the recipient must not be lost.

Circulating platelets are heterogenous with regard to size and density (1-4). There is much evidence suggesting that a small fraction of platelets with a very low density are senescent cells, and it is possible that platelet density increases during the life-time of the platelet (2,3,5-7). The results of some investigations, however, do not support this (4,8-11). Although a certain degree of correlation exists between platelet volume and platelet density (3,6,9,12-14), there is some uncertainty as to whether young platelets are larger than old platelets. Some findings support the latter conception (7,15), while others do not (1,4).

The isolation of platelets from the blood for labelling is almost invariably carried out by differential centrifugation. The sedimentation velocity of the platelets during centrifugation at low g-values in low density media (e.g., buffer or plasma) is principally determined by cell size, and to a lesser extent by cell density (16), i.e., a fraction of large cells is likely to be lost during the centrifugation procedure. The purpose of this paper has been to study the significance of this platelet loss, i.e., to throw some light on the relationship between the efficacy of platelet isolation and the results achieved in platelet kinetic studies.

Materials and methods

Patients 38 persons were subjected to platelet kinetic studies. They consisted of 25 healthy volunteers and 13 patients with an implanted artificial aortic valve. All of the subjects studied had a normal platelet count and none had taken drugs known to inhibit platelet function for at least 8 days prior to the investigation. All were instructed to avoid the intake of such agents during the investigation itself. The material was subdivided into 5 groups: Group I consisted of 10 healty subjects (3 females and 7 males) aged 22-60 years, in whom identical platelet suspensions were labelled with ^{111}In and ^{51}Cr. Group L/S comprised 10 healthy subjects (1 female and 9 males) aged 25-55 years, in whom small platelets were labelled with ^{51}Cr and large platelets with ^{111}In (vide infra). Group A consisted of 7 male patients (aged 42-65 years) with an implanted artificial aortic valve, in whom the platelet isolation yields from blood of ^{111}In- and ^{51}Cr-labelled platelets differed less than 15%. Group B comprised 6 male patients with artificial aortic valves aged 25-59 years, in whom the platelet isolation yield of ^{111}In-platelets exceeded that of ^{51}Cr-platelets by more than 15%. Group C consisted of 5 healthy persons (2 females and 3 males) aged 18-42 years, in whom ^{51}Cr-platelets were injected 3 days prior to the injection of ^{111}In-platelets.

Isolation and labelling of platelets

Platelet isolation and labelling with ^{111}In-oxine was carried out as previously described (17,18), with minor modifications of the centrifugation steps as outlined earlier (19). Fig. 1 depicts the platelet isolation procedure, in which a small quantity of erythrocytes serves as a supporting cushion for the platelets during step-wise isolation of these from the blood.

The platelets of group I and C to be labelled with ^{51}Cr were processed as described above (for details see reference 19).

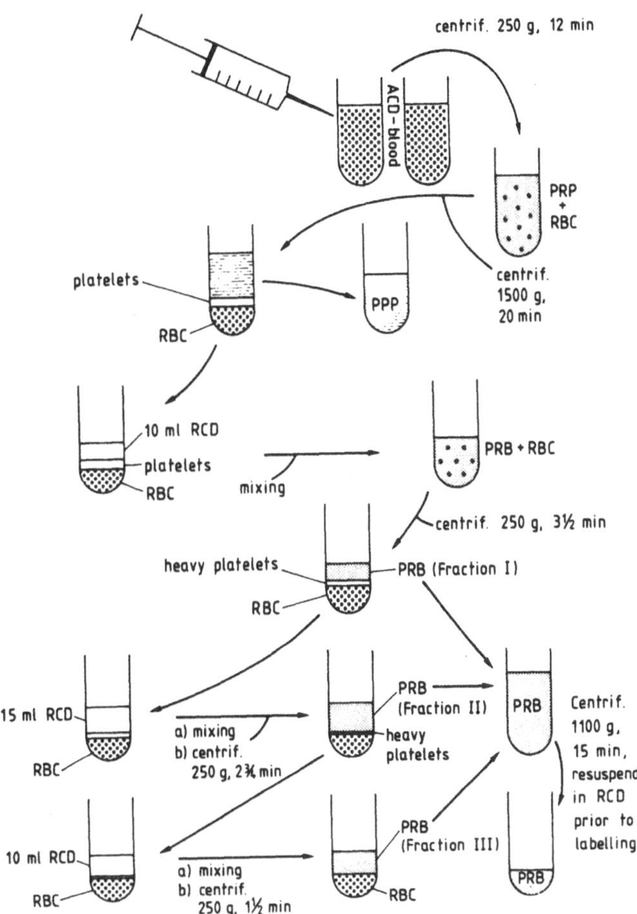

Fig. 1. The method of platelet isolation from blood. Abbreviations: PRP: Platelet-rich plasma; RBC: red blood-cells; RCD: Ringer citrate dextrose buffer; PRB: Platelet-rich buffer. (from ref. 19; with permission).

In groups A and B, ^{51}Cr-labelling of platelets separated from blood by differential centrifugation took place in plasma, as described previously (19).

In groups L/S, the platelets of fraction I (see fig. 1) were labelled with ^{51}Cr (in buffer) and those of fraction II and III were labelled with ^{111}In.

Platelet isolation and labelling was carried out at room temperature under aseptic conditions in a laminar flow hood. The time interval between blood-sampling and injection of the labelled platelets was approximately 4 hours. The volumes of blood drawn were 54-56 ml in group L/S. In the other groups they were 26-28 ml for ^{111}In-labelling and 54-56 ml for ^{51}Cr-labelling.

The platelet isolation yields, the labelling efficiencies, the fractions of platelet- and erythrocyte-bound activities, and the numbers of erythrocytes and leukocytes in the injected platelet suspensions were calculated as previously described (19).

Supplementary in vitro studies

The ^{111}In and ^{51}Cr-labelled platelets of group L/S were subjected to ultrastructural morphometric analysis. The relative platelet volumes were estimated by quotients of platelet areas and micrograph areas by linear analysis (20) of randomly photographed platelets at a final magnification of 19.200 x. 7 Micrographs from each specimen were studied. In 5 of these cases the mean platelet volumes (MPV) were also measured electronically with a Coulter Counter (R), model S-Plus II (21). MPV-determinations on fractions I, II and III were repeated 4 hours to 5 days later.

In 4 cases, labelled platelets of fraction I and fraction II and III from healthy individuals (^{111}In-labelling in 2 cases, ^{51}Cr-labelling in the other 2), suspended in ACD-platelet-poor plasma (PPP), were subjected to centrifugation on a discontinuous gradient of Percoll (R) (22). From a 90% stock solution of Percoll, iso-osmolar suspensions of Percoll at densities of 1.080, 1.066 and 1.046 g/ml were prepared by dilution with Ringer-Citrate-Dextrose buffer, and the pH adjusted to 7.0

1.5 ml of the Percoll suspensions were layered in a 12 ml polycarbonate centrifuge tube. 1 ml portions of the labelled platelets were layered on the gradients, which were centrifuged at 2000 g for 30 min at room temperature in a Heraeus Christ Makrofuge 6-4, fitted with a swing-out rotor.

We isolated fraction I and fraction II and III platelets from 5 healthy donors with the intention of comparing the efficiency of labelling of larger and smaller platelets. The platelet concentrations in these 2 fractions were adjusted to identical levels, and the platelets labelled with ^{111}In and ^{51}Cr at two platelet concentration levels.

Platelet kinetic studies

The labelled platelet suspensions were injected intravenously in succession through a 19 or 21 gauge butterfly needle; the interval between the injection of ^{111}In-platelets (always injected first) and that of the ^{51}Cr-platelets being approximately 20 sec).

Doses: ^{111}In: mean 232 µCi, range 163-340 µCi; ^{51}Cr: mean 27 µCi, range 10-70 µCi.

Blood-sampling and counting of the radioactivity of the blood-samples was carried out as previously described (19).

Calculation of the platelet mean life time (MLT) and in vivo recovery (IVR) were based on the multiple hit model (23,24), as previously described (19).

In the 10 subjects of group L/S, in whom the platelets of fraction I were labelled with ^{51}Cr and those of fraction II and III with ^{111}In, platelets were isolated 2-10 min post-injection (p.i.), according to the method depicted in fig. 1. The platelet numbers and both platelet-bound activities of fraction I and fraction II and III were calculated and the distribution of these labelled platelets expressed as the ratio fraction I/fraction II and III. In 7 cases this procedure was repeated 4-7 days later. The same procedure was carried out in the 5 subjects in group C the day following the injection of ^{111}In-platelets (corresponding to 4 days after the injection of ^{51}Cr-platelets).

In 5 cases in group L/S, lymphocytes were isolated from 3 min to 6 days p.i., according to the Ficoll-Hypaque $^{(R)}$ method (25). Contaminating platelets were removed by 3 consecutive centrifugations at 200 g for 6 min and the cells were washed in physiological saline. Activity corresponding to the residual platelets (if any) was corrected for.

Results

In vitro studies Fraction I and fraction II and III platelets were prepared from 5 healthy donors. The total platelet isolation yield averaged 74%; the platelets of fraction I represented, on average, 42% of the blood's platelets, those of fraction II and III 32%. The platelets were labelled at 2 concentration levels, averaging $570 \times 10^9/l$ and $285 \times 10^9/l$. Labelling efficiencies: at the high concentration level: ^{111}In: $\bar{x}$ = 82.2% and 82.9% (fraction I and fraction II and III, respectively); ^{51}Cr: $\bar{x}$ = 20.9% and 20.1%. At the low concentration level: ^{111}In: $\bar{x}$ = 68.4% and 71.5%; ^{51}Cr: 15.1% and 13.9%.

In the density gradient experiments the platelets sedimented in 3 distinct bands. By far the largest band was seen between the layers of densities 1.046 and 1.066 g/ml (b-2). Narrow bands were found above the 1.046 layer (b-1) and between the layers 1.066 and 1.080 (b-3). On average, 94.3% (range 91.8-98.0%) of the platelets applied to the 8 gradients were harvested by careful aspiration with a Mantoux syringe equipped with a flat-tipped 21 gauge needle. Percentage of harvested platelets found in b-1: fraction I-platelets: $\bar{x}$ = 3.4% (range 2.6-4.8%); fraction II and III-platelets: $\bar{x}$ = 1.3% (range 0.6-2.2%. Percentage in b-2: fraction I-platelets: $\bar{x}$ = 89.4% (range 85.5-92.4%) fraction II and III-platelets: $\bar{x}$ = 88.9% (range 87.6-90.8%). Percentage in b-3: fraction I-platelets: $\bar{x}$ = 7.3% (range 3.6-11.6%): fraction II and III-platelets: $\bar{x}$ = 9.8% (range 8.2-11.8%). The ratios between platelet-bound activities in b-1 and b-3: fraction I-platelets: 0.25, 0.27, 1.33 and 0.69. The corresponding ratios of fraction II and III-platelets were 0.05, 0.12, 0.23 and 0.14, thus distinctly lower than the ratios of fraction I-platelets. These results indicate that the most dense platelet fraction (b-3) was enriched with platelets from fraction II and III, and the least dense fraction (b-1) was enriched with platelets from fraction I.

Characterization of the injected platelet suspensions

The platelet isolation yields in the various groups were as follows: group I: $\bar{x}$ = 77% (range 64-93%). Group L/S: ^{111}In-platelets: $\bar{x}$ = 34% (range 24-52%); ^{51}Cr-platelets: $\bar{x}$ = 36% (range 26-46%); total: $\bar{x}$ = 70% (range 62-85%). Group A: ^{111}In-platelets: $\bar{x}$ = 73% (range 49-96%); ^{51}Cr-platelets: $\bar{x}$ = 66% (range 35-92%); mean difference between ^{111}In- and ^{51}Cr-platelets: 11% (range 6-14%)(in 2 cases the isolation yield of ^{51}Cr-platelets was superior to that of ^{111}In-platelets). Group B: ^{111}In-platelets: $\bar{x}$ = 94% (range 90-100%); ^{51}Cr-platelets: $\bar{x}$ = 66% (range 38-77%); mean difference between ^{111}In- and ^{51}Cr-platelets: 28% (range 18-52%);. Group C: ^{111}In-platelets: $\bar{x}$ = 81% (range 68-99%); ^{51}Cr-platelets: $\bar{x}$ = 76% (range 65-85%).

The labelling efficiencies averaged 86% (range 82-89%) for ^{111}In-platelets and 18% (range 13-26%) for ^{51}Cr-platelets in group L/S. In the remaining groups the corresponding values were: ^{111}In-platelets: $\bar{x}$ = 90% (range 82-96%, ^{51}Cr-platelets: $\bar{x}$ = 17% (range 9-29%).

The numbers of erythrocytes and leukocytes per 1000 platelets in the injected platelet suspensions were: group L/S: erythrocytes: ^{111}In-platelets (corresponding to fraction II and III): $\bar{x}$ = 2.0 (range 0.8-3.1), ^{51}Cr-platelets (corresponding to fraction I): $\bar{x}$ = 0.5 (range 0-1.2); leukocytes: ^{111}In-platelets: $\bar{x}$ = 0.6 (range 0-1.4), ^{51}Cr-platelets: $\bar{x}$ = 0.3 (range 0-1.5). In the groups I, A, B and C the corresponding values were: ^{111}In-platelets: $\bar{x}$ = 1.6 (range 0-6.3) for erythrocytes, and $\bar{x}$ = 0.6 (range 0-2.9) for leukocytes; ^{51}Cr-platelets: $\bar{x}$ = 0.9 (range 0-2.5) and $\bar{x}$ = 0.3 (range 0-2.9) (erythrocytes and leukocytes, respectively).

The fraction of platelet-bound ^{111}In-activity in the injected suspensions (all groups) averaged 98% (range 97-99%), that of platelet-bound ^{51}Cr-activity averaged 93% (range 87-97%). Erythrocyte-bound ^{111}In-activity was seen in 1 case in the L/S group (being 0.9%), and in one of the remaining 28 cases (being 2.0%). Erythrocyte-bound ^{51}Cr-activity was seen in 3 cases in the L/S group (1.1, 0.5 and 0.4%) and in 14 of the remaining 28 cases

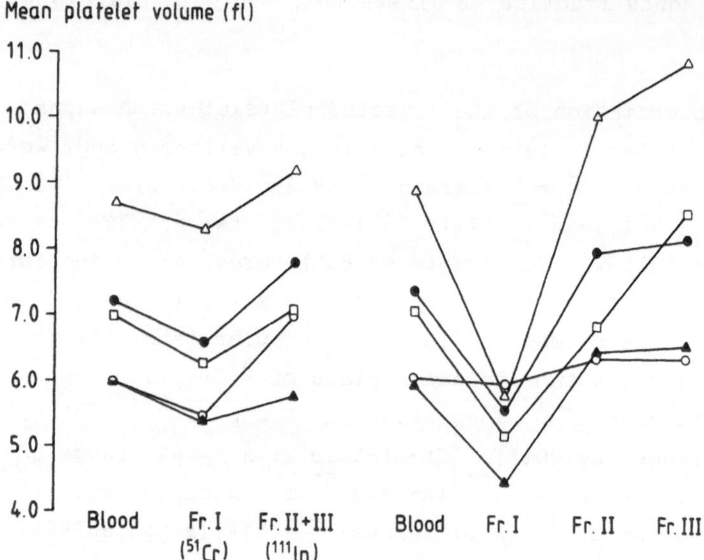

Fig. 2a. Left: Mean platelet volumes (MPV) from 5 subjects in group L/S (ACD-anticoagulated blood, ^{51}Cr-labelled fraction I-platelets, and ^{111}In-labelled fraction II and III-platelets). Right: MPV of ACD-blood and platelet fractions I, II and III isolated from the same subjects 4 hours to 5 days later.

($\bar{x}$ = 1.2%, (range 0-4.0%).

Morphometric analysis of the platelet volumes in group L/S revealed a difference between the ^{111}In-platelets of fraction II and III and the ^{51}Cr-platelets of fraction I. Relative volumes of ^{111}In- and ^{51}Cr-platelets averaged 0.487 and 0.452, respectively; this difference is significant ($0.01 < p < 0.02$, two-tailed paired t-test). The same conclusion holds for the electronically determined mean platelet volume. Fig. 2a shows the results of MPV determinations in 5 subjects from group L/S. The left part of this figure depicts MPV values of ACD-blood, ^{51}Cr-labelled fraction I-platelets and ^{111}In-labelled fraction II and III-platelets. Fraction I-platelets were smaller than fraction II and III-platelets throughout. The right part of the figure shows the results of repeatedly performed MPV determinations on platelet fraction (I,II and III), isolated from 4 hours to 5 days later. A similar pattern is seen, i.e., the platelets of fraction I are smaller than those of fraction II and fraction

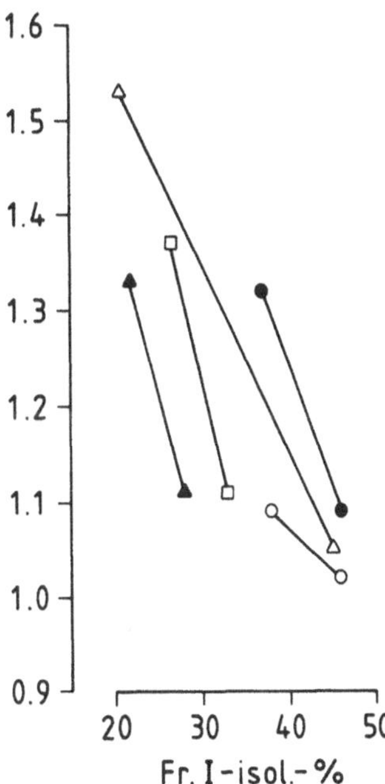

Fig. 2b. Corresponding values of isolation yield of platelets in fraction I, and the ratio between MPV in blood and fraction I.

III. The smaller volumes of fraction I-platelets in these experiments may be explained by the lower isolation yields of fraction I-platelets in comparison to the experiments of the left part of the figure (2a). Fig. 2b shows the corresponding values of blood/fraction I-MPV ratio and yield of platelets in fraction I. It can be seen that isolation of a low fraction of platelets in fraction I corresponds to a low MPV.

In vivo platelet kinetics

The results of the comparative in vivo kinetic studies in groups I, A, L/S and B are summarized in table 1. When identical platelet suspensions are labelled (group I), the platelet MLT of ^{51}Cr-platelets surpassed that of ^{111}In-platelets. In contrast, the IVR of ^{111}In-platelets was higher than that of ^{51}Cr-platelets. This difference also applies to group A in which the isolation yields of ^{111}In- and ^{51}Cr-platelets were

Table 1. Platelet mean life time (MLT) and in vivo recovery (IVR of ^{111}In- and ^{51}Cr-labelled platelets in the groups studied (see under Material and Methods). Mean value and standard errors of the means are shown. p-values refer to two-tailed t-tests.

		Group I (n=10)		Group A (n=7)		Group I+Group A (n=17)		Group L/S (n=10)		Group B (n=6)		Group L/S+Group B (n=16)	
		^{111}In	^{51}Cr	^{111}In	^{51}Cr	^{111}In	^{51}Cr	^{111}In	^{51}Cr	^{111}In	^{51}Cr	^{111}In	^{51}Cr
MLT	$\bar{x}$	182.1	189.9**	180.8	187.2	181.6	188.8***	185.1	183.9	194.4	193.1	188.6	187.3
	SE	7.6	7.2	7.7	5.4	5.4	4.7	9.9	10.0	9.2	9.3	7.0	7.0
IVR	$\bar{x}$	57.3*	55.0	64.8**	59.3	60.4***	56.8	52.5	53.4	54.2	52.0	53.1	52.9
	SE	3.6	3.4	4.5	4.9	2.9	2.8	2.8	3.2	3.1	2.1	2.0	2.1

* $0.005 < p < 0.01$

** $0.001 < p < 0.005$

*** $p < 0.001$

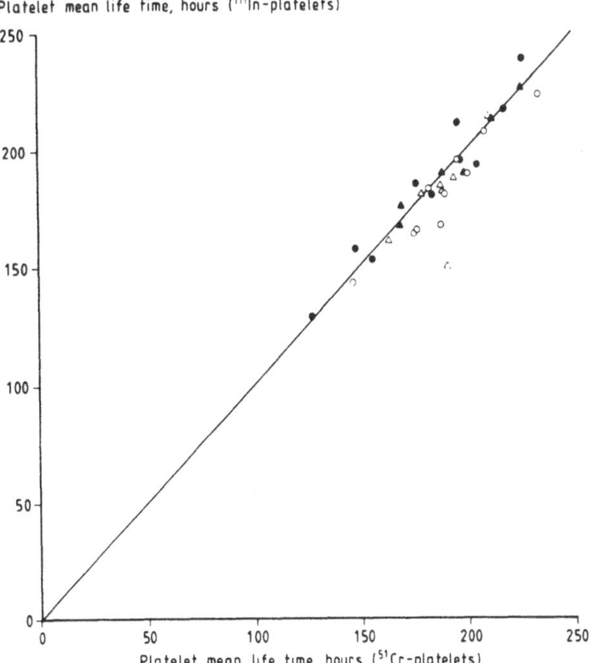

Fig. 3. Corresponding mean life time values of ^{51}Cr and ^{111}In-labelled platelets in group I, L/S, A and B (multiple hit model). The line of identity is shown. Symbols: o: identical platelet populations labelled with ^{51}Cr and ^{111}In (group I). ●: fraction I-platelets ("small platelets") labelled with ^{51}Cr; fraction II and III-platelets ("large platelets") labelled with ^{111}In (group L/S). △ :group A (platelet isolation yields of ^{111}In- and ^{51}Cr-labelled platelets differing less than 15%). ▲: group B (platelet isolation yields of ^{111}In-platelets exceeding those of ^{51}Cr-platelets by more than 15%).

almost identical. Comparison of the kinetics of ^{111}In- and ^{51}Cr-platelets from groups L/S and B revealed no differences in MLT or IVR.

Detailed presentation of the results of MLT and IVR determinations are given in figs. 3 and 4, which depict corresponding MLT and IVR values for ^{111}In- and ^{51}Cr platelets in the above mentioned four groups. It should be noted that the MLT was rather low (about 128h) in 1 subject belonging to group L/S. This might be ascribed to a hepatic disease, diagnosed after termination of the platelet kinetic study. The MLT and values of group L/S seemed to be unaffected by the isolation yield of fraction I-platelets, but it is difficult to draw

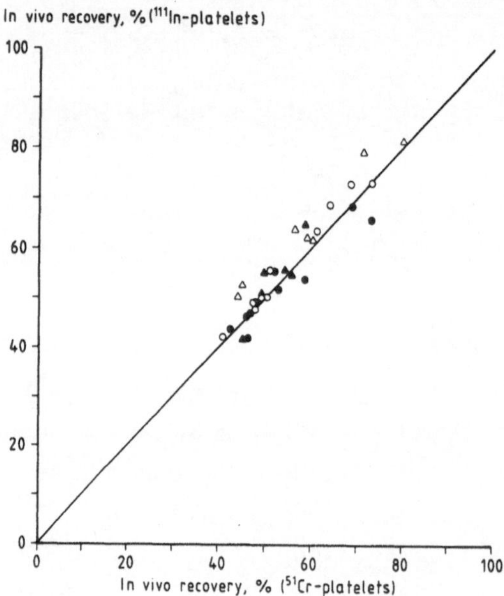

Fig. 4. Corresponding in vivo recovery values of ^{51}Cr- and ^{111}In-labelled platelets in groups I, L/S, A and B (multiple hit model). The line of identity is shown. Same symbols as in fig. 3.

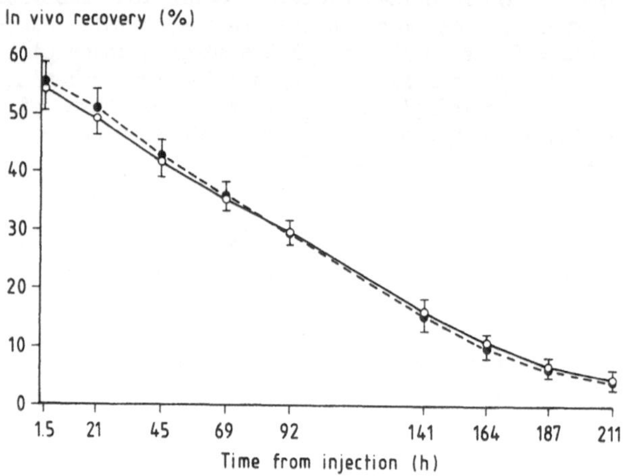

Fig. 5a. Platelet survival curves of ^{51}Cr-labelled (open symbols) and ^{111}In-labelled (filled symbols) platelets in group I (identical platelet populations labelled with ^{51}Cr and ^{111}In. Mean values and standard deviations of the means are shown.

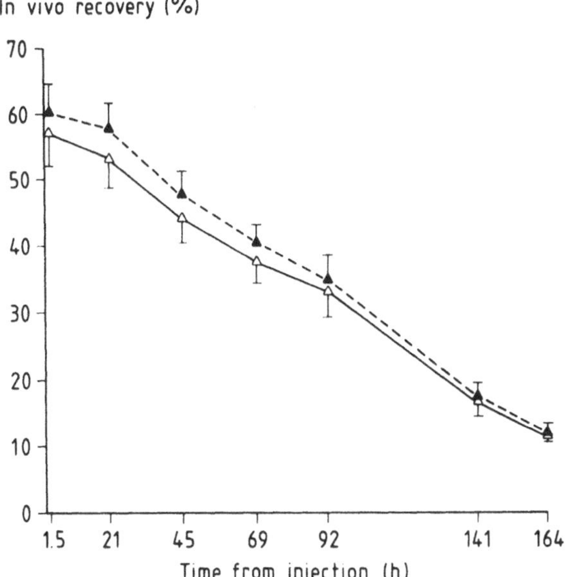

Fig. 5b. Platelet survival curves of ^{51}Cr-labelled (open symbols) and ^{111}In-labelled (filled symbols) platelets in group A (< 15% difference in platelet isolation yields). Mean values and standard errors of the means are shown.

conclusions regarding this matter because of the small dispersion around the mean value of this yield.

In order to determine further what differences in survival pattern are responsible for the observed differences in MLT and IVR in groups I and A, their in vivo recovery values from 90 min to 211 hours p.i. were calculated and the "mean survival curves" constructed (figs 5a and 5b). It may be seen that the ^{111}In-activity lies initially slightly higher as well as terminally slightly lower than of ^{51}Cr-activity, which can explain the slightly steeper course of the ^{111}In-curve and with this the differences in MLT and IVR. The corresponding curves of groups L/S and B (figs 6a and 6b) show these differences in survival pattern to be eliminated when ^{111}In-platelets were larger (and maybe denser) or were more representative of the total platelet population than were ^{51}Cr-platelets.

The precision of the multiple hit model was assessed by

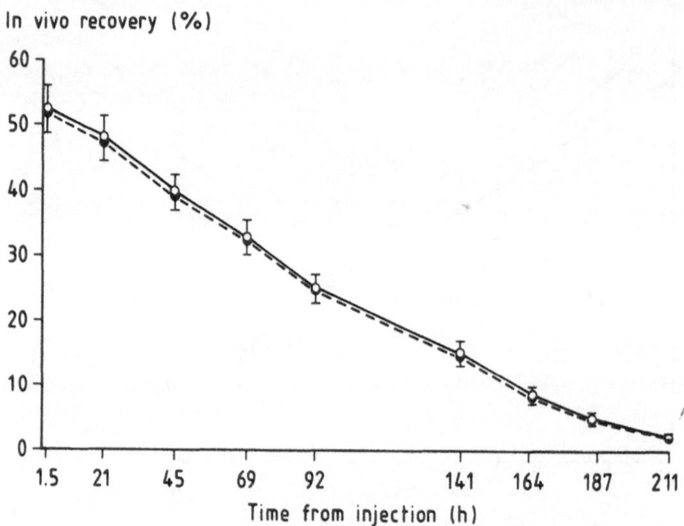

Fig. 6a. Platelet survival curves of ^{51}Cr-labelled (open symbols) and ^{111}In-labelled (filled symbols) platelets in group L/S (^{51}Cr-labelled fraction I-platelets and ^{111}In-labelled fraction II and III-platelets). Mean values and standard errors of the means are shown.

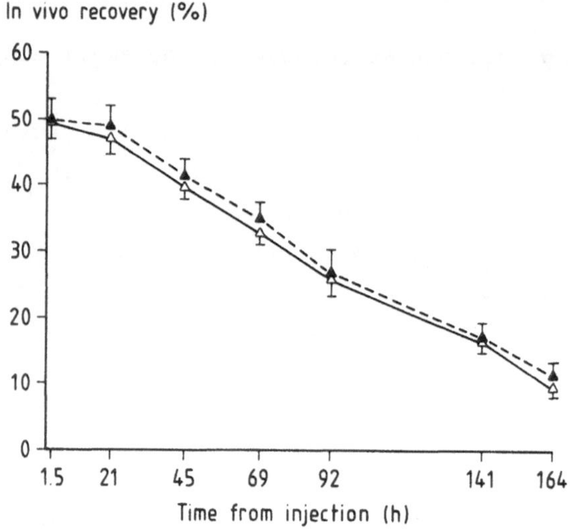

Fig. 6b. Platelet survival curves of ^{51}Cr-labelled (open symbols) and ^{111}In-labelled (filled symbols) platelets in group B (>15% difference in platelet population yields). Mean values and standard errors of the means are shown.

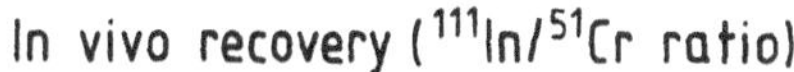

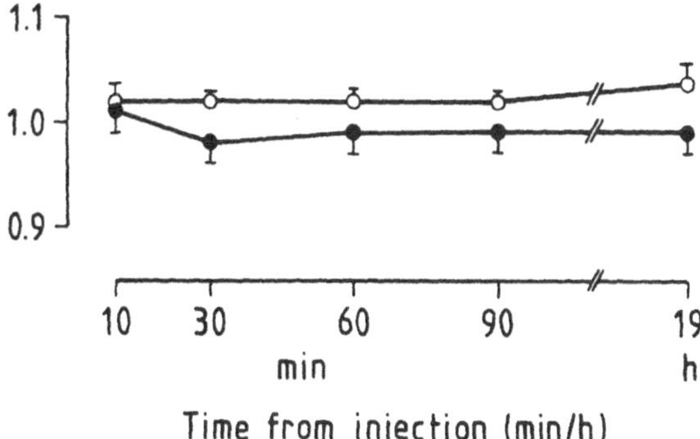

Fig. 7. ^{111}In/^{51}Cr-activity ratios in the early post-injection period of group I (open symbols) and group L/S (closed symbols).

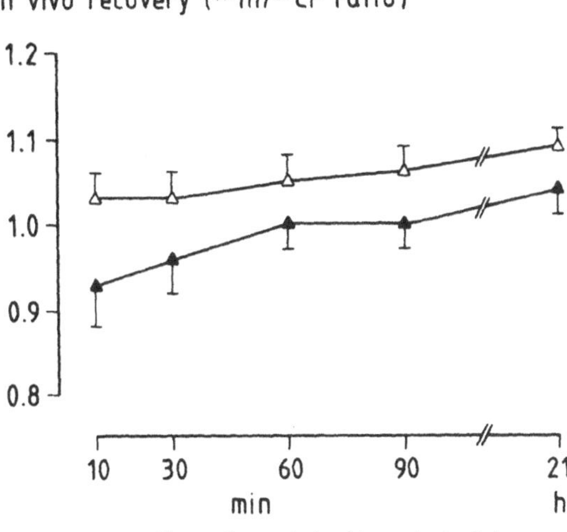

Fig. 8. ^{111}In/^{51}Cr activity ratios in the early post-injection period of group A (open symbols) and group B (closed symbols).

calculation of the residual sum of squares (RSS) (26). In all cases this model fitted the data better than the linear and exponential models. Except for 1 case (a healthy woman aged 22, in group I, the linear model fitted the data better than did the exponential model. No differences in RSS (all 3 models tested) were seen between ^{111}In- and ^{51}Cr-platelets in any of

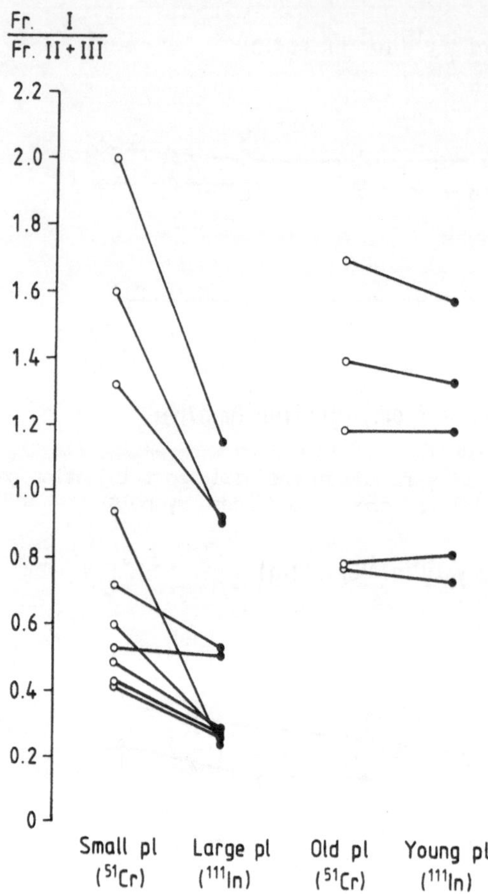

Fig. 9. Results of platelet isolation experiments carried out 3-10 min. post-injection in group L/S. Corresponding fraction I/II and III ratios of ^{51}Cr-labelled ("small") and ^{111}In-labelled ("large") platelets are shown. Right: Results of platelet isolation experiments in group C ^{51}Cr-labelled platelets injected 3 days prior to ^{111}In-labelled platelets. Corresponding fraction I/II and III ratios of ^{51}Cr-labelled and ^{111}In-labelled platelets (platelet isolation experiments performed 1 day after injection of ^{111}In-platelets).

the groups, and no difference in the number of hits (multiple hit model) was seen either.

The course of activity during the early post-injection period

The course of activity within the first 19-21 hours of the

injection, corresponding to ^{111}In- and ^{51}Cr-platelets of groups I and L/S, and of groups A and B are shown in figs 7 and 8, respectively. The courses are expressed as ^{111}In/^{51}Cr-activity ratios. The ratios of group I were found to be higher than those of group L/S ($p < 0.005$), and those of group A to be higher than group B ($p < 0.005$), by applying two-way analysis of variance (27). When platelets of fractions II and III or platelets being representative of the blood's platelet population were injected, the circulating platelet-bound activity was thus lower than that of fraction I-platelets or of a platelet population lacking in a percentage of large platelets.

In order to study the reproducibility of the platelet isolation procedure, platelets were isolated from ACD-anticoagulated blood drawn from 3 to 10 min p.i. of ^{111}In-labelled fraction II and III-platelets in the 10 subjects of group L/S. It can be seen (left part of fig 9) that the partition of the labelled platelets in the platelet fractions I and II and III, ex vivo, corresponds rather well to that occurring prior to injection, i.e. the ratio fraction I / fractions II and III was higher for ^{51}Cr-labelled ("small") platelets than for ^{111}In-labelled ("large") platelets. In 8 cases this experiment was repeated from 4 to 7 days p.i. The ratios between the ^{111}In-fraction I/ fraction II and III ratios and the ^{51}Cr-fraction I/fraction II and III ratios were calculated. Almost identical ratios were thus found (3-10 min p.i.: $\bar{x} = 0.57$, SE = 0.05; 4-7 days p.i.: $\bar{x} = 0.62$, SE = 0.08). The isolation yield in these 18 experiments averaged 76.0% (range 63.2-99%). Platelet isolation yields 3-10 min p.i. (n=10): fraction I: $\bar{x} = 31.9\%$, SE = 3.6; fractions II and III: $\bar{x} = 42.6\%$, SE = 2.5. Platelet isolation yields 4-7 days p.i. (n=8): fraction I: $\bar{x} = 36.3\%$, SE = 4.7; fractions II and III: $\bar{x} = 41.6\%$, SE = 2.7.

The right part of fig 9 shows the results of platelet isolation experiments in the 5 subjects of group C. ^{51}Cr-labelled platelets had been injected 4 days and ^{111}In-platelets 1 day prior to this platelet isolation experiment. It can be seen that almost identical fraction I/fraction II and III ratios were observed, thus indicating that platelet age does not influence the platelet partition pattern. Fraction I constituted, on average, 45% (range 37-54%), and fractions II and III 38% (range 27-43% of the blood's platelets in these 5 experiments.

The lymphocyte isolation experiments in group L/S revealed a slight degree of lymphocyte labelling. Expressed as a percentage of platelet-bound activity, the lymphocyte-bound ^{111}In-activity averaged 0.8% (range 0.2-1.1%) and the lymphocyte-bound ^{51}Cr-activity averaged 0.5% (range 0-1.1%) in the 5 subjects studied.

Discussion

As earlier demonstrated (19) in studies of a larger patient material, we have found in the present investigation evidence to the effect that after simultaneous injection of identical platelet populations labelled with ^{111}In and ^{51}Cr, there is a higher in vivo recovery (IVR) and shorter mean life time (MLT) of ^{111}In-labelled than of ^{51}Cr-labelled platelets. The reasons for these differences are not known. The lower ^{51}Cr-level initially can perhaps be attributed to elution of ^{51}Cr-activity from the platelets, and the higher ^{51}Cr-level terminally can possibly be caused by stronger labelling of younger than older platelets (28). The differences in the survival pattern of the other platelet populations investigated must be viewed in the light of the above mentioned differences. Thus, we have shown that when larger and smaller platelets are labelled with respectively ^{111}In and ^{51}Cr and injected simultaneously, the differences in IVR and MLT are eliminated, i.e., the results indicate that large platelets have a lower IVR and longer MLT than smaller platelets. The difference in IVR can be most clearly seen within the first 19-21 hours after the injection. Irrespective of whether it is larger platelets or a total platelet population which are compared with respectively small platelets or platelets lacking in a percentage of large platelets, the IVR was found to lie lower with regard to the former.

With the described centrifugation method for step-wise isolation of platelets from the blood, there is no doubt that the platelets first harvested are smaller than those obtained at the end of the procedure. The results of density gradient experiments indicate that there is a correlation between platelet size and platelet density, when the platelets are isolated from the blood in the manner described. Such a relationship has also been described previously (3,6,9,12-14).

The results of Mezzano et al (29) are contrary to our own findings. They were unable to demonstrate any difference in platelet volume (or density) between total populations and platelets isolated by a single centrifugation step, and containing an average of 74% of the total platelet population. It is logical to expect preferential sedimentation of large platelets under the described conditions of centrifugation (16). Others (14,30) have also observed that the platelets lost during differential centrifugation are larger than the platelets contained in platelet-rich plasma. Neither did Mezzano et al (29) find any difference in MLT or IVR between the above mentioned 2 platelet populations in a sequential study of 4 healthy subjects. In a study published earlier by the same group (4), no difference was found in IVR when large-dense and small-light platelets from 4 healthy subjects were compared in a similar manner. The MLT of small-light platelets was found to be longer than that of large-dense platelets. In a sequential study of 3 rhesus monkeys, Corash et al (2) found the same IVR for both dense and light platelets, isolated by isopycnic centrifugation. In that study the MLT of dense platelets surpassed that of the light platelets.

In order to achieve pure platelet suspensions without contamination by leukocytes and erythrocytes, we were reticent to harvest platelets close to the buffy-coat layer. The slight contamination of the injected platelet suspensions by these cells and the results of the activity measurements on them show that the platelet suspensions were of acceptable purity. We did not carry out cross experiments involving ^{51}Cr-labelling of platelets from fractions II and III, due to the risk involved of contamination by ^{51}Cr-labelled erythrocytes (a problem that becomes negligible when ^{111}In is used for platelet labelling (18)).

There is no agreement as to whether dense platelets are younger than light ones, or as to whether large platelets are younger than small ones. Many studies relating to this subject have been carried out on animals under stress conditions with stimulated thrombopoiesis, and the results may not be relevant to the situation in the healthy human organism. Several different methods have been used for platelet separation from blood. Experiments with isopycnic centrifugation of rhesus monkey or rabbit platelets and extrinsic (population) labelling with ^{51}Cr support the concept that dense platelets are younger than light platelets, and that platelets loose weight during ageing in the circulation (2,5). These findings are supported by the results of intrinsic (cohort) labelling experiments (3,6,7,13), even if the mapping of the platelet density distribution was carried out using a velocity sedimentation method (7). Other studies do not support the concept that dense platelets are younger than light ones (4,8-11), and the whole subject appears to be rather confused.

Whether or not larger platelets are younger than small platelets is unknown, but some evidence suggests that they are not (1.4). One of the problems is that due to the correlation between size and density it can be difficult to stratify platelets experimentally in respect of these properties.

With regard to the centrifugation methods, irrespective of whether it applies to velocity sedimentation or isopycnic sedimentation, standardization is difficult, and it is often arduous to compare the results of various investigators, due to the uncertainty of whether the platelet sedimentation has been carried out according to the size or density (or both).

Our findings regarding IVR are compatible with the concept that the spleen preferentially sequestrates large platelets (31). Whether or not our MLT findings can be accepted as supporting the idea that large platelets live longer than the smaller ones is uncertain. The results of our studies with platelet isolation after staggered injections of ^{51}Cr- and ^{111}In-labelled platelets do not suggest that the age of the platelets is a determinant in respect of their distribution in fractions I and II and III. The observed tendency to a longer life time of large platelets as compared to the small could be a consequence of the difference in IVR, in other words, sequestration of large platelets in the spleen could provide protection against trauma which would occur in the circulation. Such a transient sequestration with subsequent release of large (and dense?) platelets may perhaps explain the observations of other investigators of a transient increase in the number of labelled dense platelets in the circulation after injection of ^{51}Cr-labelled platelets (4), as well as the finding of a delay in the malondialdehyde reappearance in dense platelets after aspirin ingestion (11). The results of our in vitro experiments with the simultaneous labelling of platelets in fraction I and fractions II and III suggest that the tendency to the in vivo activity of the latter fraction being higher terminally is not due to stronger labelling of this fraction.

In conclusion, it may be said that with the described centrifugation method for step-wise isolation of platelets from the blood, small platelets are harvested first and larger platelets last. The recovery of larger platelets in vivo is lower than that of the smaller platelets, presumably due to preferential sequestration of large platelets in the spleen. This phenomenon is probably the explanation of the tendency for larger platelets to live longer than the small platelets rather than this difference being dependent on an actual difference in age between large and small platelets.

Acknowledgement

This study was supported by grants from Fonden for Laegevidenskablig Forskning m.v. ved Fyns Amts Sygehusvaesen.

The authors are grateful to Dorrit Østergaard Nielsen, Kirsten Thaisen and Mette Clausen for skilful technical assistance during platelet isolation and labelling, and to Kirsten Hansen for valuable help in processing specimens for electron microscopy.

REFERENCES

1. Paulus JM, Platelet size in man. Blood 46:321, 1975.

2. Corash L, Shafer B, Perlow M, Heterogeneity of human whole blood-platelet subpopulations. II. Use of a subhuman primate model to analyze the relationship between density and platelet age. Blood 52:726, 1978.

3. Rand ML, Greenberg JP, Packham MA, Mustard JR, Density subpopulations of rabbit platelets: size, protein, and sialic acid content, and specific radioactivity changes following labeling with ^{35}S-sulfate in vivo. Blood 57:741, 1981.

4. Mezzano D, Hwang KI, Catalano P, Aster RH, Evidence that platelet buoyant density, but not size, correlates with platelet age in man. Amer. J. Hemat. 11:61, 1981.

5. Corash L, Shafer B, Use of asplenic rabbits to demonstrate that platelet age and density are related. Blood 60:166, 1982.

6. Charmatz A, Karpatkin S, Heterogeneity of rabbit platelets. I. Employment of an albumin density gradient for separation of a young platelet population identified with Se^{75}-selenomethionine. Thrombos. Diathes. haemorrh. Stuttg. 31:485, 1974.

7. Karpatkin S. Heterogeneity of rabbit platelets. VI. Further resolution of changes in platelet density, volume, and radioactivity following cohort labelling with ^{75}Se-selenomethionine. Brit. J. Haemat. 39:459, 1978.

8. Busch C, Olson PS, Density distribution of ^{51}Cr-labelled platelets within the circulating dog platelet population. Thromb. Res. 3:1, 1973.

9. Penington DG, Lee NLY, Roxburgh AE, McCready JR, Platelet density and size: The interpretation of heterogeneity. Brit. J. Haemat. 34:365, 1976.

10. Mishory B, Danon D, Structural aspects of in vivo aging rabbit blood platelets. Thromb. Res. 12:893, 1978.

11. Boneu B, Sie P, Caranobe C, Nouvel C, Bierme R, Malondialdehyde (MDA) re-appearence in human platelet density subpopulations after a single intake of aspirin. Thromb. Res. 19:609, 1980.

12. Karpatkin S, Charmatz A, Heterogeneity of human platelets. I. Metabolic and kinetic evidence suggestive of young and old platelets. J. clin. Invest. 48:1073, 1969.

13. Amorosi E, Garg SK, Karpatkin S, Heterogeneity of human platelets. IV. Identification of a young platelet population with ^{75}Se-selenomethionine. Brit. J. Haemat. 21:227, 1971.

14. Corash L, Tan H, Gralnick HR, Shafer B, Heterogeneity of human whole blood platelet subpopulations. I. Relationship between buoyant density, cell volume, and ultrastructure. Blood 49:71, 1977.

15. Blajchman MA, Senyi AF, Hirsh J, Genton E, George JN, Hemostatic function, survival, and membrane glycoprotein changes in young versus old rabbit platelets. J. clin. Invest. 68:1289, 1981.

16. De Duve C, Berthet J, Beaufay H, Gradient centrifugation of cell particles. Theory and applications. Prog. Biophys. Biophysic. Chem. 9:325, 1959.

17. Schmidt KG, Rasmussen JW, Preparation of platelet suspensions from whole blood in buffer. Description of a method which gives a large platelet yield. Scand. J. Haemat. 23:88, 1979.

18. Schmidt KG, Rasmussen JW, Labelling of human and rabbit platelets with ^{111}Indium-oxine complex. Scand. J. Haemat. 23:97, 1979.

19. Schmidt KG, Rasmussen JW, Rasmussen AD, Arendrup H, Comparative studies of the in vivo kinetics of simultaneously injected ^{111}In- and ^{51}Cr-labelled human platelets. Scand. J. Haemat. 1983 (submitted for publication).

20. Williams MA, Quantitative methods in biology. In: Practical methods in electron microscopy. Glauert AM (ed), Elsevier/North-Holland Biomedical Press, Amsterdam Vol. 6, 5:84, 1977.

21. Bessman JD, Williams LJ, Gilmer PR Jr, Platelet size in health and hematologic disease. Amer. J. Clin. Path. 78:150, 1981.

22. Pertoft H, Laurent TC, Låås T, Kågedal L, Density gradients prepared from colloidal silicia particles coated by polyvinylpyrrolidone (Percoll). An. Biochem. 88:271, 1978.

23. Murphy EA, Francis ME, The estimation of blood-platelet survival. II. The multiple hit model. Thrombos. Diathes. haemorrh. 25:53, 1971.

24. Scheffel U, McIntyre PA, Evatt B, Dvornicky Ja Jr, Natarajan TK, Bolling DR, Murphy EA, Evaluation of Indium-111 as a new high photon yield gamma-emitting "physiological" platelet label. Johns Hopk. Med. J. 140-285, 1977.

25. Böyum A, Isolation of mononuclear cells and granulocytes from human blood. Scand. J. Clin. Lab. Invest.21:77, 1968 (suppl. 97).

26. Scheffel U, Tsan MF, Mitchell TG, Camargo EE, Braine H, Ezekowitz MD, Nickoloff L, Hill-Zobel R, Murphy E, McIntyre PA, Human platelets labeled with In-111 8-hydroxyquinoline: Kinetics, distribution, and estimates of radiation dose. J. nucl. Med. 23:149, 1982.

27. Wallenstein S, Zucker CL, Fleiss JL, Some statistical methods useful in circulation research. Circ. Res. 47:1, 1980.

28. Tsukada T, Steiner M, Baldini MG, Chromium^{51} uptake as a function of platelet age. Scand. J. Haemat. 8:270, 1971.

29. Mezzano D, Hwang K, Aster RH, Characteristics of total platelet populations and of platelets isolated in platelet-rich plasma. Transfusion 22:197, 1982.

30. Karpatkin S, Khan Q, Freedman M, Heterogeneity of platelet function. Correlation with platelet volume. Amer. J. Med. 64:542, 1978.

31. Freedman ML, Karpatkin S, Heterogeneity of rabbit platelets. V. Preferential splenic sequestration of megathrombocytes. Brit. J. Haemat. 31:255, 1975.

14
^{111}In-OXINE LABELLED PLATELETS AND HOMOLOGOUS ^{51}CR LABELLED PLATELETS SIMULTANEOUS KINETICS AND EXTERNAL COUNTINGS OF AUTOLOGOUS

N. VIGNERON, Y. NAJEAN

The labelling of platelets with ^{111}In-oxinate was first introduced for imaging procedures. Autologous platelets labelled with this pure γ-emitting agent could be suitable for location of vascular thrombi in humans (1,2). Moreover, ^{111}In-oxinate presents clear advantages over currently used sodium (^{51}Cr)-chromate for platelet kinetic studies.

Up to now, it was well established that autologous plasma seems to be the best medium for suspension of platelets during in vitro handling (3-5). In spite of the high affinity of Transferrin for Indium (6), labelling of platelets in plasma medium keeps them functionally normal as judged by in vitro aggregation tests and in vivo initial recovery and platelet life span. The low rate of labelling related to the Transferrin interference in plasma medium is not affected by the platelet count and this allows us the kinetic study of autologous platelets in severe thrombocytopenia (up to 10.10^9 platelets per 1).

In cases of thrombocytopenia of obscure origin, simultaneous kinetic study of autologous (^{111}In)-platelets and homologous (^{51}Cr)-platelets can reveal a corpuscular abnormality (7) (fig 1 and 2). In such conditions of double labelling in plasma medium, 2 important remarks are to be pointed out:

1. In various geometrical conditions of counting (4Π for blood-sample countings, 2Π for external countings) a sum peak appears from the 2 photopeaks of 171 keV, and 245 keV which is superimposed to the ^{51}Cr-photopeak of 320 keV. Analysis of data from blood-sample countings in ^{111}In-^{51}Cr double labelling studies needs a careful calibration of the spectometre used.

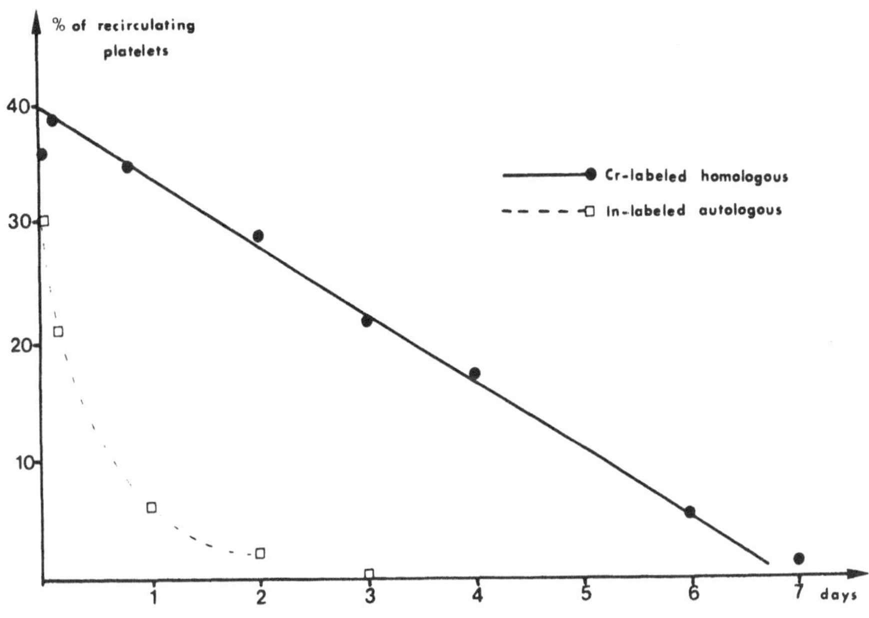

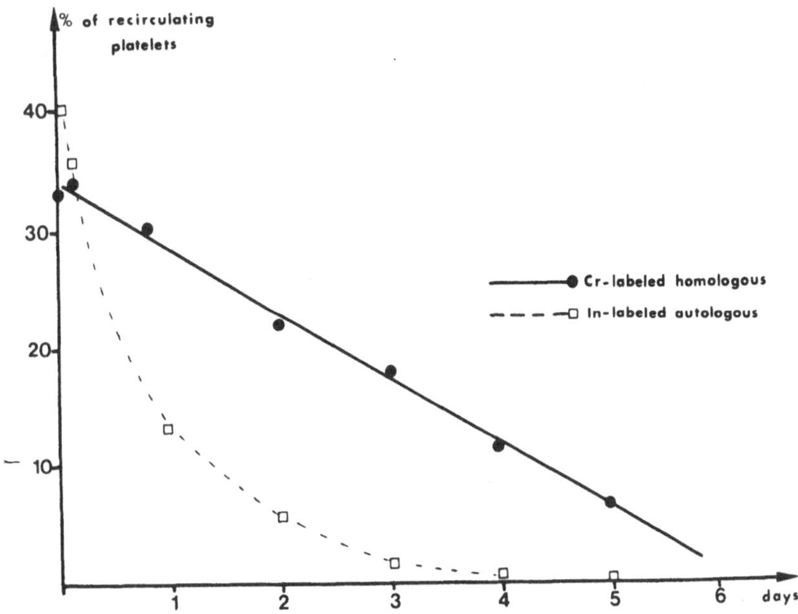

Fig. 1 and 2. Platelet life span studied by (^{111}In-^{51}Cr) double labelling in 2 patients with a familiar corpuscular platelet abnormality.

Table 1. Correlation between mean survival time values of simultaneous kinetic study with ^{111}In. Autologous platelets and ^{51}Cr-homologous platelets.

IDENTIFICATION DIAGNOSIS	PLATELET COUNT PER µL	MEAN SURVIVAL TIME	
		111IN	51CR
1 LAC. I T P	50 000	2 D.	1.5 D.
2 BEN. "	10 000	1.5 D.	2 D.
3 HAO. "	60 000	3 D.	2.5 D.
4 PRA. "	154 000	2 D.	2.5 D.
5 MAY "	48 000	2 D.	24 H.
6 KAR. "	110 000	3.5 D.	3 D.
7 MAL. "	55 000	3 D.	3 D.
8 MER. PRODUCTION DEFECT	52 000	7 D.	7 D.
9 LEG. "	97 000	8 D.	8 D.
10 VOL. "	119 000	6 D.	6 D.
11 MAR. "	30 000	7 D.	7 D.
12 DUT. "	36 000	10 D.	10 D.
13 DAU. "	56 000	7 D.	7 D.
14 APA. SPLENOMEGALY	100 000	6 D.	6 D.
15 DUF. "	117 000	6 D.	6 D.
16 DEM. HYPERCONSUMPTION	250 000	8 D.	8 D.

Table 2 and 3. Splenic sequestration versus hepatic sequestration on the same day of maximum sequestration values by external counting - Comparison of ^{111}In and ^{51}Cr-data.

NR	S/H (51CR)	S/H (111IN)	S/H (51CR) / S/H (111IN)
1	12.20	5.04	2.40
2	15.17	7.17	2.11
3	26.68	12.28	2.17
4	20.63	4.48	4.60
5	58.73	6.90	8.51
6	24.40	7.36	3.31
7	3.89	1.79	2.17

Table 3.

NR	S/H (51CR)	S/H (111IN)	S/H (51CR) / S/H (111IN)
8	14.17	3.30	4.30
9	14.30	11.40	1.20
10	22.82	7.71	2.90
11	8.26	3.09	2.67
12	4.88	1.85	2.64
13	16.70	6.07	2.75
14	35.07	16.30	2.15
15	16.66	4.08	4.08
16	10.62	4.94	2.15

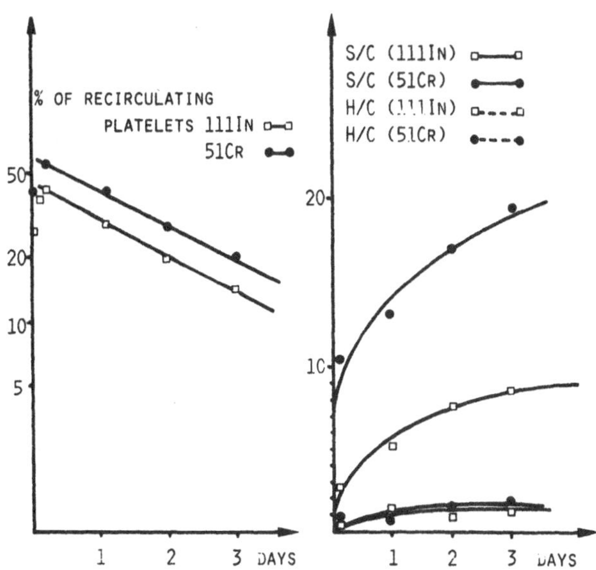

Fig. 3. Platelet survival study and external counting data in ITP (splenic and hepatic area versus precordial area count ratio).

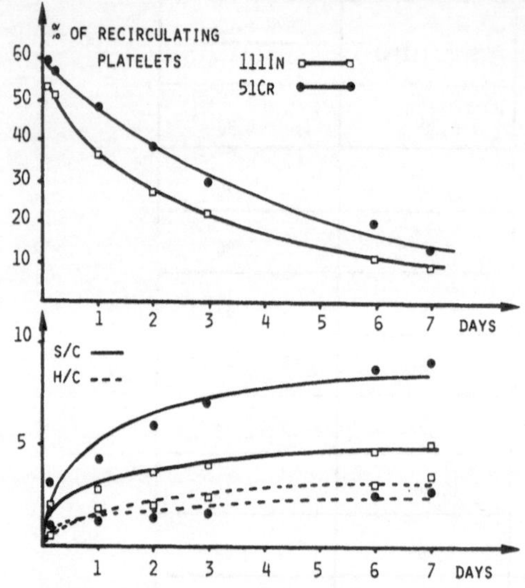

Fig. 4. Platelet survival study and external counting data in production defect. (Splenic and hepatic area versus precordial area count ratio).

2. Indium-oxine is a rather weak complex compared with Indium Transferrin. In routine studies using plasma medium in normal subjects, even after careful cell washing, about 5% of the total radioactivity is infused as labelled Transferrin, and 10-15% of the total radioactivity immediately reaches the liver. The data from external countings are so modified, and need correction for analysis of the platelet distribution.

It was previously established that the platelet life span obtained with ^{111}In-labelled cells is identical to that obtained with ^{51}Cr labelled cells (5,7) (table 1). Considering the 2 previous remarks, the external countings in 16 patients (7 ITP, 6 production defects, 2 splenomegalies and 1 hyper-consumption by arteritis) with double labelling show some differences between Chromium and Indium results. When the spleen-liver ratio (S/H) is calculated from the ^{111}In-energy window, the result differs from that calculated from the ^{51}Cr-energy window by a dividing factor of 2.3 (± 0.46) whatever the pathology studied (table 2 and 3). This factor is considerably enhanced by any loss of care in the labelling method.

So, it can be stated that the sequestration site of the platelets is the same whether provided by ^{111}In or ^{51}Cr external countings (fig 3 and 4) but that the spleen-liver ratio is closely dependant on: first, the counting spectrometry, and second, the quality of labelling procedure.

REFERENCES

1. Davis HH, Siegel BA, Joist JH et al, Scintigraphic detection of artherosclerotic lesions and venous thrombi in man by Indium-111 labelled autologous platelets. Lancet 1:1185, 1978.

2. Goodwin DA, Bushberg JT, Doherty PW et al, Indium-111 labelled autologous platelets for location of vascular thrombi in humans. J. nucl. Med. 19:626, 1978.

3. Bang NU, Sandbjerg HM, Heidenreich RO, The influence of plasma proteins on platelet function and metabolism. In: Platelets, recent advances in basis research and clinical aspects. Ulutin ON (ed), Excerpta Medica, Int. Congr. Series, Amsterdam, pp 118-126, 1975.

4. Recommended methods for radioisotope platelet survival studies. The panel on diagnostic application of radioisotopes in hematology. International Committee for standardization in Hematology. Blood 50:1137, 1977.

5. Scheffel U, Min-Fu Tsan, McIntyre PA, Labelling of human platelets with (III-In) 8-hydroxyquinoline. J. nucl. Med. 20:524, 1979.

6. Hosain F, McIntyre PA, Poulose K et al, Binding of trace amounts of ionic Indium 113 m to plasma transferrin. Clin. Chim. Acta 24:69, 1969.

7. Vigneron N, Dassin E, Najean Y et al, Double marquage des plaquettes par 51 Cr et 111-In. Application à l'ètude simultanée de la durée de vie des plaquettes autologues et homologues. Nouv. Presse Méd. 9:1835, 1980.

15 PLATELET SURVIVAL TIME (^{51}CR) AND PLATELET PRODUCTION TIME (ASPIRIN-MDA METHOD): A SIMULTANEOUS EVALUATION IN PATIENTS AFFECTED WITH CANCERS

A. BONEU, R. BUGAT, P. SIE, B. BONEU

INTRODUCTION

Aspirin irreversibly inhibits platelet cyclooxygenase and thus the synthesis of thromboxanes and of malondialdehyde (MDA) in the circulating platelets (1). This property has been proposed to determine the platelet production time (PPT) after a single intake of aspirin (2). From a theoretical point of view, this non-isotopic method can constitute an alternative to the routine isotopic techniques for platelet kinetic measurements in stationary states.

We report preliminary results concerning a simultaneous evaluation of the PPT and of the platelet survival time (PST) after autologous labelling with ^{51}Cr. This study was conducted in patients affected with various types of cancer in which the platelet life-span was expected to be normal or moderately reduced. Mean platelet volume as an index of megakaryocyte hyperstimulation was also determined (3).

Patients and methods

Patients: 13 patients hospitalized for various advanced solid malignant tumours were investigated. Their platelet count ranged from 215 to 450 X 10^3/cuµm and did not vary significantly during the time course of the study. The results of PPT and PST were compared to those of 13 and 15 normal healthy volunteers respectively.

Methods:

- Determination of PST. Autologous platelets were labelled with ^{51}Cr according to the recommendations of the International Committee for Standardization in Haematology (4). EDTA-K3 blood-samples (vacutainer-system) were obtained twice a day during the five first days and daily during the five following days. The residual circulating radioactivity corresponding to labelled red cells determined 15 days after injection was substracted from the proceeding values. The mean platelet recovery in the patient group was 55.5% and ranged from 32 to 83%.

The data were computerized and analyzed according to the three following mathematical methods: linear, exponential and multiple hit. The mean PST was provided by the method which gave the best fit (minimal sum of least squares).

- Determination of PPT. The PPT was determined according to the method of Stuart et al (2). Patients or volunteers were instructed not to take aspirin for at least ten days before the test. The basal level of MDA was determined twice before the prescription of 0.50 g per os of aspirin. The MDA level was first evaluated 36 hours after aspirin administration and then daily until the basal level was reached. The pattern of MDA re-appearance was always linear, so the determination of the PPT was a graphical evaluation as indicated in fig 3. The details for the MDA determination have been reported elsewhere (5): in brief, 4 ml of blood were taken on 1 ml of Aster-Jandl solution. Platelets were isolated by differential centrifugation and resuspended in a tyrode, albumin buffer. MDA synthesis was induced by sodium arachidonate (final concentration: 500 µM); the MDA level was evaluated using the thiobarbituric assay. Each blood-sample allowed a triplicate evaluation and the variation coefficient was 2.6%. With this method, the mean MDA level was founds to be 15.7 µmoles/10^9 platelets in the controls and 14.03 µ moles/10^9 platelets in the patient group (non-significant difference).

- Platelet count and platelet volume. The platelet count was carried out with a manual method at least three times during the course of each kinetic determination to assess the stationary state of the patient.

The mean platelet volume (MPV) was determined on Aster-PRP with a Coulter counter Z BIC coupled with a channelyser C 1000 (6).

Table 1. Platelet survival time, platelet production time and mean platelet volume (mean ± SD) in controls and in patients

	P S T days	P P T days	M P V cu µm
Controls	9.5 ± 0.5	9.9 ± 1.5	6.9 ± 0.5
Patients	3.8 ± 1.7	8.02 ± 1.9	6.5 ± 0.8
Student's T Test	P <0.001	P <0.05	P >0.05

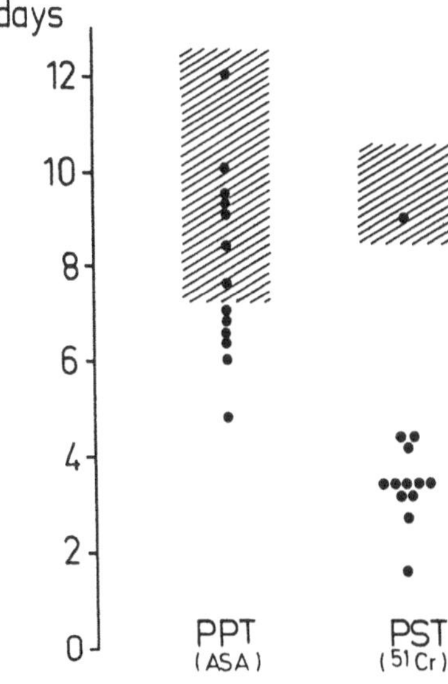

Fig. 1. Comparative results of platelet production time (PPT) and of platelet survival time (PST) in the patient group. The hatched areas delineate the normal range for the controls (mean ± 2 SD).

Results

The results are summarized in table 1. In the normal healthy volunteers the values of PST and of PPT were not significantly different. In the patient group, there was a significant reduction in the PST and in the PPT in comparison with the control values.

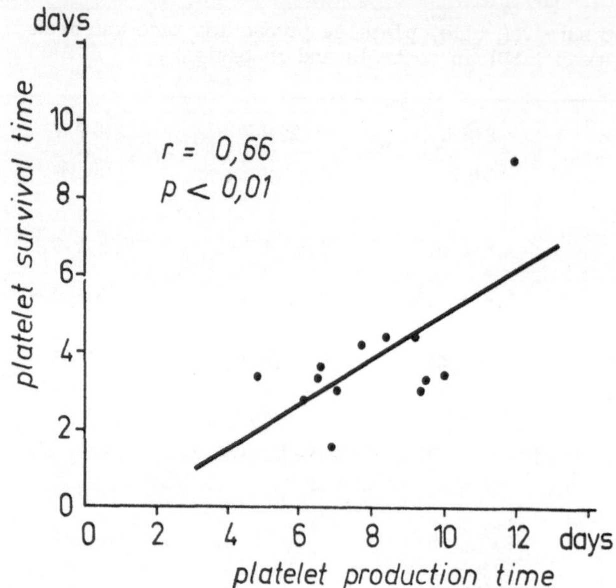

Fig. 2. Correlation between PPT and PST in the patient group.

Fig 1 shows that the reduction of the PST is greater than that of the PPT; all the results, except one, are below the normal range for the PST while seven patients are in the normal range for the PPT. The weak, but significant correlation between the two methods is indicated in fig 2.

The pattern of radioactivity disappearance was always curvilinear in all the patients except in the one case where the PST was in the normal range. This patient excepted, the best fit for the calculation of the PST was given by the multiple hit model. In contrast, the pattern of MDA re-appearance was always linear in cases of very short PPT. Fig 3 gives a typical example of this discrepancy.

Discussion

In normal subjects, where the pattern of radioactivity disappearance is linear, the mean PST is comparable to the mean PPT; unfortunately we did not have the possibility of simultaneously performing the two methods on the same control subjects, but in the patient where the radioactive disappearance was linear,

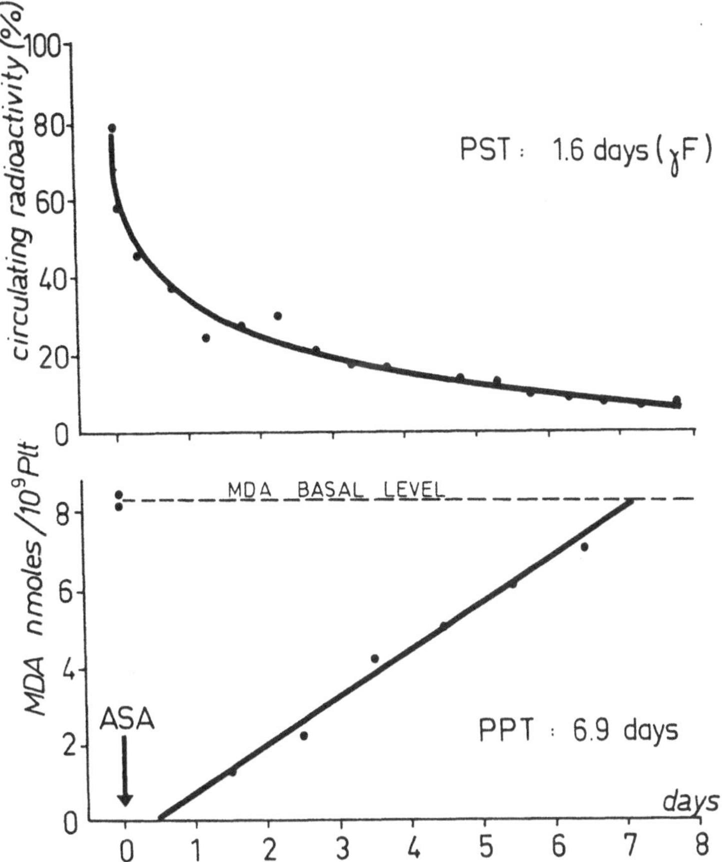

Fig. 3. A typical example of the discrepancy between ^{51}Cr PST and aspirin PPT. PST was calculated by the multiple hit model and PPT by graphical extrapolation.

indicating normal PST (9 days), the PPT was also in the normal range (12 days). In the other cases, where the best fit was provided by the multiple hit model and where the PST was significantly reduced, the results of the two methods are clearly different in spite of steady state platelet kinetics as indicated by the absence of modifications of the platelet count throughout the study. Such a discrepancy has already been reported (7) and several factors can account for this difference.

The MDA-PPT method presents certain theoretical and practical advantages - non-irradiation, autologous method, in vivo labelling avoiding platelet manipulations - but in spite of this there are also several drawbacks. One of them concerns the 24-48 hour lag-phase before the increase in the MDA level. This delay may be due to an inhibition of the megacaryocyte cyclooxygenase as demonstrated in rat (8). More recently, it was suggested that albumin, present in the suspending medium where the platelets are stimulated, could impair MDA or thromboxane synthesis by platelets newly released from the bone marrow (7). In the present study this lag-phase was not taken into account since the first blood-sample was made 36 hours after aspirin intake. The PPT was calculated by a graphical linear extrapolation of the MDA levels to the x axis intersection. Another problem concerns the specificity of the MDA-thiobarbituric assay as an indicator of prostaglandin synthesis (9). A few hours after aspirin ingestion, or on _in vitro_ aspirin treatment, the MDA level ranges between 10 to 15% of the pre-aspirin value. If this value, which was not determined in this study, is substracted from the pre-aspirin MDA level, the PPT would be reduced by approximately one day. Even with this correction, the MDA-PPT is longer than the chromium PST. Lastly, preferential utilization of newly released platelets at the tumour site could result in a false prolongation of PPT by reducing the apparent rate of renewal of circulating platelets. This phenomenon cannot be presently excluded.

The chromium method, which is widely used in human clinical investigations, has also to be discussed. _In vitro_ chromium labelling requires several steps where the functional properties of the platelets can be modified; one cannot exclude the possibility that these labelled platelets may be preferentially removed in cases of moderate platelet hyperconsumption. It is known that platelets can loose membrane glycoprotein throughout their survival (10) and that thrombin-treated platelets survive normally even though they have lost a large part of their granular content (11). The interaction between platelets and tumour cells could lead to such phenomena and we do not know whether, in this _in vivo_ situation, there is a premature loss of the cytoplasmic radioactive marker leading to an enhanced reduction of the PST.

In conclusion, in spite of the above mentioned possible

restrictions, the chromium PST method appears to be more sensitive to detect moderate platelet hyperconsumption. Nevertheless, the results provided by the aspirin method seem more compatible with the other haemostatic data: normal platelet count, absence of macrothrombocytosis suggesting that megakaryocytes are not hyperstimulated and absence of biological symptoms of consumption coagulopathy (data not shown).

Work is in progress to compare PPT with Indium-labelled PST.

Acknowledgements

We are indebted to Mrs. A.M. Gabaig for her invaluable technical assistance. This work was supported in part by a grant from Université Paul Sabatier.

REFERENCES

1. Koesis JJ, Hernandovich J, Silver MJ, Smith JB, Ingerman C, Duration of inhibition of platelet prostaglandin formation and aggregation by ingested aspirin or indomethacin. Prostaglandins 3:141, 1973.

2. Stuart MJ, Murphy S, Oski FA, A simple nonradioisotope technique for the determination of platelet life span. New Engl. J. Med. 292:1310, 1975.

3. Paulus JM, Platelet size in man. Blood 46:321, 1975.

4. The panel on diagnostic application on radioisotopes in hematology, International Committee for standardization in Hematology: Recommended methods for radioisotope platelet survival studies. Blood 50:1137, 1977.

5. Boneu B, Sie P, Caranobe C, Nouvel C, Bierme R, Malondialdehyde (MDA) re-appearance in human platelet density subpopulations after a single intake of aspirin. Thromb. Res. 19:609, 1980.

6. Boneu B, Corberand J, Plante J, Bierme R, Evidence that platelet density and volume are not related to aging. Thromb. Res. 10:475, 1977.

7. Catalano PM, Smith JB, Murphy S, Platelet recovery from aspirin inhibition in vivo; differing patterns under various assay conditions. Blood 57:99, 1981.

8. Dejana E, Barbieri B, Cerletti C, Livio M, De Gaetano G, Impaired thromboxane production by newly formed platelets after aspirin administration to thrombocytopenic rats. Brit. J. Haemat. 46:465, 1980.

9. Pryor WA, Stanley JP, A suggested mechanism for the production of malondialdehyde during the autoxidation of polyunsaturated fatty acids. Nonenzymatic production of prostaglandin endoperoxides during autoxidation. J. Org. Chem. 40:3615, 1975.

10. George JN, Lewis PC, Morgan RR, Studies on platelet plasma membranes. III. Membrane glycoprotein loss from circulating platelets in rabbits: inhibition by aspirin - dipyridamole and acceleration by thrombin. J. Lab. clin. Med. 91:301, 1978.

11. Reimers HJ, Kinlough-Rathbone RL, Cazenave JP, Senyi AF, Hirsch J, Packham MA, Mustard JF, In vitro and in vivo functions of thrombin treated platelets. Thrombos. Haemost. 35:151, 1976.

LABELLED PLATELETS: SCINTIGRAPHIC STUDIES

16 SURVIVAL TIME AND ORGAN DISTRIBUTION OF ^{111}IN-OXINE-LABELLED HUMAN PLATELETS IN NORMAL SUBJECTS

H.W. WAHNER, W.L. DUNN, M.K. DEWANJEE, V. FUSTER

INTRODUCTION

^{111}In-oxine was introduced in 1976 (1) as a platelet marker for imaging platelet deposition. The new label is of equal interest for kinetic and organ distribution studies. The value of the ^{111}In-oxine marker for the latter purpose has not been well established. It was the objective of this effort to establish a normal data base with respect to platelet kinetics and organ distribution.

Material and methods

Survival time and organ distribution were studied in 28 healthy volunteers (20 females, 8 males). Mean age was 37.5 years (females 39.5, males 32.5 years), and ages ranged from 22 to 63 years. The subjects were nonsmokers, had no family history of coronary artery disease, were free from hypertension and diabetes mellitus, and were not taking antiplatelet drugs or hormone treatment. Platelets were labelled by the method of Heaton and colleagues (2). Details of the quality of the injected platelet preparation are given in table 1.

Table 1. Quality of injected ^{111}In-labelled platelet preparation

			Total cells injected (%)	
	Mean	2SD	Mean	2SD
Total cells ($\times 10^9$ cells)	4.24	4.31		
Platelets ($\times 10^9$ cells)	4.18	4.14	96.3	4.04
White cells ($\times 10^9$ cells)	2.61	3.86	0.14	0.30
Red cells ($\times 10^9$ cells)	0.12	0.11	3.50	3.80
Labelling efficiency (%)	72.8	14.2		

Recovery of injected platelets (10 min) was 54.2 ± 10.3% (mean ± SD). Injected ^{111}In-activity was 178.8 ± 57.2 μCi, volume was 4.8 ± 0.5 ml, and labelling efficiency was 64.2 ± 13.5%. Consistently throughout the study, about 5% of ^{111}In-activity in the blood was associated with plasma proteins.

Venous blood-samples were drawn at 10 min, 20 and 27 hours and once or twice each succeeding 24 hour period for 165 hours. All patients had gamma camera images of the anterior chest (blood-pool of the heart), anterior abdomen (liver, spleen), and posterior abdomen (spleen) at 1 hour and daily for 7 days. Data were acquired on an MDS, A^2 computer for quantitative analysis. Imaging time was 5 min. Quantitation was performed with the use of correction factors established experimentally for organ depth, crossover from one organ to the other, blood-activity, and tissue background.

Results

Survival time. Disappearance curves of activity from blood were fitted to an exponential and a linear regression, and the goodness of fit was tested. In 21 of 28 cases the better fit was linear (fig 1). 4 of the patients in whom the exponential fit was better were females (ages 30.2 ± 11.9 years).

For the entire population study, the mean value of radioactivity, expressed as percent of the dose, declined from 56 ± 10% at t=O (intercept) to 13.7 ± 3.7% at 165 hours (table 2). The distribution of the mean survival time was normal for both models used. No significant correlation was found between mean survival time and variables such as age, body surface, blood-volume, injected activity, or y-intercept.

Organ distribution

Activity was seen in the blood-pool, spleen, and liver (fig 2). Mean activity in the spleen was 34.7 ± 10.2% (mean ± 1 SD) at 1.5 hours and increased to 40.4 ± 13.2% at 167 hours. Initial activity in the spleen is due to platelet pooling. In support of this finding, our data suggest a weak negative correlation between recovery of injected platelets (10 min)

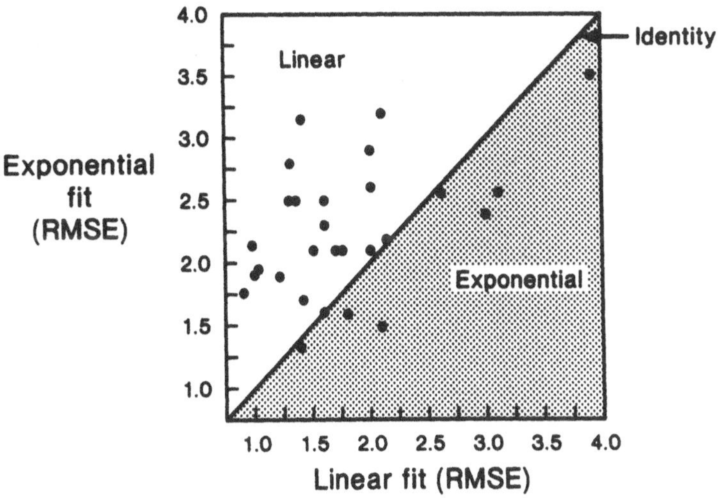

Fig. 1. Distribution of the root mean square error (RMSE) (index of the goodness of fit) for linear fit (abscissa) and exponential fit (ordinate). In white area, better fit is linear; in shaded area, better fit is exponential.

Table 2. Survival of ^{111}In-labelled platelets in 28 normal subjects

	Linear regression	Exponential regression	
Mean survival time			
All subjects ($\bar{x}$ ± SD)	211.92 ± 14.16 h	122.4 ± 14.4 h	
Males (8)	205.8 ± 14.8 h	117.6 h	} P >0.05
Females (20)	214.2 ± 13.4 h	125.8 h	
Half-life (T½)	...	84.8 ± 10.0 h	

and spleen size on the scintigram (r= -0.40, P<0.07). In addition, a highly negative correlation was found between recovery and initial spleen uptake (r= -0.76, P<0.05). Hepatic activity increased from 5.8 ± 3.4% at 1.5 hours to 24.9 ± 8.5% at 167 hours. Liver activity is due mainly to sequestration of damaged platelets and fragments of labelled platelets (fig 3).

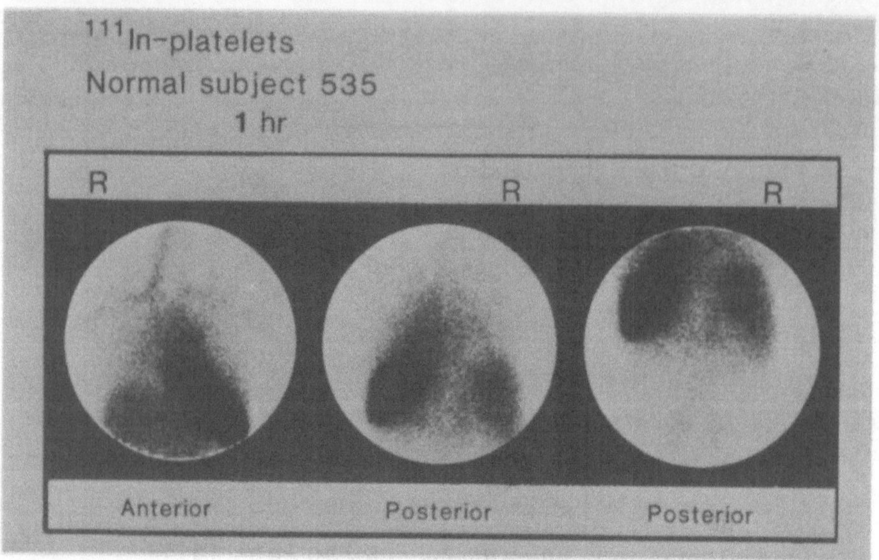

Fig. 2. Anterior and posterior gamma camera images of chest and abdomen after injection of ^{111}In-oxine-labelled platelets.

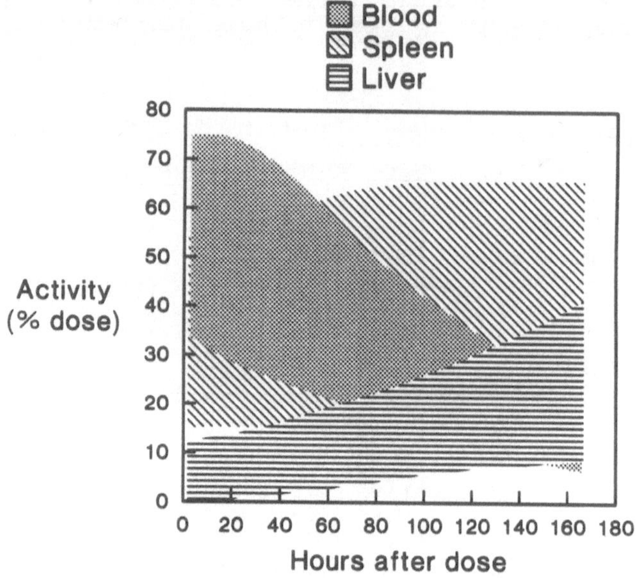

Fig. 3. Activity in liver, spleen, and blood after injection of ^{111}In-labelled platelets. Range of values was obtained in 28 normal subjects.

Comment and conclusions

As with ^{51}Cr, survival curves obtained with ^{111}In-oxine are, in general, linear (3). This suggests absence of elution of the label from platelets and an aging process as the causes of platelet removal in normal subjects. Survival time for ^{111}In-labelled platelets was equal to that reported by Heaton and others (2) but somewhat shorter than that found for ^{51}Cr in our laboratory (3). The difference between sexes shown for ^{51}Cr was not demonstrated with ^{111}In. Great variability in uptake of ^{111}In-labelled platelets was found in the spleen and liver, even in this normal population.

Splenic size is a determining factor in splenic uptake in this normal population. This feature may restrict the value of splenic uptake measurements in patients with platelet diseases and splenomegaly when splenic sequestration is considered. ^{111}In-labelled platelets appear to be suitable for kinetic studies, which were heretofore reserved only for ^{51}Cr-labelled platelets.

REFERENCES

1. Thakur ML, Welch MJ, Joist JH, Coleman RE, Indium-111 labelled platelets: studies on preparation and evaluation of in vitro and in vivo function. Thromb. Res. 9:345, 1976.

2. Heaton WA, Davis HH, Welch MJ, Mathias CJ, Joist JH, Sherman LA, Siegel BA, Indium-111: a new radionuclide label for studying human platelet kinetics. Brit. J. Haemat. 42:613, 1979.

3. Fuster V, Chesebro JH, Frye RL, Elveback LR, Platelet survival and the development of coronary artery disease in the young adult: effects of cigarette smoking, strong family history and medical therapy. Circulation 63:546, 1981.

17 ^{111}IN-LABELLED PLATELETS IN THE DIAGNOSIS OF KIDNEY TRANSPLANT REJECTION

M.R. HARDEMAN, J. VREEKEN, S. SURACHNO, J.H. TEN VEEN, J.M. WILMINK, E.A. VAN ROYEN, J.B. VAN DER SCHOOT

INTRODUCTION

Deterioration of kidney graft function shortly after surgery occurs frequently due to various disorders. Often it may be difficult to differentiate the diagnosis of graft rejection from other complications like acute tubular necrosis, vascular or urological problems or viral infections. A similar problem exists in determining the different types of rejection, i.e. vascular or cellular.

Clinical signs most often encountered during rejection are a swelling and tenderness of the kidney, a rise in temperature and blood-pressure, a decrease in sodium and water excretion, a general diminution of renal function and proteinuria. Besides these clinical and biochemical parameters, scintigraphy (employing Tc^{99m}-DTPA and/or ^{131}I-hippuran) is often performed in post-operative management, to determine perfusion and function of the graft. However, no specific non-invasive methods are available to establish graft rejection definitely. Although lymphocytes and monocytes are predominantly found in the interstitial tissue of the rejection graft, accumulation of neutrophilic granulocytes and platelets also occur. The availability of a very efficient labelling technique for these latter cells with ^{111}In-oxinate prompted us to investigate the role of granulocytes and platelets in graft rejection, in particular the early stages of that proces (1).

The results with granulocytes, published elsewhere, showed just a slight increased accumulation of apparently viable granulocytes during a florid kidney graft rejection and could thus not sustain the preliminary results of Frick et al (2,3) that these cells might be a useful tool in the diagnosis of graft rejection. Therefore it was decided to proceed the study using autologous ^{111}In-labelled thrombocytes, the results of which are reported in this paper.

Compared to the "classical" cell-marker ^{51}Cr, ^{111}In permits more photons per mrad absorbed dose. Moreover, the gamma-energies emitted by the latter radionuclide (173 and 247 KeV) makes it very suitable for in-vivo detection with a gamma camera. Finally, the radioactive half-life of ^{111}In (2.8 days) combines favourably with the biological half-life of both granulocytes (4-6 hours) and thrombocytes (4 days).

Patients

Selection of patients. Only patients with immediate graft function were submitted to this study. Informed consent was obtained in every case. All patients received cadaveric kidneys placed retroperitoneally in the fossa iliaca. Standard surgical procedures were employed under epidural anaesthesia (4). Conventional immunosuppressive therapy, consisting of prednisolone and azathioprine was administered.

Rejection. The clinical diagnosis of rejection was establishe upon a combination of several signs and symptoms such as fever, enlargement and tenderness of the graft, gain in bodyweight, hypertension, salt and water retention, decrease of creatinine clearance, eosinophilia in peripheral blood, proteinuria with casts, lymphocyturia and decrease in renal perfusion and function as monitored by dynamic renal scintigraphy. In addition in every case histological confirmation was obtained by percutaneous graft biopsy. Rejections were treated with 3 or more pulses of 1000 mg methylprednisolone, occasionally dipyridamole, heparin and dactinomycin was administered.

Methods

^{111}In-oxinate. The ^{111}In-oxinate complex was prepared as described by Thakur et al (1). In the last and largest part of this study, however, a commercial preparation of the complex, purchased from Byk-Mallinkrodt CIL BV (Petten, The Netherlands) was used. At activity reference time the specific activity was 1 mCi per 25 μg 8-hydroxyquinoline (oxine).

Thrombocyte isolation and labelling. The procedure has been described in detail in this volume.

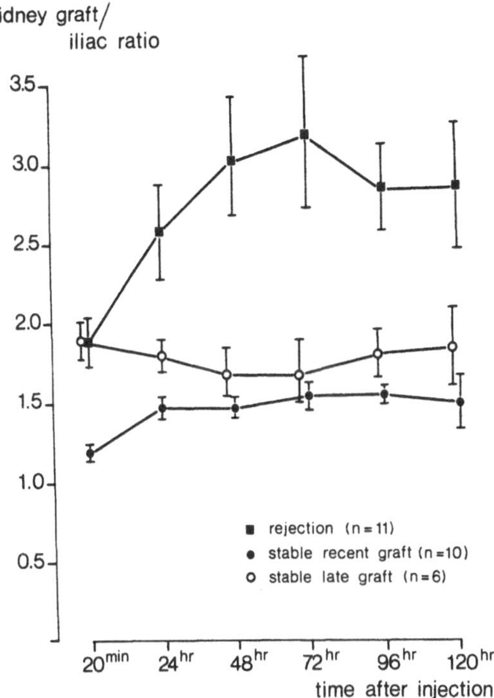

Fig. 1. Radioactivity (mean ± SEM) accumulated over the stable or rejecting kidney graft, relative to the activity measured over the opposite iliac region, various times after injection of ^{111}In-thrombocytes.

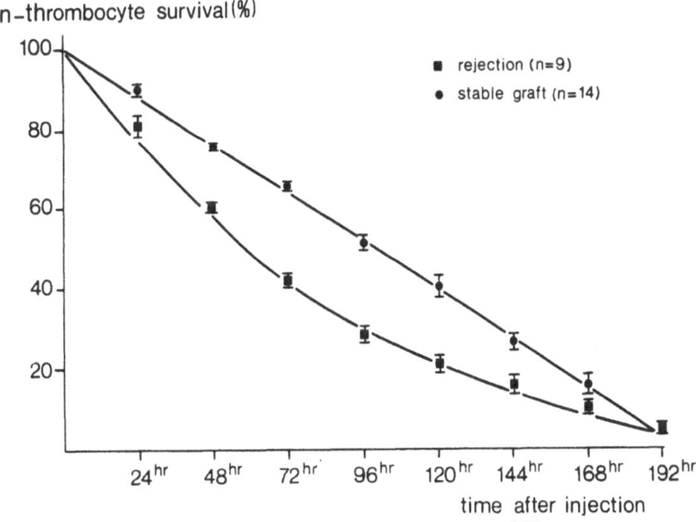

Fig. 2. In-vivo survival (mean ± SEM) of re-injected ^{111}In-labelled thrombocytes in patients with stable and rejecting kidney grafts.

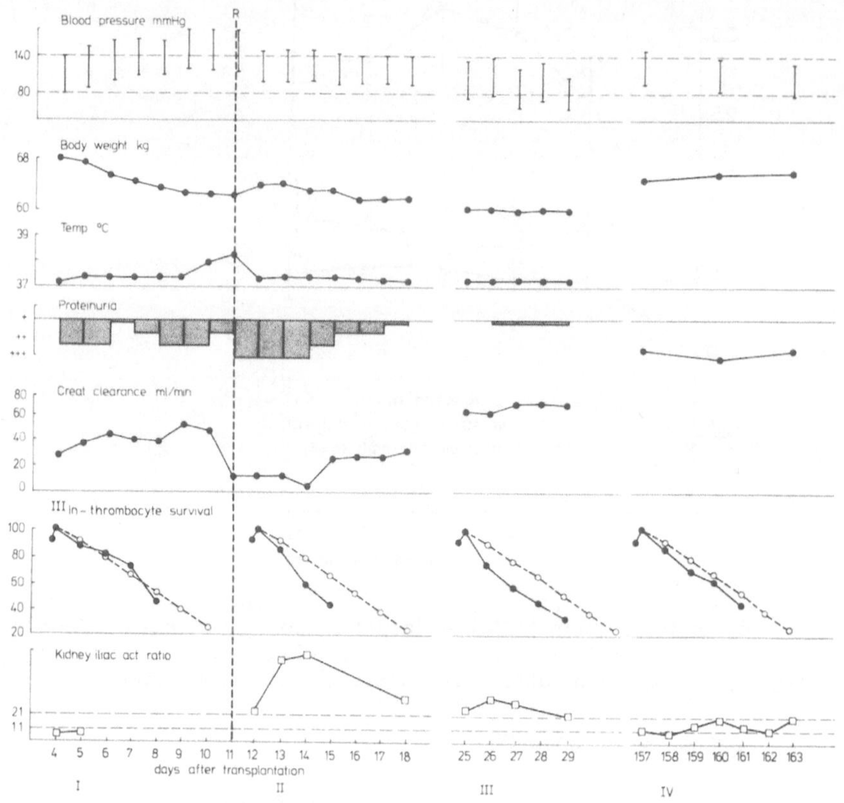

Fig. 3. Longitudinal survey of various clinical and biochemical parameters, ^{111}In-thrombocyte survival and the accumulation of radioactivity over the kidney graft, relative to the activity measured over the opposite iliac region of patient A (see text). The occasions on which the scintigrams, shown in fig. 4 I-IV were made are marked with I-IV, respectively. R= antirejection therapy.

Thrombocyte survival study. EDTA blood samples (5 ml) are collected at known time intervals for several days. Whole blood and platelet free plasma are counted in a well-type gamma counter. It can be stated that at least in our hands the lable did not elute from the platelets after injection, because: 1) measurements after blood-cell fractionation showed that the

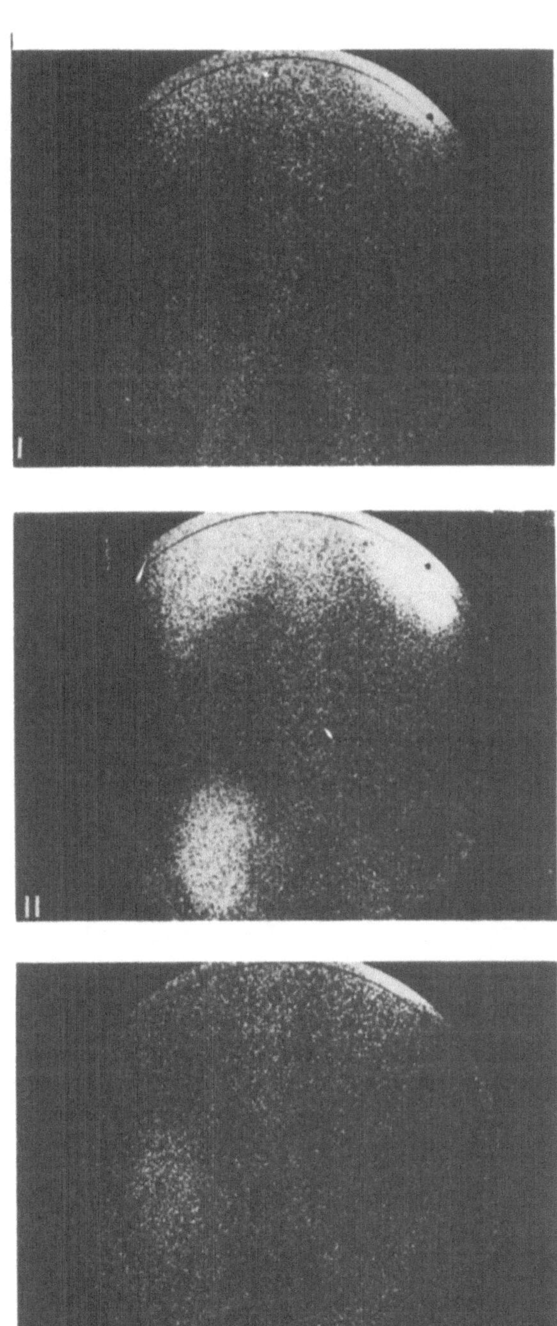
I
II
III

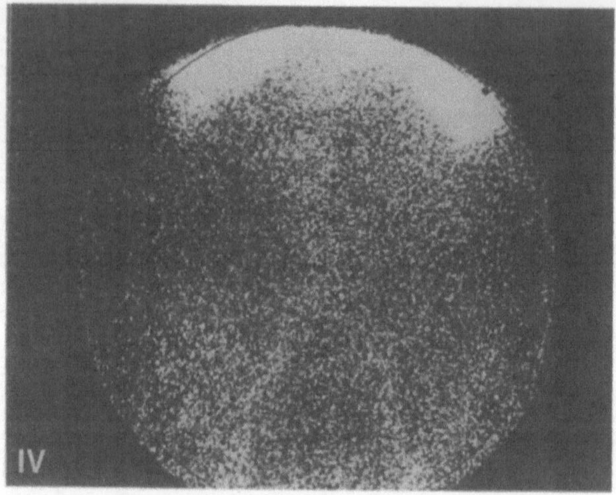

Fig. 4. I-IV. Scintigrams made on various occasions of patient A. (see text and fig. 3).

radioactivity was confined to the platelet fraction, 2) any radioactivity in the plasma fraction disappeared within 2-3 days, 3) in 24 hours urines only very small quantities of radioactivity i.e. less than 1% of the injected dose could be found. This makes isolation of thrombocytes, for the radioactivity measurements unnecessary.

Nevertheless, a correction should be made for any injected, non-platelet bound, activity during the first 2 or 3 days. For an exact calculation the hematocrit has to be measured also daily. If the activity measured in 1.0 ml EDTA-blood = x, the activity measured in 1.0 ml EDTA-cell free plasma = y and the hematocrit =z%, than it is possible to calculate the radioactivity in the blood-cell fraction as:

$$x - \frac{(100 - z)\ y}{100}$$

Scintigraphy. In all patients scintigrams were performed at 20 min and 24 hours after the injection of the labelled cells. In the thrombocyte studies, additional daily scintigrams were made up to 5-8 days. The aquisition time was 10 min using a large field of view gamma camera linked on line to a computer. Irregular

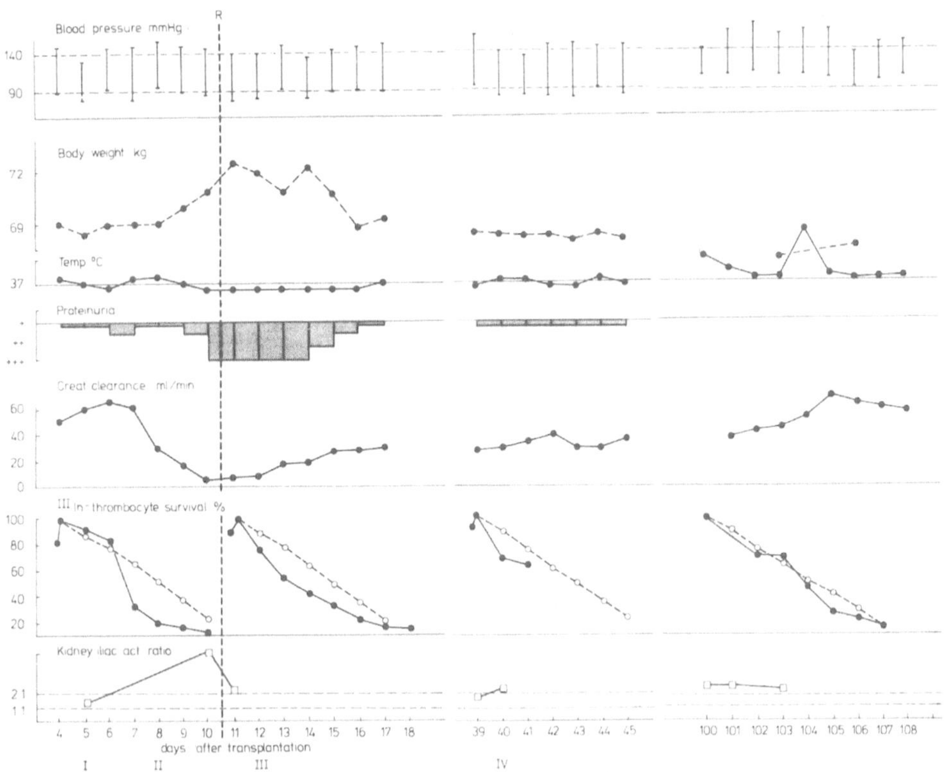

Fig. 5. Longitudinal survey of various clinical and biochemical parameters, ^{111}In-thrombocyte survival and the accumulation of radioactivity over the kidney graft relative to the activity measured over the opposite iliac region of patient B (see text). The occasions on which the scintigrams, shown in fig. 6 I-IV were made are marked with I-IV, respectively. R= antirejection therapy.

regions of interest were defined around the renal graft and the opposite iliac region, the aorta, abdomen, liver and spleen. The integrated counts in each region were corrected for injected activity and physical decay and expressed in units: counts / 10 min / 100 µCi / pixel. Relative graft activity was calculated by the kidney graft/iliac region ratio.

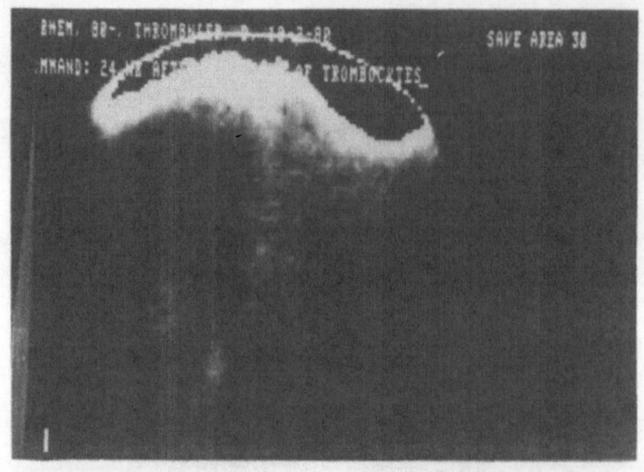
SAVE AREA 38
TROMBOCYTES_
I

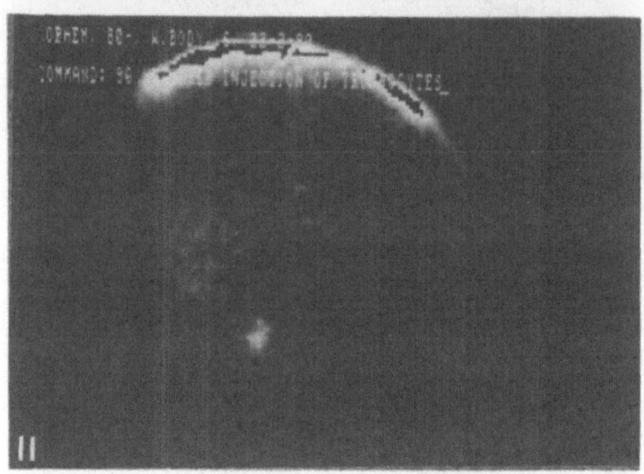
INJECTION OF
II

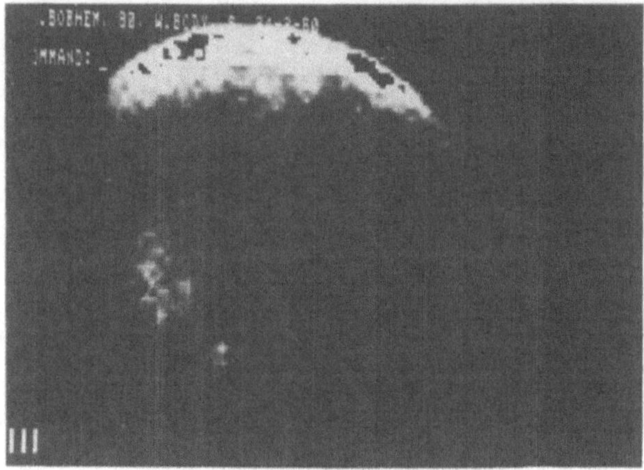
.BOBHEM. 80. W.BODY
MMAND: _
III

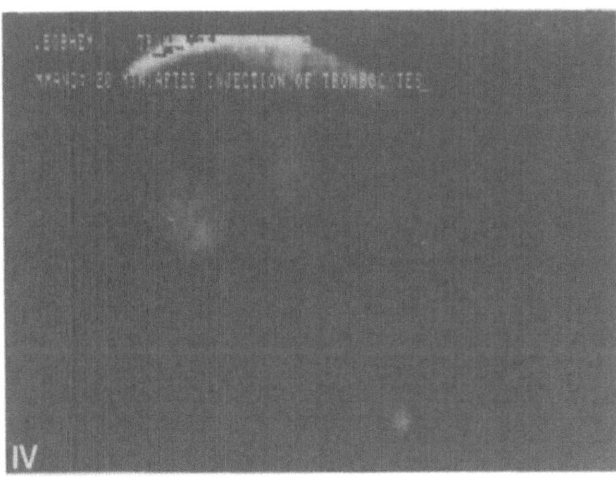

Fig. 6. I-IV. Scintigrams made on various occasions of patient B (see text).

Results

Thrombocyte studies. In total 38 patients were studied, most of them on several occasions. In fig 1 the kidney graft iliac region ratio's are plotted of:

- 6 studies in 6 patients who underwent transplantation at least 6 months earlier and were in a stable condition: "stable late grafts".
- 10 studies in 10 patients, made within 2 weeks after transplantation and considered, retrospectively, as normal since no signs of rejection presented at the time the study was performed: "stable recent grafts".
- 11 studies performed in 10 patients during rejection episodes, as defined under "patients selection". Thrombocyte survival curves are shown in fig 2; since there were only minimal differences between the two "stable" groups they were, for the sake of clarity, combined.
- 4 patients were studied also after successful anti-rejection therapy. Both kidney graft iliac region ratio and thrombocyte disappearance rate were still slightly above normal in 3, whereas in 1 study all values had returned towards the normal ranges (not shown).

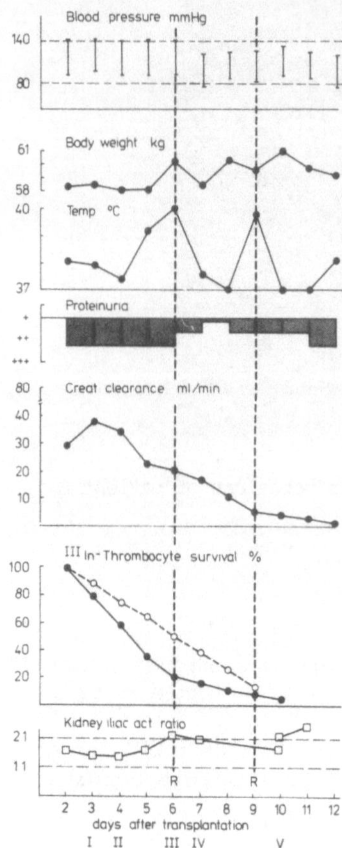

Fig. 7. Longitudinal survey of various clinical and biochemical parameters ^{111}In-thrombocyte survival and the accumulation of radioactivity over the kidney graft relative to the activity measured over the opposite iliac region of patient C (see text). The occasions on which the scintigrams, shown in fig. 8 I-V were made are marked with I-V, respectively. R= anti-rejection therapy.

The remaining studies could not be conclusive due to:

- Clinical complications other than, or in addition to, rejection e.g. renal artery thrombosis, pyelonephritis, acute pancreatitis, shunt thrombosis and DVT.
- Interference of other radionuclides used in routine diagnostic procedures i.e. Tc^{99m}-DTPA and/or ^{131}I-hippuran.

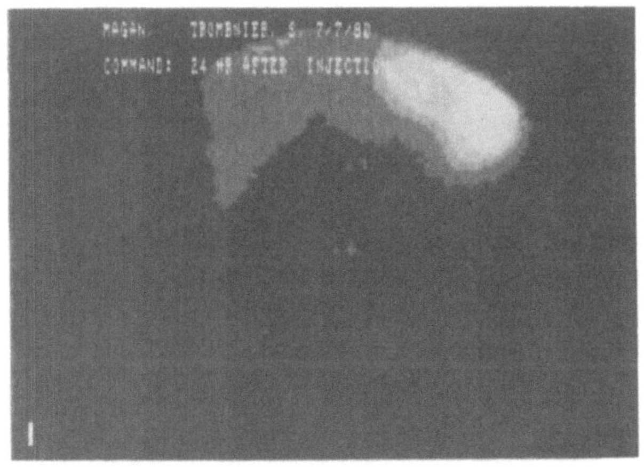
MAGAN
COMMAND: 24 HR AFTER
I

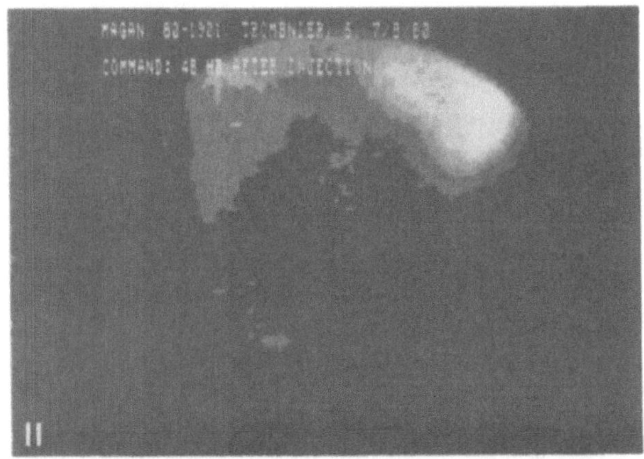
MAGAN
COMMAND: 48 HR
II

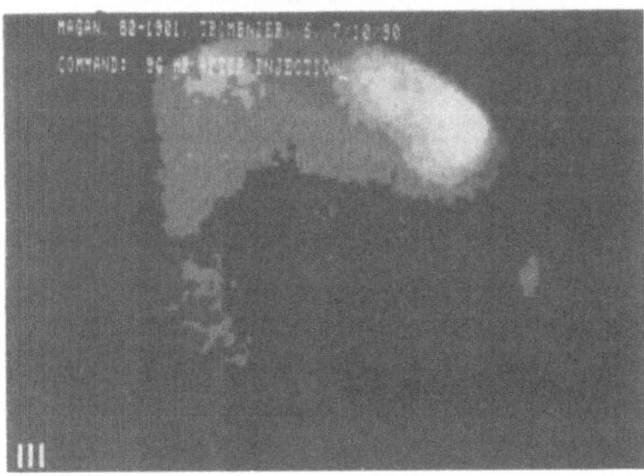
MAGAN
COMMAND: 96 HR
III

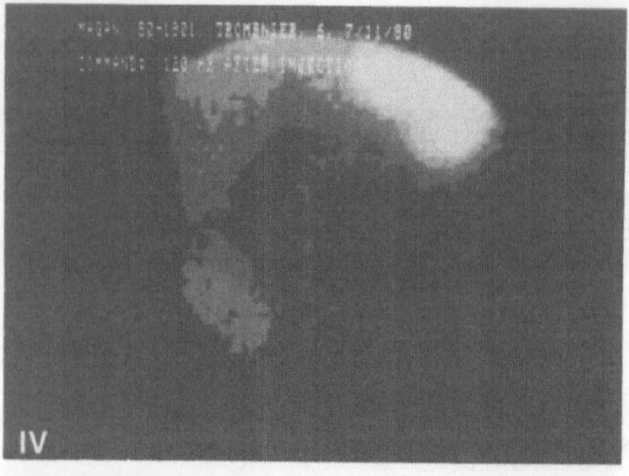

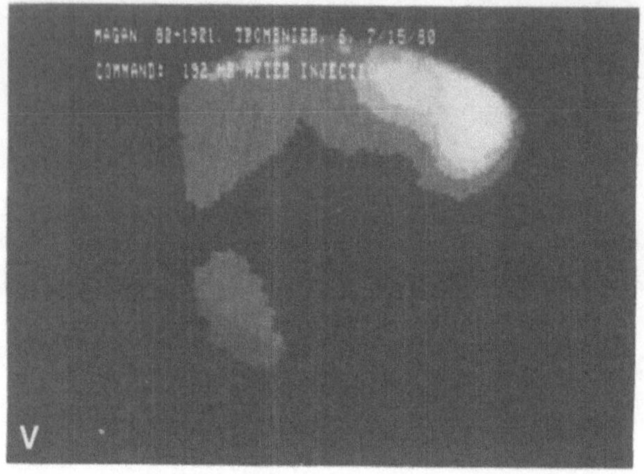

Fig. 8. I-V. Scintigrams made on various occasions of patient C (see text and fig. 7). VI scintigram made after nephrectomy of a sagittal slice of the kidney graft of patient C.

<u>Case reports</u> (longitudinal study). Patient A is a 43 year female with a lg A nephropathy. Fig 3 shows the various parameters in this patient during 4 episodes in which ^{111}In-thrombocytes were injected. Fig 4 I-IV are scintigrams made in this patient 24 hours after each injection, respectively on 4, 12, 25 and 157 days after transplantation.

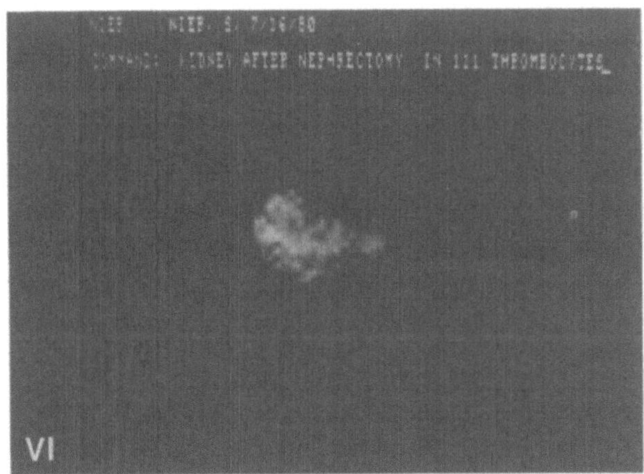

At the time of the first injection there were no signs of rejection. On day 12, a rejection episode was strongly suspected on clinical grounds (proteinuria, decrease of renal function etc) and confirmed histologically as an acute vascular rejection. Scintigrams then showed accumulation of ^{111}In (fig 4 II), reflected by an increased kidney-iliac ratio and decreased thrombocyte survival. Anti-rejection therapy was started (indicated by "R").

Scintigrams made after the third injection of ^{111}In-thrombocytes on day 25, when renal function demonstrated no further deterioration, showed diminished accumulation of ^{111}In (fig 4 III); kidney iliac ratio had decreased, although thrombocyte survival was still shortened. On day 157, renal function had improved and no signs of rejection were observed. There was minimal accumulation of ^{111}In (fig 4 IV), resulting in a normal kidney iliac ratio; also a normal thrombocyte survival time was found.

Patient B, a 48 year old male with end stage renal failure as a result of diabetic nephropathy received a cadaveric kidney on day 0. The kidney graft had three main renal arteries which ended on one aortic patch and one renal vein.

During the first days after injection of ^{111}In-thrombocytes on day 4, no clinical signs of rejection, were apparent (fig 5). Scintigrams made 24 hours after injection, however, showed obvious abnormalities (fig 6 I). A "hot spot" was localized at the site of the vascular anastomosis, also an area of decreased activity in the upper pole of the graft was seen. Kidney iliac ratio as well as ^{111}In-thrombocyte survival were normal in this phase. On day 7 there was a sharp increase of the ^{111}In-thrombocyte disappearance rate. Renal function deteriorated, although no clinical signs of rejection appeared yet. Another scintigram was made on day 8 (fig 6 II).

Renal arteriography was then performed to substantiate the suspicion of occlusion of one or more renal arteries; indeed a complete occlusion of one main renal artery could be demonstrated. On day 10 anti-rejection therapy (R) was initiated as various signs and symptoms of rejection appeared (fig 5). A new dose of ^{111}In-thrombocytes was administrated on day 11. The scintigram made hereafter (fig 6 III) showed clearly the perfusion defect of the upper pole of the graft and apparent activity at the vascular anastomosis. Kidney iliac ratio was still higher than normal as was the thrombocyte disappearance rate.

On day 39, a third dose of ^{111}In-thrombocytes was given. The perfusion defect of the upper pole remained unchanged but there was no activity observed anymore at the vascular anastomosis (fig 6 IV). Kidney iliac ratio had almost normalised. Another "hot spot" appeared over the left leg; deep venous thrombosis of the left leg was proven by phlebography.

Patient C, a 36 year old woman with end stage renal disease due to focal glomerulosclerosis received a cadaveric kidney graft implanted in the right iliac fossa. On day 2 after transplantation ^{111}In-thrombocytes were injected while graft function was improving (fig 7).

The scintigrams made 24 hours after injection (fig 8 I) did not show any abnormal accumulation of radioactivity by the graft. On the scintigrams made 48, 96 and 120 hours after injection (fig 8 II, III, IV) the accumulated amounts of radioactivity gradually increased. In the mean time there was an increased disappearence rate of ^{111}In-thrombocytes (fig 7). Rejection was evident on day 6 after transplantation and anti-rejection therapy (R) was given. Although several of the measured parameters e.g. temperature, bodyweight and proteinuria improved, the deterioration of kidney function could not be stopped. Intra-venous therapy with anti-thymocyte globulin was started on day 9 (R), however with no success. The scintigram (fig 8 V) made 24 hours after a second injection with ^{111}In-thrombocytes given on day 10 after transplantation, showed an abnormal high accumulation of radioactivity over the graft.

Histological investigations, on material obtained by needle biopsy on day 12, showed predominantly a cellular rejection with an initiating vascular component as well. Nephrectomy was performed the next day and a scintigram was made of a sagittal slice of the kidney (fig 8 VI).

Discussion

Because of the uncertainty in the exact assessment of the start (and the end) of a kidney graft rejection episode, it is difficult to evaluate a method based on the commitment of injected labelled short living cells in such a rejection. The moment of injection in relation to the onset of rejection is rather critical for obtaining conclusive results.

Furthermore, since clinical manifestations are probably late reflections of the actual (immunological) rejection crisis, radiolabelled blood-cells should, in the ideal situation, circulate before the clinical symptoms become evident. This will make a potential rejection diagnosis possible at an earlier time. Depending upon the survival time of the cells under study, more or less subsequent injections are necessary in order to fulful this requirement, possibly resulting in an unacceptably high radiation for the patient.

The fact that granulocytes have a biological half-life of only 4-6 hours might be the cause for the inconsistency in the results when these kind of cells are used (3). Thrombocytes, normally circulating 8-10 days, fulfil these requirements much better. Therefore, the results reported in this study, employing ^{111}In-labelled thrombocyte suspensions were more consistent and significant.

First of all we established the normal ranges at the site of the graft and the opposite iliac region during several days following injection of labelled thrombocytes. Subjects who underwent successful transplantation at least 6 months prior to this study ("stable late grafts") showed a rather narrow range of activity values.

Patients studied shortly after transplantation, without complications at that time ("stable recent grafts") did not differ significantly from the first group except, interestingly enough, after injection! The reason for this deviation from the stable late grafts is not quite clear; the cause might well be a suboptimal blood-perfusion of the fresh implanted graft at this time. If this is true, one might argue whether it is necessary to correct for the latter factor. Apparantly surgery as such did not appreciably increase thrombocyte accumulation at the graft and its vascular anastomosis.

It is clear from fig 2 that the kidney iliac ratio could distinguish the patients with rejection as a group from patients without complications after transplantation. In the individual patient, however, a decisive diagnosis based on the kidney-iliac ratio seems not (yet) possible due to the high standard deviation of the values measured in patients with rejection.

Factors that could cause the wide range of kidney iliac values are:

- differences in the severity of the rejection,
- differences in the type of rejection,
- problems in a close timing of the thrombocyte injection related to the onset of a graft rejection,
- variations in the quantitive interpretation of the scintigraphic results.

Regarding thrombocyte survival curves, there was hardly any difference between the two "stable" groups. During rejection a decreased survival time was found. However, one should realize that this is not a specific finding; apart from rejection other thrombotic complications elsewhere could influence the results as well. If an increased disappearance rate of ^{111}In-thrombocytes is found in the absence of rejection other "hot spots" may be found.

From the generalized results and the longitudinal case studies reported here, we may conclude that gamma-camera scintigraphy, kidney iliac ratio and ^{111}In-thrombocyte survival are useful indicators for rejection and during follow-up after therapy, either successful (patient A) or unsuccessful (patient C). As has been illustrated with patient B it is possible using ^{111}In-thrombocytes, to monitor various events:

- renal artery occlusion (thrombosis),
- kidney graft rejection in an early phase,
- local accumulation of thrombocytes elsewhere (DVT).

Several questions, however, remain unanswered.

What is the earliest possible time a rejection can be diagnosed with this method in relation to other parameters and is this of clinical significance? As has been stated before, the time of injection relative to the onset of rejection may be important. Possibly frequent measurements, using a sensitive portable NaI crystal detector, might give the answer. Such a method is now under investigation in this department.

Another question that still remains open concerns the potential of this method to discriminate between various types of rejection. More extensive histological studies of biopsy material and extirpated grafts in combination with ^{111}In-thrombocyte studies is urgently needed.

Acknowledgements

The authors would like to thank Mrs. E.G.J. Eitjes-van Overbeek and Miss A.J.M. van Velsen for their skilful assistance. This study has been made possible with financial aid from the Dutch Kidney Foundation, grant no. C 186.

REFERENCES

1. Thakur ML, Lavender JP, Anot RN, Silvester DJ, Segal AW, ^{111}In-labeled autologous leukocytes in man. J. nucl. Med. 18:1014, 1977.

2. Frick MP, Henke CE, Forstrom LA, Simmons RA, McCullough J, Loken MK, Use of In-111 labeled leukocytes in evaluation of renal transplant rejection: A preliminary report. Clin. Nucl. Med. 4:24, 1979.

3. Van Royen EA, Van der Schoot JB, Hardeman MR, Surachno S, Ten Veen JH, Vreeken J, Wilmink JM, Use of Indium-111 oxinate labelled granulocytes and thrombocytes in kidney transplantation. In: Medical Radionuclide Imaging, Vol. 1. 1980. Intern. Atomic Energy Agency, Vienna pp 449, 1981.

4. Dabhoiwala MT, Ten Cate HW, Linschoten H, Wilmink JW, Ten Veen JH, Conservative surgical managements of urological complications after cadaveric renal transplantation. J. Urol. 120:290, 1978.

18 CONTINUOUS MONITORING OF HUMAN KIDNEY TRANSPLANTS BY AUTOLOGOUS LABELLED PLATELETS

H. SINZINGER, Ch. LEITHNER, R. HÖFER, L. BOLTZMANN

INTRODUCTION

Platelets seem to participate in nearly all types of kidney transplant rejection, but the degree of involvement differs considerably. Peracute (hyperacute) rejection starts with an aggression of the host's performed antibodies on the endothelial layer of graft vessels. This severe damage induces platelet deposition followed by the formation of a fibrin network (1). The rapidly ongoing process ends within minutes or hours in a total thrombosis of the transplant.

In the vascular type of acute rejection the endothelium can be regarded as the primary battlefield too. Exactly here the immunologic aggression, in part by antibodies directed against endothelial-monocyte antigens, as well as the naturally provided defence mechanisms of the blood-vessels, mainly the release of prostacyclin, exert their opposing effects (2,3). However, the thrombotic alterations develop much slower than in peracute rejection. Besides the histological picture is characterized by proliferative arterial lesions (4). Platelet deposition probably enhances these proliferations by the release of a mitogenic factor (5). The degree of platelet involvement in the rare, interstitial types of acute rejection has not been studied.

Chronic rejection is characterized by obliterative arterial/arteriolar lesions similar as in acute rejection, but showing a higher fibre content due to the slow progression of this disease. Platelets may play here a harmful role by release of mitogenic factor, too.

In 1976 Thakur et al developped a new platelet labelling technique. They used a complex between oxine and ^{111}In, which was avidly phagocytozed by platelets. The short half-life time (67.4 hours) of the γ-rays emitter ^{111}In enabled repeated applications in humans. Therefore this method gained widespread clinical application, also in the field of kidney transplantation (6,7).

In the publication presented here we describe our methodological modification, which allows by quantification of the platelet uptake a higher accuracy and reliability in the diagnosis of graft rejection.

Material and methods

The collective consisted of 75 patients (44 men, 31 women), 8-60 years old (X±SD; 36.2±12.4). The basic renal disease was chronic glomerulonephritis in 70, chronic pyelonephritis in 2, polycystic kidneys in 2, and bilateral Wilms tumours in 1 case. The majority of patients, namely 69, underwent the first transplantation. We collected 25 patients each in one of 3 groups, which were statistically comparable concerning age and sex. In group I the patients were examined during the first 4 weeks after transplantation. For immunosuppression antilymphocyte globulin, prednisolone and azathioprin were applicated. Diagnosis of acute graft rejection was made by observation of clinical symptoms, as fever, swelling of the graft (documented by ultrasonic scan), by decrease of transplant function, as well as by percutaneous or open biopsy in the severe acute rejections. Alterations of transplant function by other diseases, as hydronephrosis, bacterial or viral infections were excluded.

In group II patients with histologically proven chronic transplant rejection* were examined 12-119 months (61±35.4) after transplantation. Clinically the graft function had decreased rather slowly in these cases, showing a plasma creatinine of 4.2±1.7 mg/dl. In this group II, other transplant alterations, which could be misinterpreted as chronic rejection, namely stenosis of the transplant artery anastomosis, hydronephrosis, bacterial and viral infections

---

*Histological diagnosis was kindly provided by Dr. G. Syré, Dept. of Pathology, University of Vienna.

were excluded too.

In group III patients with good and stable graft function were collected at least 9 months (74.5±49.4) after transplantation. The plasma creatinine was in a range of 1.0-2.0 mg/dl at the time of study. For immunosuppression the patients of group II and III were treated with prednisolone and azathioprine. No patient of all groups received aspirin-like drugs.

The platelet labelling was performed in the patients in group I in weekly intervals, in group II and III at least once in each patient. For this purpose 17 ml of blood were drawn by venipuncture with a 1.2 mm needle into 2 syringes (Monovette, Sarstedt, Rommelsdorf, FRG), which contained each 1.5 ml of ACD as anticoagulant and 250 ng prostacyclin (kindly provided by Dr. John E. Pike, The Upjohn Company, Kalamazoo, Michigan, USA). Then platelet-rich plasma (PRP) was obtained and used during separation of the platelet pellet from platelet-poor plasma (PPP). Then a suspension of platelet pellet in 1.0 ml Tyrode-albumin buffer (pH 6.35) was produced. The next step was an incubation of this suspension with 400 µl of ^{111}In-oxine (250 µCi ^{111}In; 50 µg oxine) at 37°C for 5 minutes. ^{111}In-oxine was purchased from Research Center Seibersdorf, Austria. A dilution of the suspension with stored PPP provided a radiolabelled platelet suspension, which was ready for injection.

The patients were examined 2-3 times daily under the gamma camera. This was performed by a computerized static study of 5 minutes duration. At least 20.000 counts each were measured. A constant region of interest was defined for each patient and compaired with the contralateral region having the same size. The quotient of counts (transplant region / control region) termed as platelet uptake index (PUI) served for quantification of platelet trapping. Blood-samples were drawn thrice daily for measurement of platelet half-life time (t/2) by means of surviving curves. For statistical comparison Student's-t-test for paired and unpaired data were used.

Results

In 12 patients of group I 13 episodes of acute rejection were

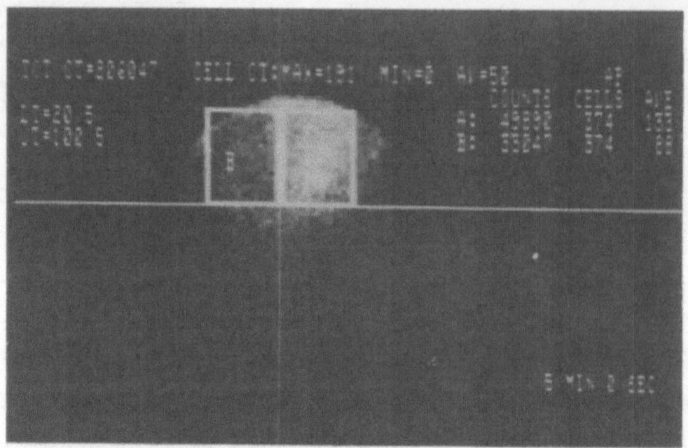

Fig. 1. Platelet trapping by a transplant in the left fossa iliaca region in case of an acute rejection (PUI=1,50).

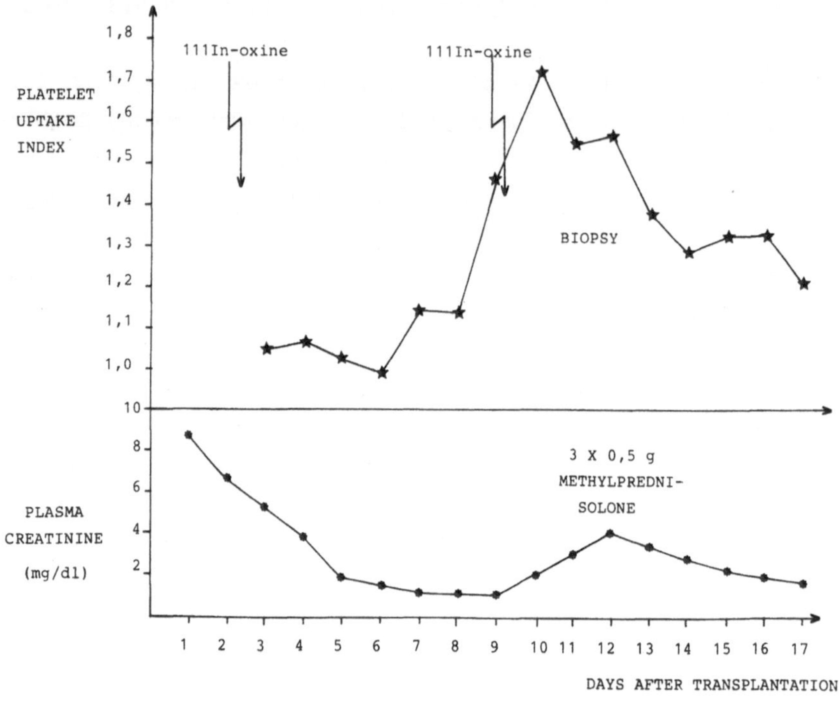

Fig. 2. Postoperative course in a patient demonstrating that the PUI increases much earlier than the rise in plasma creatinine.

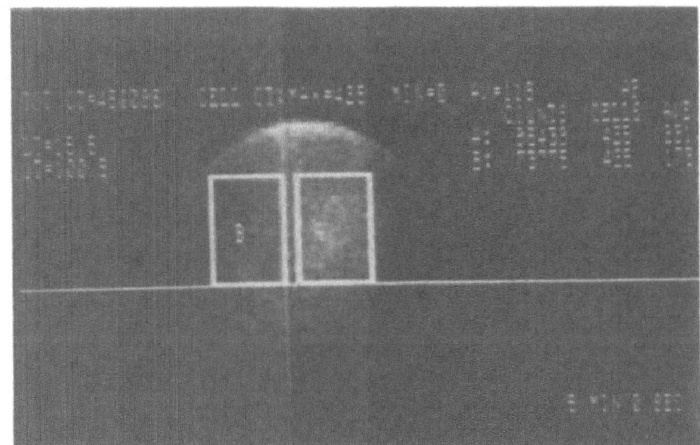

Fig. 3. Patient with chronic transplant rejection, transplant on the left side: (PUI=1,33).

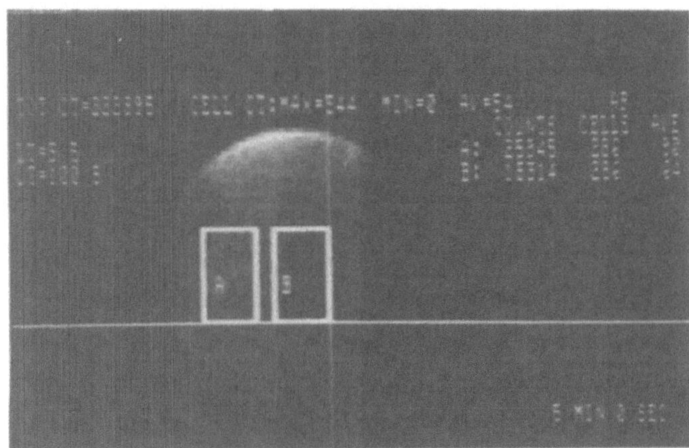

Fig. 4. Stable transplant function, transplant on the right side.

observed. These 12 patients included 2 cases, were oligo-/anuria persisted during the whole observation period. Histological confirmation of clinical diagnosis of rejection was performed in 6 rejections. Biopsy specimen showed 5 acute vascular rejections and 1 acute interstitial rejection. Usually after transplantation there was nearly no platelet trapping by the graft. Up to 24 hours before the onset of clinical symptoms of rejection, the increased platelet trapping occured, resulting in a clear visualization of the graft under the gamma camera. The PUI increased significantly ($p<0.01$) in 12 of 13 acute rejection episodes from 1.13±0.11 to 1.74±0.17 (fig. 1). This increase was observed 0-48 hours (15.5±12.0) before the clinical diagnosis of rejection (fig. 2). The acute interstitial rejection exhibited only a small increase of PUI from 1.3-1.5. The outcome of graft rejection manifested itself in changes of PUI too. Reversible rejections resulted in a decrease c PUI to a level of 1.34±0.10; irreversible rejections showed a high range of 1.76±0.18. One false positive increase of PUI was observe in a transplant haematoma. In 2 other cases an acute rejection was supposed because of clinical symptoms, but the PUI showed normal values. Some days later it became evident that the malfunction of the transplant was caused by a severe pyelonephritis and an absces surrounding the graft respectively. 10 cases of group I showed no graft rejection during the whole observation period and had PUI values of 1.19±0.14.

The cases with chronic transplant rejection (group II) showed only a mild to moderate platelet trapping (fig. 3) by the graft, which became evident in a PUI of 1.33±0.15. The higher the values of PUI in this group the more progressive was the chronic graft re jection. In group III the platelet trapping was usually mild (fig. 4) or missing, resulting in a PUI of 1.08±0.13. This level was statistically significant ($p<0.01$) lower than the PUI values of group II.

The platelet survival correlated usually well with PUI. The platelet half-life (t/2) measured 87.9±18.6 hours before the onset of rejection. Coincidently with the increase of PUI, t/2 fell to 42.4±21.0 hours ($p<0.01$). The outcome of rejection influenced the t/2 values markedly. After reversible rejection t/2 rose again to 83.0±26.8 hours. On the other hand t/2 remained in the low range (47.6±29.9 hours, when rejection became irreversible. The 10 cases in group I without rejection exhibited a nearly normal t/2 of 93.1±21.0 hours. In group II (chronic rejections) the t/2 of 62.2±22.4 hours differed significantly ($p<0.01$) from the t/2 of group III (103.1±18.2 hours).

Discussion

The platelet labelling provided a good diagnostic tool for the early diagnosis of acute transplant rejection. This was particular ly important in cases with oligo- / anuria where diagnosis of acute rejection with non invasive methods is usually difficult.

However, one case of acute intersitial rejection exhibited only a minor increase of PUI. Further studies seem to be necessary for clarification of the question, whether platelets are involved in this type of rejection too. The platelet t/2 was in good accordance with the PUI in acute rejection, which gave a further argument for the reliability. Another method, which uses the involvement of platelets in acute rejection is the immunological demonstration of immunereactive thromboxane B2 (TXB2) in urine (8). Here the urinary excretion of TXB2 which is a sign of platelet activation precedes the onset of clinical symptoms of rejection in a similar way as PUI. However, in our opinion the platelet labelling has the advantage that this diagnostic approach can be performed in oligo- / anuric cases too. False positive increases of PUI can occur in transplant haematoma, but theoretically in recurrence of haemolytic-uraemic syndrome after transplantation too (9). False negative results are possible in thrombocytopenia and due to insufficient platelet labelling.

The increased PUI in chronic rejection confirms earlier observation of an enhanced platelet trapping by such grafts (10). This phenomenon supports our hypothesis that the obliterative arterial lesions of this rejection type are promoted by the platelet-derived growth factor (5). Some patients of group III with good and normal transplant function showed a relatively high PUI of 1.13. It seems possible that these three cases are prone to develop chronic rejection in the future, because they are subjected to harmful platelet deposition.

Summary

^{111}In-oxine labelled autologous platelets were prepared and injected in 75 renal transplant patients, who were collected in 3 groups of 25 persons each. Group I consisted of cases examined during the first 4 weeks after transplantation, group II of patients suffering from histologically proven chronic rejection and group III of cases with good and stable grafts a long time after transplantation. The grafts were monitored by gamma camera imaging and the calculation of a platelet-uptake index (PUI), as well as by estimation of platelet t/2. For diagnosis of acute rejection the platelet scan was of great help, when PUI rose from 1.13±0.11 to 1.74±0.17. The further outcome of graft rejection, reversible or irreversible, documented itself in a decrease or a sustaining high level of PUI respectively. The PUI of patients with chronic rejection differed significantly from those of cases with long-term stable grafts. The platelet t/2 correlated well with PUI. The possible pitfalls of this method giving a false positive result are haematomas and theoretically the recurrence of haemolytic-uraemic syndrome after transplantation. All in all we regard this method as a number of important and conclusive stones in the rather complex mosaic of rejection diagnosis.

REFERENCES

1. Leithner Ch, Piza-Katzer H, Kruzik P, Winter M, Mayr WR, Stachelberger H, Sinzinger H, A study of hyperacute rejection of renal transplants using scanning electron microscopy. Dialysis & Transplantation 10:336, 1981.

2. Claas FHJ, Paul LC, Van Es LA, Van Rood JJ, Antibodies against donor antigen on endothelial cells and monocytes in eluates of rejected kidney allografts. Tissue Antigens 15:19, 1980.

3. Leithner Ch,Sinzinger H, Silberbauer K, Wolf A, Stummvoll HK, Pinggera W, Enhanced prostacyclin synthesis in acute human kidney transplant rejection. Proc. Europ. Dial. & Transpl. Assoc. 17:424, 1980.

4. Kincaid-Smith P, Histological diagnosis of rejection of renal homografts in man. Lancet 11:849, 1967.

5. Ross R, Glomset JA, The pathogenesis of atherosclerosis. New Engl. J. Med. 295:369, 1976.

6. Thakur ML, Welch MJ, Joist JH, Coleman RE, Indium-111-labelled platelets: Studies on preparation and evaluation of in vitro and in vivo functions. Thromb. Res. 9:345, 1976.

7. Smith N, Chandler S, Hawker LM, Barnes AD, Indium-111 labelled autologous platelets as diagnostic aid after renal transplantation. Lancet 11:1241, 1979.

8. Foegh ML, Zmudka M, Cooley C, Winchester JF, Helfrich GB, Ramwell PW, Schreiner GE, Urine i-TXB2 in renal allograft rejection. Lancet 11:431, 1981.

9. Fenech A, Bennet B, Catto GRD, Edward N, Douglas AS, Smith FW, Sharp PF, Parry-Jones D, Diagnosis of post-transplant renal haematoma with autologous Indium-111 labelled platelets. Lancet 1:1250, 1980.

10. Leithner Ch, Sinzinger H, Angelberger P, Syre G, Indium-111-labellet platelets in chronic kidney transplant rejection. Lancet 11:213, 1980.

19 USE OF ^{111}IN-LABELLED PLATELETS IN CARDIOVASCULAR DISEASE

J. VREEKEN, M.R. HARDEMAN, G.D.C. VOSMAER, E.A. VAN ROYEN, J.B. VAN DER SCHOOT, D.R. DÜREN

INTRODUCTION

Blood platelets play a key role in haemostasis, thrombosis and in all probability in atherosclerosis. Labelling autologous blood platelets with ^{111}In by means of complexing ^{111}In with the lipid soluble compound oxine makes it possible after reinjection of the platelets to study their in-vivo role in atherosclerosis and thrombosis by means of a gamma camera. In the human, ^{111}In-oxine is bound to the cytoplasm of the platelet when the label is brought together with a platelet suspension. So even after release of alpha granulae and dense bodies from the platelets a positive ^{111}In labelled platelet scan can theoretically still be obtained. It is clear that for a positive scan a certain minimal amount of ^{111}In labelled platelets is necessary. The role of blood platelets in different thrombi (e.g. venous, arterial and in aneurysms) is different. At forehand, therefore, it can be anticipated that the contribution of the blood platelet scan for the study of the pathogenesis of thrombosis in those different thrombi is not the same.

Venous thrombi

Venous thrombi are supposed to originate in the valve pockets of veins starting with a relative small platelet nidus which develops without a clearly visible local vessel wall abnormality. When venous stasis takes place sometimes a rather long venous thrombus may develop of which the tail is "clot like". In this clot like tail blood platelets, like other blood cells, are captured more or less at random. Clinical symptoms develop when veins are largely occluded, when clinical inflammation of the vessel wall occurs or when a pulmonary embolus suddenly develops. Therefore one may expect a positive ^{111}In-oxine labelled platelet scan only under certain circumstances (e.g. during the early development of the thrombus) and perhaps often no longer at the moment when the patient presents himself with symptoms of venous thrombosis, provided that the injection is given at that time. In cases of venous stasis one must always be aware of the possibility that every element of the blood (also blood platelets) may be present in an area of intensive pooling of blood by stasis without representing a thrombus mass. One may anticipate that only in the situation when marked platelets are circulating before venous thrombosis develops hot spots can be obtained. Compared with the ^{125}I-fibrinogen method the advantage of ^{111}In-labelled platelets is that the latter can be made visible with the gamma camera also in the upper extremities and the pelvic area. One can assume that the amount of fibrinogen as fibrin in a venous thrombus is relatively more than the amount of platelets. However, ^{125}I has a low gamma energy and besides that the specific activity of the preparation has to be taken into account.

Fenech and co-workers (1) indeed showed in 33 post-operative patients, who got ^{111}In-labelled platelets as a routine procedure (so there were "marked" platelets circulating at the moment of the development of the thrombosis), a good positive correlation between phlebographic results and ^{111}In scan. Remarkable enough, however, they also found a similar correlation in 15 patient who were suspected for chronic thrombosis. Even in a patient in which the thrombus was supposed to be 5 weeks old at the moment of investigation. Therefore the use of ^{111}In-labelled platelets in clinical venous thrombosis has to be evaluated further in order to find the real place of this technique in diagnosis. Regarding venous thrombosis we have had only one occasional observation: when studying a patient with ^{111}In-labelled platelets for renal transplant rejection the patient developed a hot spot (outside the region of interest) which turned out to be thrombosis of the vena femoralis as could be demonstrated by phlebography. However, as can be seen at the phlebogram the thrombus is much larger than the platelet hot spot.

Arterial thrombosis

Artherial thrombosis platelets are supposed to play a much more important role than in venous thrombosis, although the clinical presentation does not correlate with the amount of thrombus in the nourishing artery. Especially in early phases of cardiac ischaemia spasm of the coronary artery can contribute to the clinical picture As has been shown (2) the release of platelet granular concent is an intermittent phenomenon in cardiac ischaemia. It seems plausible therefore that the contribution of platelets to cardiac ischaemia is early and intermittent. Whereas the time for a patient to reach the hospital after a heart attack is about 3 hours, at least in our town, it does not seem very probable that ^{111}In-labelled platelet scan can contribute very much to the solution of the question: what happened in the early phases of coronary artery occlusion, provided that the resolving power of the technique is large enough. However there are no studies on this point.

Contribution of platelet scanning can be expected, however, in the study of large arterial lesions at which surface thrombi are formed and platelets are taken up as a more or less continuous process. In this way one can think of extensive ulcerative atherosclerotic lesions in big arteries (e.g. carotids) and of atherosclerotic aneurysms and aneurysma cordis. Positive results with ^{111}In labelled blood platelets in these categories are mentioned in the literature. Our own experience is in agreement on this point. David et al (3,4,5) reported ^{111}In platelet deposition on 20 of the 33 arteriographically found carotic atherosclerotic lesions in 23 patients. As found by Powers (6) there was no relation between platelet positive scans in cerebrovascular disease and prognosis of the patients. Ritchie et al (7) found in 12 of 18 patient with abdominal aortic aneurysms positive platelet scans. Although the presence of a thrombotic mass in the other 6 patients was also suspected. This suggests that incorporation of platelets is not a continuous process in the aneurysm of the abdominal aorta or, alternatively, sometimes presents as such a low level that it cannot be made visible with this technique. However ^{111}In-labelled blood platelets are in general taken up in aortic aneurysm in a relative high degree.

With regard to arterial thrombi our own results include 9 aortic aneurysms of which 6 were positive and 3 dissecting aneurysms, all three were positive.

Left ventricular aneurysms

In left ventricular aneurysms positive ^{111}In platelet scans have been reported by Stratton and co-workers (8), Ezekowitz and co-workers (9) and Hardeman and co-workers (10). Platelet studies do not always give the same results as 2 dimensional echocardiography studies. Stratton (8) reports 6 discrepancies in 15 patients. Ezekowitz (9) does not find any discrepancy between the results found by ^{111}In platelet scanning and those proven by surgery or at post mortem in 17 patients /5 positive scans, 12 negative scans). It seems to be so that the single presence of a thrombotic mass in a ventricular wall aneurysm does not guarantee that platelets are taken up all the time, so such a mass is not always "active". Our own results include: 14 cardiac aneurysms of which 4 had a positive ^{111}In-labelled platelet scan, 3 of them were operated and all had a thrombus mass, 1 patient with a negative scan had a thrombus mass at operation. In this patient the thrombus was shown with 2D-echography, on the other hand one of the patients with a positive scan (shown with operation) had a negative 2D-echography.

A problem in the study of the presence of a thrombus in an aneurysm is that a non-specific pooling of blood in the aneurysm may also cause a concentration of activity without representing the presence of a thrombus. Non-specific blood pooling can be corrected for by a blood pool scan with Tc^{99m} labelled erythrocytes performed at the same time. After subtraction of this activity a still positive ^{111}In scan can be obtained rather soon after injection of the platelets (fig. 1a, 1b, 1c). Another possibility is the delay of at least 48 hours between injection and scintigraphy during which time circulating ^{111}In platelets become in equilibrium with all physiological body spaces and eventually more ^{111}In platelets have had time to accumulate in the region of interest. Thus the study of ^{111}In-labelled platelets seem to teach us something about thrombogenesis under certain circumstances.

An interesting possibility is to study the influence of drugs

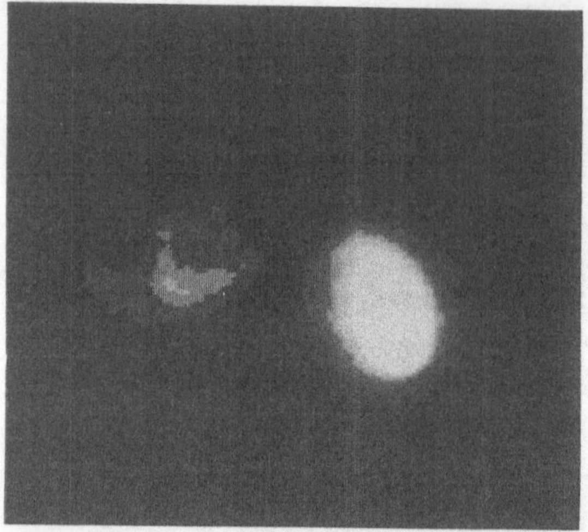

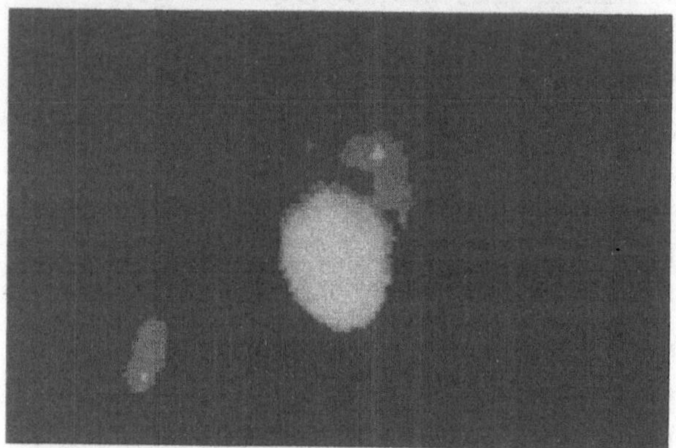

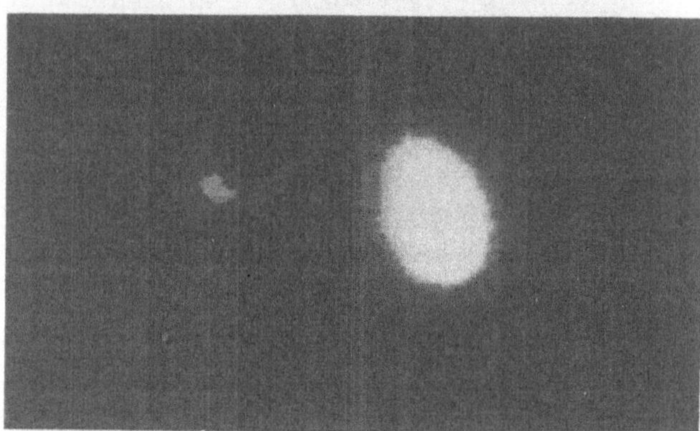

Fig. 1. Scintigraphy of a patient with an aneurysm cordis; a) 24 h after injection of ^{111}In thrombocytes. b) Immediately after injection of Tc^{99m} erythrocytes (blood pool background). c) result of the ^{111}In thrombocyte scan after computer-assisted subtraction of blood-pool background

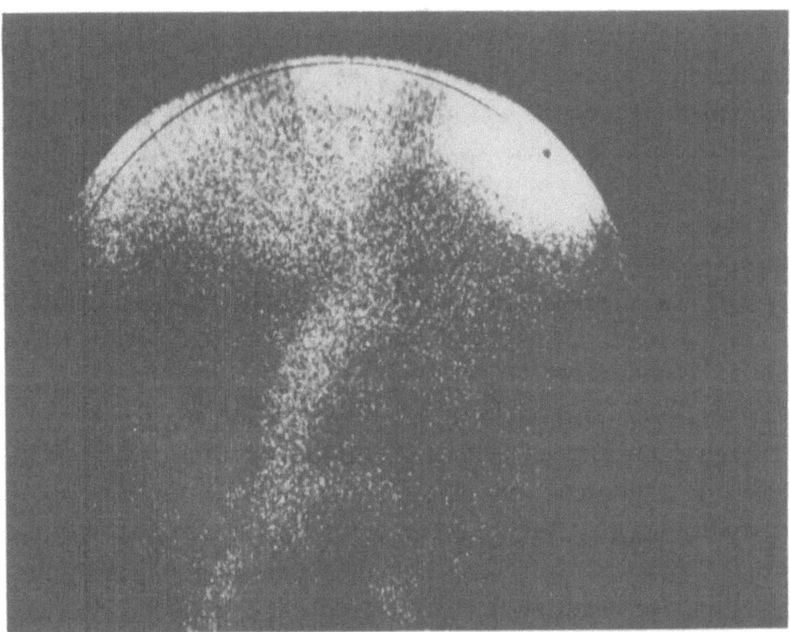

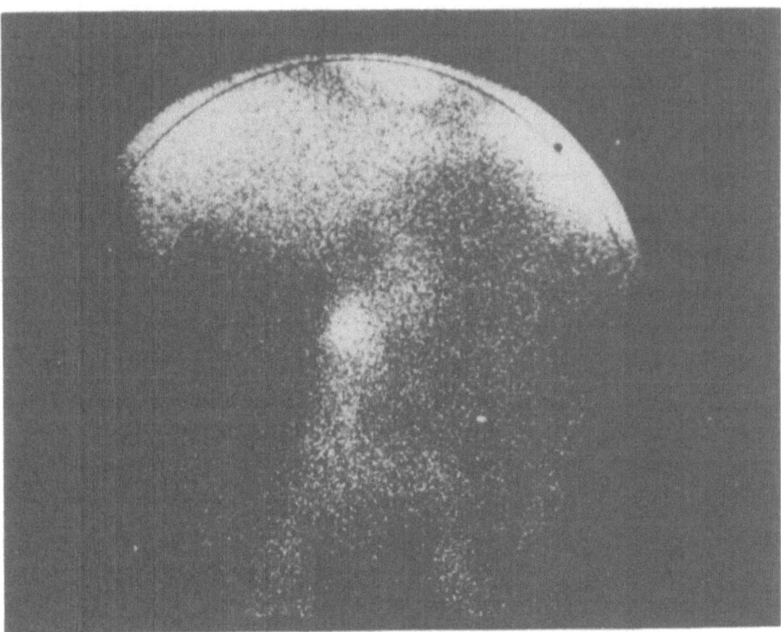

Fig. 2. Scintigraphy of a patient with an aneurysm aorta; a). 24 h after injection of ^{111}In thrombocytes. b) The same, however, after treatment with ASA.

on the accumulation of platelets in this situation. We found a great therapeutic dosis of coumarin does not prevent the accumulation of platelet at aortic and cardiac aneurysms. This does not imply that coumarins are not usefull in those patients. Because a luxurious formation of fibrin around the platelet nidus can perhap be prevented or reduced by coumarin treatment and therefore emboli may be prevented or reduced in frequency by coumarin, in spite of the fact that the incorporation of platelets in the nidus is not altered. Still more interesting is the possibility to study the influence of drugs which are supposed to have their main action on platelet function on the accumulation of platelets.

We studied the influence of aspirin (dose 500 mg/day) on the accumulation of platelets at aortic aneurysm and found that after aspirin the quantity of platelets accumulated in an aneurysm at least did not decrease (fig. 2a, 2b). The same was found by Ritchi et al (7), who also combined aspirin with dipyridamole. These investigators found in two of the four patients with abdominal aneurysms a decrease of ^{111}In platelet incorporation after sulfinpyrazone. So the study of ^{111}In-labelled platelets seems to enable us to deepen the insight in the pathogenesis of certain thrombotic processes, especially thrombi in aneurysms and at gross atherosclerotic lesions. Besides that is possible to study the factors which influence this incorporation especially also the influence of platelet active drugs.

REFERENCES

1. Fenech A, Hussey JK, Smith FW, Bendey BP, Bennett B, Douglas AS, Diagnosis of deep vein thrombosis using autologous Indium-111 platelets. Br. med. J. 1:1020, 1981.

2. De Boer AC, Beta-thromboglobuline. Studies in arterial venous thrombo-embolism. Thesis Amsterdam, 1982.

3. Davis HH, Heaton WA, Siegel BA, Mathias CJ, Joist JH, Sherman LA, Welch MJ, Scintigraphic detection of atherosclerotic lesions and venous thrombi in man by Indium-111 labelled autologous platelets. Lancet 1:1185, 1978.

4. Davis HH, Siegel BA, Sherman LA, Heaton WA, Welch MJ, Scintigraphy with III-In-labelled autologous platelets in venous thrombo-embolism. Radiology 136:203, 1980.

5. Davis HH, Siegel BA, Sherman LA, Heaton WA, Naidich TP, Joist JH, Welch MJ, Scintigraphic detection of carotid atherosclerosis with Indium-111-labelled autologous platelets. Circulation 61: 982, 1980.

6. Powers WJ, Siegel BA, Mathias CJ, Davis HH, Welch MJ, Scintigraphy with Indium-111 platelets in cerebrovascular disease. Neurology (Minneap.) 31:55, 1981 (abstract).

7. Ritchie JL, Stratton JR, Thiele B, Hamilton GW, Warrick LN, Huang TW, Harker LA, Indium-111 platelet imaging for detection of platelet deposition in abdominal aneurysms and prosthetic arterial grafts. Amer. J. Cardiol. 47:882, 1981.

8. Stratton JR, Ritchie JL, Hamilton GW, Hammermeister KE, Harker LA, Left ventricular thrombi: In vivo detection by Indium-111 platelet imaging and two dimensional echocardiography. Amer. J. Cardiol. 47:874, 1981.

9. Ezekowitz MD, Leonard JC, Smith EO, Allen EW, Taylor FB, Identification of left ventricular thrombi in man using Indium-111-labelled autologous platelets. Circulation 63:803, 1981.

10. Hardeman MR, Vreeken J, Van der Schoot JB, The detection and localization of arterial thrombotic processes with autologous Indium-111-labelled thrombocytes: first results.In: Progress in Radiopharmacology, Vol.2. Cox PH (ed), Elsevier/North-Holland Biomedical Press, Amsterdam,1981.

20 HOMOCYSTINURIA: KINETICS AND DISTRIBUTION OF ^{111}IN-LABELLED PLATELETS

R.L. HILL-ZOBEL, R.E. PYERITZ, U. SCHEFFEL, O. MALPICA, S. ENGIN, E.E. CAMARGO, M. ABBOTT, T.R. GUILARTE, J. HILL, P.A. McINTYRE, E.A. MURPHY, MIN-FU TSAN

INTRODUCTION

The pathogenesis of thromboembolism, a major cause of morbidity and mortality, in patients with homocystinuria due to cystathionine beta-synthase deficiency remains unclear. Two previous studies of platelet survival using the ^{51}Cr label have produced conflicting results. In this study, we have investigated the kinetics and biodistribution of ^{111}In-oxine labelled platelets in 11 normal volunteers and 12 homocystinuric patients, none of whom had clinical evidence of acute thrombosis at the time of the study. Six of the patients were pyridoxine resistant and had homocystinemia. There were no statistical differences in mean platelet survival times between pyridoxine responders and non-responders, and pyridoxine responders or non-responders and normals, regardless of whether a linear, exponential, weighted mean, or multiple-hit model was used to analyze the kinetic data. By the multiple-hit estimate model, which best fitted the kinetic data, the mean platelet survival time (MPS)for homocystinuric patients was 7.92 days (SEM = 0.30 days) compared with 8.40 days (SEM = 0.25 days) for the normals ($p>0.1$). Plasma homocystine levels had no apparent effect on mean platelet survival time. There was no abnormal accumulation of platelets in any of the patients and the distribution of platelets in liver and spleen was similar to that in normal controls. Our results suggest that the kinetics and distribution of platelets in patients with homocystinuria who have no clinical evidence of thromboembolism are normal. Thus, the data do not provide evidence for disordered platelet function or for an ongoing interaction of platelets with vessel wall in this condition.

Homocystinuria due to cystathionine beta-synthase deficiency is an inborn error of metabolism involving the transsulfuration of amino acids (1-9). Affected individuals accumulate homocystine and methionine in plasma and tissues and excrete homocystine and mixed disulfides in the urine. The untreated condition is characterized by clinically variable, pleiotropic features: ectopia lentis, skeletal deformity, osteoporosis, mental retardation and a high frequency of thromboembolism. Some patients with this disorder are responsive to pharmacologic doses of pyridoxine (vitamine B_6), while others are resistant (6,8-10).

Whether platelets are involved in the pathogenesis of thrombosis in this disorder remains uncertain. Harker and co-workers (11,12) reported a marked decrease in ^{51}Cr-platelet survival time in four homocystinuric patients without clinical evidence of acute thrombosis at the time of the study (mean = 4.3 days, SD = 0.6 days, as compared to normal figures of mean = 9.5 days, SD = 0.6 days). Treatment with pyridoxine in two pyridoxine-responsive patients and with dipyridamole in two pyridoxine-unresponsive patients restored platelet survival times to near-normal. In contrast, Uhlemann and co-workers (13) studied six homocystinuric patients using ^{51}Cr-platelets and found normal mean platelet survival times. Confronted with these conflicting data and the potentially devastating consequences of thromboembolism, clinicians have frequently opted for treating homocystinuric patients with medications that interfere with platelet function (8,9,11). Abnormal turnover or sequestration of platelets, such as might occur during active thrombosis or in response to homocystine-induced endothelial injury, would strengthen the rationale for antiplatelet therapy.

Recently introduced as a platelet label, ^{111}In-oxine offers several advantages over ^{51}Cr-sodium chromate (14-16). The labelling efficiency of ^{111}In-oxine for platelets is higher than that of ^{51}Cr. Gamma photons with energies of 173 keV (84%) and 247 keV (94%) are emitted by ^{111}In as compared to

320 keV (9%) for ^{51}Cr. Because of these emissions, it is possible to quantitate the in vivo distribution of ^{111}In-platelets by external imaging.

We have studied the survival and in vivo distribution of ^{111}In-platelets in homocystinuric patients and normal volunteers (16,17), as part of our attempt to define the causes, natural history, and therapy of thromboembolism in cystathionine beta-synthase deficiency.

Methods

Patients. 12 homocystinuric patients (table 1), between 16 and 61 years of age, were admitted to the Clinical Research Unit of the Johns Hopkins Hospital for this study. All patients had previously documented homocystinemia, homocystinuria, and clinical findings compatible with cystathionine beta-synthase deficiency. 4 patients (2,5-7) had cystathionine beta-synthase deficiency established by enzyme assay of cultured skin fibroblasts (18,19). Patients 1-6 were considered pyridoxine-responsive because plasma methionine and homocystine levels were normalized at least 2 weeks after beginning oral treatment with pyridoxine 500 mg and folic acid 10 mg daily. Patients 7-12 showed no response to this regimen. Accordingly, patients 1-5 continued on pyridoxine and folic acid. Patient 6 continued on pyridoxine but, inadvertently, not folic acid. 2 patients, 5 and 9, were taking phenobarbital for past episodes of seizures. Patient 3 was taking thyroid hormone replacement and patient 12 was taking methyldopa and chlorothiazide for hypertension. Alcohol consumption, cigarette smoking, and all other medications, including those containing aspirin, were discontinued 2 weeks before and throughout the 12-day study period.

Clinical histories of cerebral thromboembolic events were present in patients 1,2,5,7 and 9. Four patients, 3,4,7 and 10 had histories of lower limb thrombophlebitis. At the time of this study, none of the 12 patients had acute thrombosis evident by history or examination.

The diet during the study was patient-selected from an

TABLE 1. PATIENT PROFILE

HOMOCYSTINURIC PATIENT #	AGE	SEX	TAKING B_6	TAKING FOLATE	HISTORY OF THROMBOEMBOLIC EPISODE: CVA *	HISTORY OF THROMBOEMBOLIC EPISODE: THROMBOPHLEBITIS	NORMAL CONTROL #	AGE	SEX
1	41	F	+	-	+	-	1	20	M
2	29	F	+	+	+	-	2	32	M
3	61	M	+	+	-	+	3	23	M
4	40	F	+	+	-	+	4	23	M
5	24	M	+	+	+	-	5	23	M
6	22	F	+	-	-	-	6	39	M
7	41	F	-	-	+	+	7	31	M
8	27	M	-	-	-	-	8	26	M
9	16	M	-	-	+	-	9	23	M
10	32	M	-	-	-	+	10	23	M
11	24	F	-	-	-	-	11	21	M
12	48	M	-	-	-	-			

* Cerebral Vascular Accident.

unmodified regular hospital menu. Daily calory, protein, methionine, and cystine intake were determined by a dietician; the range of average values for all patients over the 12-day study were: 1215-3160 calories, 45-150 grams protein, 1050-4000 mg methionine, and 700-2000 mg cystine per day.

Controls for platelet survival studies were normal male volunteer outpatients whose ages ranged from 20 to 39 years (table 1).

Written informed consent was obtained from all volunteers, and patients or their parents and the study was approved by the Joint Committee on Clinical Investigation of the Johns Hopkins Medical Institutions.

Platelet survival studies. The method of platelet labelling with ^{111}In-oxine in autologous plasma and survival curve analysis have been described previously (14-16,20,21). Briefly, ^{111}In-Cl_3 (Mediphysics, Emeryville, California) was chelated with 8-hydroxyquinoline (oxine), extracted, evaporated to dryness, and dissolved in a mixture of ethanol and normal saline containing approximately 16 µg oxine in a final volume of 100 µl.

Platelets from 50 ml of venous blood were harvested with acid-citrate-dextrose (ACD) as the anticoagulant and labelled in an aseptic open test-tube system as described previously (16). All patients and controls had platelet counts within normal ranges. Briefly, all procedures were done in a laminar flow hood with sterile equipment and supplies. Platelet-rich plasma (PRP) was obtained by centrifuging the blood for 10 min at 220 g. The platelets were sedimented into a button by spinning the PRP for 10 min at 1000 g. The platelet button was then resuspended in 2 ml of platelet-poor plasma (PPP) and incubated with 750-1300 µCi (28-48 megabecquerels-MBq) 111In-oxine for 60 min at room temperature. Unbound ^{111}In was removed by washing the platelets with 5 volumes of PPP. The supernatant PPP was removed and the radiolabelled platelets resuspended in 7-10 ml PPP. Contaminating red blood cells were removed by centrifugation at 150 g for 5 min. The platelet suspension, with a maximum activity of 160 µCi (5.9 MBq), was drawn into a syringe. (This is equivalent to a radiation dose of 5 rads (0.05 grays) to the spleen (16)). A dose calibrator (Mediac, Nuclear-Chicago, Des Plaines, Illinois) was used to determine the activity injected by measuring the syringe before and after infusion of the ^{111}In-labelled platelets. The volume injected was determined by weighing the syringe before and after the infusion.

Following intravenous infusion of 115-160 µCi (4.3-5.9 MBq) ^{111}In-platelets, blood-samples of 14-21 ml were obtained at 90 min post-infusion and daily thereafter for 10 days. The platelet counts, measured with a Coulter Counter (Florida), and the hematocrit were determined on each sample. Separate aliquots of 3-5 ml whole blood, lysed with saponin, and 2 ml plasma, diluted to 5 ml with water, were prepared in duplicate for measurement of radioactivity. Aliquots of 50 µl of the ^{111}In-platelet injectate in 5 ml water were used as standards. All were counted to less than 3% statistical counting error in an Auto-Gamma system (Packard Instruments Co, Downers Grove, Illinois). The results were expressed as percentages of injected dose in circulating platelets assuming a blood-volume of 65 ml/kg for females and 70 ml/kg for males. Correction of blood-volume estimation due to obesity or cachexia was done according to Wright (23). The mean of the duplicate measurements on each sample was used for analysis.

To estimate mean platelet survival time, the experimental data were subjected to computer analysis. 3 mathematical models were used for normal curve fitting: a linear model, an exponential model, and a maximum-likelihood estimate of the integer-order gamma function multiple-hit model (the first two being special cases of the latter) (20,21). Also, the weighted mean of the linear and exponential estimates was calculated (21). The residual sum of squares was used as a measure of the precision of the curve fitting. The power of a one-tailed t-test was calculated at the 0.05 significance level based on the results of the multiple-hit estimates for MPST (22).

In vivo quantification studies. For quantification of ^{111}In-activity in liver and spleen, a modification of the geometric computation for correction of photon attenuation was used. This method has previously been validated in both phantom and animal studies (16,24,25). In brief, the overall effective transmission factor (Tr) was determined before infusion of the ^{111}In-platelets. This was accomplished by placing the patient's upper abdominal and lower chest areas directly on top of a 38 inch diameter flood source containing 650-850 µCi (24-32 MBq) ^{111}In. A 500.000 (500 K) count static image was obtained with a large field-of-view camera (Technicare, Cleveland, Ohio) coupled to a 280 keV medium sensitivity parallel-hole collimator and data processing system (VIP, Technicare, Cleveland, Ohio). The pulse-height analyzer was peaked to include the 247 keV photopeak with a 20% window. A second 500 K count image was acquired of the flood source only. Liver and spleen regions were outlined using a light pen. The ratio of counts transmitted through the organ of interest to the unfiltered flood counts in the same region represents Tr.

The ^{111}In-platelets were infused with the patient positioned supine under the camera. Anterior scintigraphic images were obtained immediately after infusion. Five 60-sec and five 250-sec images were sequentially obtained. At 30 and 90 min and daily thereafter for 3 days, anterior and posterior views containing from 80 K to 170 K counts of the liver/spleen regions were acquired for each patient. No imaging was done for patient 5. Liver and spleen regions were drawn with a light pen and the counts per region were expressed as C_a (anterior) and C_p (posterior) for each organ. To determine the sensitivity (S) of the imaging system in counts per µCi, a standard was prepared in a 600 ml plastic culture flask containing 140-400 µCi ^{111}In in 100 ml of acidified ethylenediamine tetra-acetic acid (EDTA). Daily images of the standard flask were acquired. The equation used to compute the percentage of the injected dose in the organ of interest was:

$$\% \text{ Injected Dose} = 100 \left((C_a)(C_p)/Tr \right)^{\frac{1}{2}} (S^{-1}) (P^{-1}),$$

where P = µCi of ^{111}In-platelets injected. These values were used to generate time-activity curves of organ radioactivity.

In addition to images obtained for the in vivo quantification studies, anterior images of the head, upper chest, and lower extremities were acquired at 24 hours after the infusion of the ^{111}In-platelets. These were screened for any area of abnormal accumulation of ^{111}In-platelets.

Amino acid analysis. Samples of plasma, obtained after an overnight fast on the first and last days of the study, were immediately deproteinized with sulfosalicylic acid. The levels of plasma amino acids were determined with an amino acid analyzer (Beckman 121MB, Palo Alto, California), as described by Spackman (26).

Vitamin assays. Blood from fasting patients was obtained at the beginning and end of the study by venipuncture and aseptically transferred to heparinized vacutainer tubes. Exposure to light was minimized to prevent degradation of vitamin B_6 compounds. The methods for the radiometric-microbiological assay of plasma vitamin B_6, B_{12}, folate, and red blood-cell folate have been previously reported (27,28).

Results

Table 2 shows the plasma amino acid levels in the 12 homocystinuric subjects. None of the 6 pyridoxine-responsive patients who were taking vitamin B_6 (1-6) had detectable plasma homocystine, and their methionine and cystine levels were within the normal range. Of the patients taking folate (1-5), none were deficient in vitamin B_6, B_{12}, or folate. The 6 pyridoxine non-responsive patients (7-12), none of whom were taking B_6 or folate, had all detectable plasma homocystine levels at values similar to those described by Harker (11,12) and Uhlemann (13). In addition, their plasma methionine levels were abnormally high and cystine levels abnormally low. Patients 7-12 were all deficient in vitamin B_6, patients 9 and 11 had low levels of vitamin B_{12}, and patients 7-11 were deficient in folate.

The kinetics of the ^{111}In-labelled platelets were presented in table 3. Using a one-tailed t test, there were no statistically significant differences in mean platelet survival

TABLE 2: AMINO ACID AND VITAMIN LEVELS IN HOMOCYSTINURIC PATIENTS

PATIENT	PLASMA AMINO ACID LEVELS (mM) *,†			VITAMIN LEVELS *,§			
#	HOMOCYSTINE	METHIONINE	½ CYSTINE	B_6	B_{12}	FOLATE	RBC FOLATE
1	N , N	0.024, 0.130	0.130, 0.098	94, 78	387, 365	24, 29	567, 548
2	N , N	0.013, 0.033	0.090, 0.143	107, 114	383, 330	10, 6	268, 323
3	N , ND	0.036, ND	0.129, ND	61, 164	290, 300	30, 31	543, 512
4	N , N	0.035, 0.053	0.095, 0.098	128,>400	310, 217	52, 22	718, 811
5	ND , T	ND , 0.032	ND , 0.064	>200,>200	510, 480	22, 13	661, 684
6	N , N	0.028, 0.049	0.081, 0.120	380,>400	310, 217	2, 0.8	36, 37
7	0.050, 0.082	0.928, 0.805	0.025, 0.026	1.3, 1.4	170, 125	5.5, 4.4	125, 127
8	0.084, 0.106	0.296, 0.257	0.023, 0.049	2.6, 2.2	220, 198	3.5, 2.5	88, 95
9	0.118, 0.096	0.072, 0.064	0.045, 0.005	2.7, 1.2	108, 85	3.7, 2.7	53, 46
10	0.086, 0.055	0.112, 0.507	0.046, 0.030	2.4, 3.8	263, 318	1.4, 2.8	74, 78
11	0.110, 0.097	0.103, 0.451	0.025, 0.010	<1, <1	115, 110	2.7, 2.4	108, 87
12	0.028, 0.048	0.124, 0.080	0.051, 0.030	<1, 1.3	170, 170	4.1, 4.3	213, 208

* VALUES REPRESENT THOSE OF PRE-STUDY AND POST-STUDY, RESPECTIVELY. N = NONE DETECTED; ND = NOT DONE; T = TRACE.

† NORMAL CONTROL LEVELS: METHIONINE (0.001-0.049 mM); ½ CYSTINE (0.044-0.096 mM); HOMOCYSTINE (0 mM).

§ CRITERIA FOR VITAMIN DEFICIENCY: <3 ng B_6/ml PLASMA: <120 pg B_{12}/ml PLASMA; <3 ng FOLATE/ml PLASMA; <140 ng FOLATE/ml RED BLOOD CELLS.

TABLE 3. KINETICS OF ^{111}In-LABELED PLATELETS IN PATIENTS WITH HOMOCYSTINURIA AND NORMAL CONTROLS *

PATIENT	PLATELET COUNT(#/µl)†		LINEAR		EXPONENTIAL		WT'D MEAN	MULTIPLE-HIT			
#	MEAN	SEM	MPST	RSS	MPST	RSS	MPST	MPST	RSS	% RECOVERY	# HITS
Pyridoxine Responders											
1	232,000	3,200	10.25	0.0029	4.10	0.0467	9.89	9.87	0.0020	61.9	27
2	234,000	4,800	8.95	0.0023	3.57	0.0097	7.91	7.59	0.0003	39.4	7
3	115,000	1,600	8.64	0.0196	2.15	0.1446	7.87	6.88	0.0064	47.3	17
4	243,000	5,400	9.25	0.0089	3.12	0.0249	7.63	6.90	0.0019	45.3	5
5	229,000	11,700	9.16	0.0040	2.82	0.0466	8.66	7.94	0.0006	39.0	15
6	343,000	5,200	9.56	0.0021	3.21	0.0302	9.15	8.67	0.0003	36.6	19
Pyridoxine Nonresponders											
7	203,000	3,600	10.12	0.0078	3.85	0.0712	9.50	9.72	0.0067	62.7	31
8	334,000	6,500	9.81	0.0045	3.76	0.0151	8.42	7.80	0.0012	44.4	5
9	287,000	7,000	8.64	0.0062	3.13	0.0462	7.99	7.41	0.0006	62.6	9
10	262,000	13,000	9.00	0.0030	2.51	0.0344	8.48	7.38	0.0005	28.5	11
11	328,000	7,000	9.26	0.0108	3.06	0.0431	8.02	6.67	0.0017	55.9	9
12	376,000	5,000	9.83	0.0076	3.84	0.0298	8.62	8.21	0.0003	62.6	7
Normal Volunteers											
1	281,000	8,400	11.64	0.0137	4.15	0.0374	9.63	9.80	0.0039	46.8	11
2	251,000	6,300	10.08	0.0170	3.42	0.0786	8.89	8.20	0.0053	64.1	7
3	259,000	8,100	9.94	0.0161	3.03	0.1563	9.30	8.57	0.0031	60.9	17
4	213,000	5,000	10.51	0.0133	3.90	0.0383	8.81	7.48	0.0043	59.7	3
5	273,000	5,700	9.84	0.0074	3.74	0.0410	8.91	9.23	0.0063	43.3	19
6	331,000	10,200	8.92	0.0323	2.75	0.1683	7.93	6.63	0.0091	79.0	5
7	177,000	3,100	9.64	0.0071	3.48	0.0658	9.04	8.53	0.0011	59.5	12
8	217,000	3,700	9.30	0.0060	2.62	0.3031	9.17	8.76	0.0019	61.9	50
9	278,000	4,600	9.15	0.0085	2.76	0.1322	8.77	8.11	0.0018	55.0	19
10	206,000	5,700	9.27	0.0096	2.78	0.1468	8.88	8.35	0.0036	62.3	22
11	346,000	5,900	9.56	0.0054	3.13	0.1219	9.28	8.78	0.0005	66.5	23
Pyridoxine Responders (n=6)											
MEAN	233,000		9.30		3.16		8.52	7.98		44.9	15
SEM	29,500		0.23		0.27		0.36	0.47		3.8	--
Pyridoxine Nonresponders (n=6)											
MEAN	298,000		9.44		3.36		8.51	7.87		52.8	11
SEM	25,000		0.23		0.22		0.22	0.43		5.7	--
All Homocystinuric Patients (n=12)											
MEAN	266,000		9.37		3.26		8.51	7.92		48.8	13
SEM	20,900		0.16		0.17		0.20	0.30		3.8	--
Normal Volunteers (n=11)											
MEAN	257,000		9.80		3.25		8.96	8.40		59.9	17
SEM	15,700		0.23		0.16		0.13	0.25		2.9	--
Analysis 1 §											
p	>.05		>.25		>.25		>.25	>.25		>.1	>.05¶
Analysis 2 **											
p	>.2		>.05		>.25		>.05	>.1		<.0025	>.05¶
Analysis 3 ‡‡											
p	>.05		>.1		>.25		<.05	>.1		>.1	>.05¶
Analysis 4 §§											
p	>.25		>.05		>.25		<.05	>.1		<.025	>.05¶

* From (17), with permission from the publisher. Survival curves analyzed with the mathematical models indicated. MPST denotes mean platelet survival time; RSS, residual sum of squares.

† Mean and SEM calculated over the 10-day study.

§ P value for difference between pyridoxine responsive and nonresponsive patients using a one-tailed t-test. P values >.05 are considered not significant.

** Same statistical analysis, but between pyridoxine responsive patients and normal controls.

‡‡ Same statistical analysis, but between pyridoxine nonresponsive patients and normal controls.

§§ Same statistical analysis, but between all homocystinuric patients and normal controls.

¶ Statistical analysis using Mann-Whitney rank-sum non-parametric test.

times between pyridoxine responders and non-responders, and pyridoxine responders or non-responders and normals, regardless of the survival model used. The kinetic data fitted the multiple-hit model best as judged from the residual sum of squares. Similar results were obtained in normal volunteers (16). Subsequent comparison, therefore, was done using estimates derived from the multiple-hit model. Based both on the number of subjects in each of the homocystinuric and normal groups

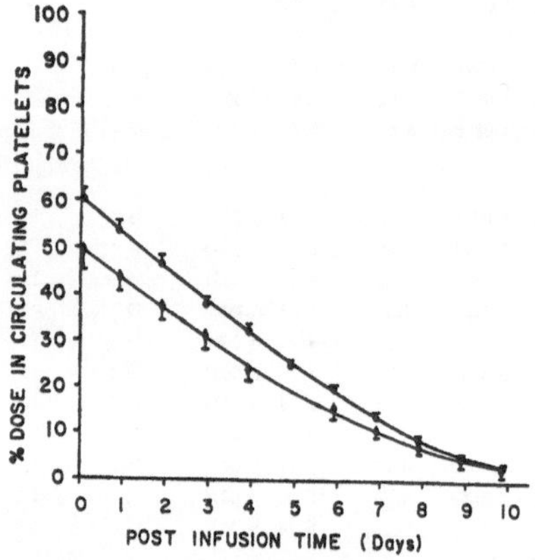

Fig. 1. ^{111}In-platelet survival curves for normal volunteers (● , n=11) and homocystinuric patients (♦ , n=12). Plotted as Mean +/- SEM. This is the maximum value of the SEM. The actual SEM will be smaller, since here it is grouped with systematic errors of data sampling). (From (17), reprinted, by permission of The New England Journal of Medicine, 307: 781-6, 1982.

and on 0.05 being the level of significance, the power of the t-test to detect a difference on MPST of 1 day or greater is 78.8% and for 2 days or greater is 99.5%. Fig 1 shows the radioactivity associated with the circulating platelets at various times after the infusion of ^{111}In-platelets in patients and controls. The initial recovery of ^{111}In-platelets in the circulation was slightly lower for homocystinurics than for the normal volunteers (mean= 48.8%, SEM= 3.8% vs mean= 59.9%, SEM= 2.9%; $p < 0.25$). However, when the initial recovery of ^{111}In-platelets was normalized to 100%, the ^{111}In-platelet survival curves of homocystinuric patients were identical to those of the normal volunteers. The mean platelet survival times (fig 2) in homocystinurics were not significantly

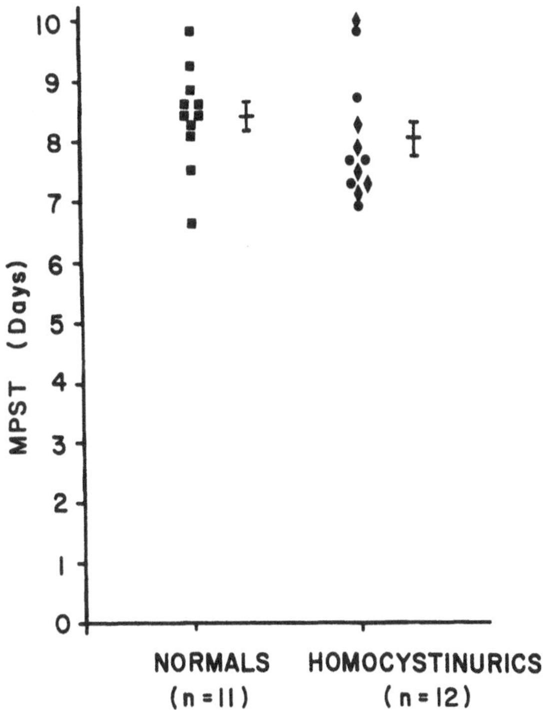

Fig. 2. The Mean Platelet Survival Time (MPST) of ^{111}In-platelets in normal volunteers (■) and homocystinuric patients both taking vitamin B_6 (● , n=6) and not taking vitamin B_6 (◆, n=6). Mean +/- SEM. (From (17), reprinted by permission of The New England Journal of Medicine 307:781-6, 1982.

different from those of normals (mean= 7.92 days, SEM= 0.30 days vs mean= 8.40 days, SEM= 0.25 days, respectively; $p > 0.1$). When these 2 variates, percent recovery and mean platelet survival time, were compared for patients taking vitamin B_6, no statistically significant difference was observed.

For ethical reasons, particularly the risks from radionuclides in young women, it was not possible to achieve perfect matching in the controls. Since age may have an impact on platelet survival, some confounding results from this mismatching and true differences between the affected and control subjects may be concealed. As a refinement, therefore, adjustments were made by linear covariance analysis. No significant

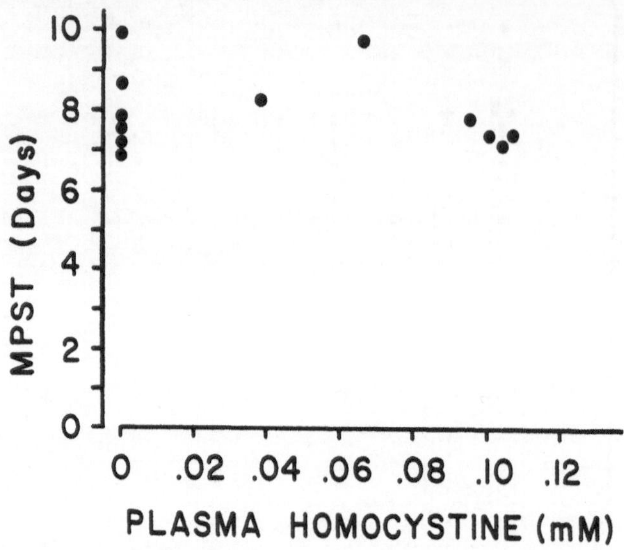

Fig. 3. The effect of plasma homocystine on Mean Platelet Survival Time (MPST). The mean of pre-study and post-study homocystine levels is plotted for each patient. (From (17), reprinted, by permission of The New England Journal of Medicine 307:781-6, 1982.

differences were found in either regression slopes or age-adjusted means.

Fig 3 shows the relationship between mean platelet survival time and plasma homocystine levels in the 12 patients. No effect of the plasma homocystine level on the mean survival time of ^{111}In-platelets was apparent.

The temporal distribution of ^{111}In-platelets in liver and spleen are shown in fig 4. The administered dose of 160 µCi (5.9 MBq) permitted in vivo quantification for 3 days only. A level of about 15% of the injected dose of ^{111}In-platelets was found in the liver after 4 min with little change over the subsequent 3 days. Furthermore, there was no perceptible difference between patients and controls. The ^{111}In-platelets accumulated in the spleen, reaching 45% of the injected dose at 30 min following infusion with little subsequent accumulation. Controls and patients did not differ in this respect either.

24 hours after injection of the ^{111}In-platelets, whole

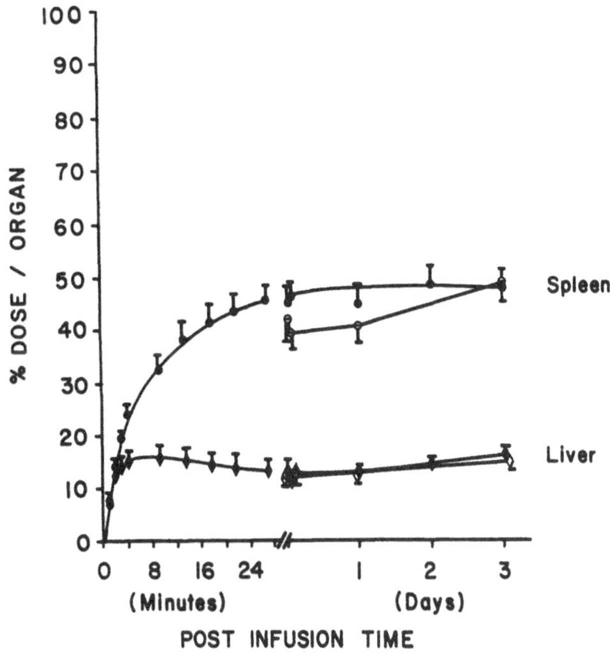

Fig. 4. Temporal distribution of ^{111}In-platelets in the liver (Diamonds) and spleen (Circles). Closed symbols = homocystinuric patients (n= 10). Open symbols = normal volunteers (n= 10). Mean +/- SEM. (This is the maximum value of the SEM. The actual SEM will be smaller, since, here it is grouped with systematic errors of data sampling). (From (17), reprinted, by permission of The New England Journal of Medicine 307:781-6, 1982.

body scanning revealed no abnormal focal accumulation of radioactivity in any of the patients.

Discussion

Homocystinuria and homocystinemia occur as a result of several different autosomal recessive defects in amino acid transsulfuration (8). While homocystinuria is therefore somewhat nonspecific as a name or a sign, it is commonly used to designate the disorder due to deficient activity of cystathionine beta-synthase, a pyridoxal phosphate-requiring enzyme (Reaction 1, fig 5). Failure to condense homocysteine with serine results in deficiency of cystathionine and cysteine, 2 compounds distal to the metabolic block, and accumulation of homocysteine, 2 molecules of which condense to form homocystine. Hypermethioninemia, secondary to folate-dependant remethylation of homocysteine (Reaction 4, fig 5), is a useful diagnostic feature because it occurs only in homocystinuria due to cystathionine beta-synthase deficiency. Thus, all 12 patients in this study likely had inadequate cystathionine beta-synthase activity to account for their disorder, a presumption confirmed in 4 subjects.

Genetic heterogeneity of cystathionine beta-synthase deficiency is evident from clinical, genetic, and biochemical studies in vivo and in vitro (7-9,30,31). Pharmacologic doses of pyridoxine in some, but not all, patients effect normalization of plasma methionine and homocystine and amelioration or prevention of clinical consequences.

Because of the morbidity and mortality associated with the cardiovascular complications of homocystinuria, means of protecting patients from thromboembolism are desirable. To this end, patients have been treated with chronic anticoagulation or agents which interfere with platelet function, despite little or conflicting evidence that coagulation (11,32) or platelets (8,11-13) are abnormal. Studies of platelet kinetics have been viewed as particularly relevant in determining both the pathogenesis of thromboembolism and the rationale for therapy.

Harker and co-workers observed a marked decrease in mean platelet survival time in 4 homocystinuric subjects; the mean platelet survival time was normalized in 2 pyridoxine responders by pyridoxine administration and in 2 pyridoxine non-responders by dipyridamole administration (11). In contrast, Uhlemann and associates (13) found normal mean platelet survival times in 6 homocystinuric patients, all of whom had homocystinemia when studied and only one of whom was a pyridoxine responder. All the patients studied by these 2 groups had no acute thrombosis at the time of the studies (11,12,13). The differences in mean platelet survival times between these 2 studies were throught originally to be due to the disparity in plasma homocystine levels of the patients studied. Harker and co-workers (12) subsequently corrected an error in their previous calcula-

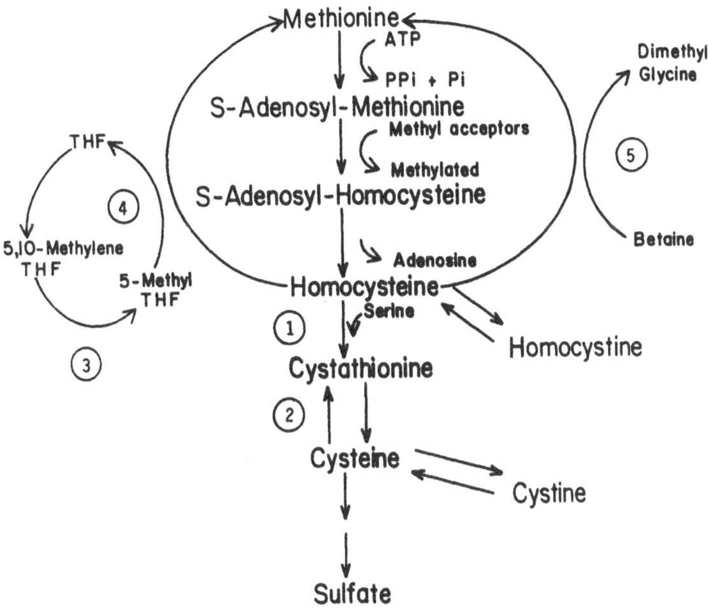

Fig. 5. The metabolic pathways of methionine and homocyst(e)ine. The enzymes and cofactors of the reactions are as follows: Reaction 1: Cystathionine beta-synthase and vitamin B_6. Reaction 2: Cystathionase and vitamin B_6. Reaction 3: 5,10-methylene tetrahydrofolate reductase and vitamin B_6. Reaction 4: 5-methyl-tetrahydrofolate-homocysteine methyl transferase and methyl-vitamin B_{12}. Reaction 5: Betaine-homocysteine-methyl transferase.

tions and the plasma homocystine levels became similar in the 2 studies. Harker also measured the platelet kinetics in 2 patients first studied by Uhleman and co-workers (13) and reported decreased mean platelet survival times as compared to those reported earlier (7.7 vs 8.5 days and 5.7 vs 10.4 days). These contradictory results have remained unresolved. It is possible that methodologic differences between the studies account for the differences in mean platelet survival time. In one study, the mean platelet survival times in some individuals were derived from the linear model, while those in other individuals were obtained from the exponential model (11); Harker and colleagues decided visually whether the linear or the exponential model would better fit their data. This approach does nothing to reduce analytic bias, a factor which can markedly affect the mean platelet survival time for a given patient (33). The impact is clear by comparing the estimates that the same data would yield when calculated using linear and exponential models (table 3).

Our study differed from the above studies in several aspects. First, we used ^{111}In instead of ^{51}Cr. The high photon yields in ^{111}In enabled more precise determinations of the radioactivity contained in blood-samples in the latter days of the kinetic studies. Second, in order to eliminate arbitrary decisions by the observer, our kinetic data were analyzed by computerized least-square fittings to 3 different mathematical models of curve analysis: linear, exponential, and multiple-hit models. Because both the exponential (or one-hit) model and the linear (or infinite-hit) model are special cases of the multiple-hit model, whether either is, in fact, the best model will be chosen by the program. In this study, in every case the best-fitting curve involved an intermediate number of hits, and the residual sum of squares was usually conspicuously less. Similar results were also seen in our normal controls (16). Third, a larger number of homocystinuric patients was studied. Nonetheless, the mean platelet survival time of none of the 12 subjects was found to deviate significantly from the group, suggesting that, despite considerable genetic heterogeneity, it is unlikely that previous studies examined a special variant of homocystinuria. Finally, the physical characteristics of ^{111}In made possible in vivo imaging studies.

Our results suggest that the mean platelet survival time in cystathionine beta-synthase deficiency is not abnormal. Plasma homocystine does not significantly affect the survival of platelets or their in vivo biodistribution. Homocystinuric patients, whether pyridoxine responsive or non-responsive, who lack clinical evidence of thromboembolism, do not have an abnormal focal platelet distribution detectable by in vivo imaging. Further studies are necessary to elucidate the pathogenesis of thromboembolism in homocystinuria.

Acknowledgements

This work was supported by US Public Health Research Grants AM-20812, AI-13004 and GCRC-00035-20 and an USDA Science and Education Administration grant 78-59-2243-01-013-1. REP is George Morris Piersol Teaching and Research Scholar of the American College of Physicians. M-FT is a recipient of a Research Career Development Award (AI-00194) from the National Institute of Allergy and Infectious Diseases. We wish to thank Daniel Koller, Steven Herda and Gerald McCormick for their technical assistance.

REFERENCES

1. Carson NAJ, Cusworth DC, Dent CE, Field CMB, Neill DW, Homocystinuria: A new inborn error of metabolism of methionine associated with mental deficiency. Arch. Dis. Child. 38:425, 1962.
2. Carson NAJ, Neill DW, Metabolic abnormalities detected in a survey of mentally backward individuals in Northern Ireland. Arch. Dis. Child. 37:505, 1962.
3. Mudd SH, Finkestein JD, Irreverre F, Laster L, Homocystinuria: An enzymatic defect. Science 143:1443, 1964.
4. Spaeth GL, Barber GW, Homocystinuria in a mentally retarded child and her normal cousin. Trans. Amer. Acad. Ophthalmol. Otolaryngologia 69:912, 1965.
5. Schimke RN, McKusick VA, Huard T, Pollack AD, Homocystinuria: Studies of 20 families with 38 affected members. Jama 193:711, 1965.
6. McKusick VA, Homocystinuria. In: Heritable disorders of connective tissue. 4th ed. Mosby CV, St. Louis, pp 224-281, 1972.
7. Grieco AJ, Homocystinuria: Pathogenetic mechanisms. Amer. J. Med. Sci. 273:120, 1977.
8. Mudd SH, Levy HL, Disorders of transsulfuration. In: The metabolic basis of inherited diseases. Stanbury JB, Wyngaarden JB, Fredrickson DS (eds), McGraw-Hill, New York, pp 458-503, 1978.
9. Valle D, Shashidar Pai G, Thomas GH, Pyeritz RE, Homocystinuria due to cystathionine beta-synthase deficiency: Clinical manifestations and therapy. Johns Hopk. Med. J. 146:110, 1980.
10. Barber GW, Spaeth GL, The successful treatment of homocystinuria with pyridoxine. J. Pediat. 75-463, 1969.
11. Harker LA, Slichter SJ, Scott CR, Ross R, Homocystinuria: Vascular injury and arterial thrombosis. New Engl. J. Med. 291:537, 1974.
12. Harker LA, Scott CR, Platelets in homocystinuria. New Engl. J. Med. 296:818, 1977.
13. Uhlemann ER, TenPas JH, Lucky AW, Schulman JD, Mudd SH, Shulman NR, Platelet survival and morphology in homocystinuria due to cystationine synthase deficiency. New Engl. J. Med. 295:1283, 1976.
14. Scheffel U, McIntyre PA, Evatt B, Dvornicky JA, Natarajan TK, Bolling DR, Murphy EA, Evaluation of Indium-111 as a new high photon yield gamma-emitting "physiological" platelet label. Johns Hopk. Med. J. 140:285, 1977.
15. Scheffel U, Tsan MF, McIntyre PA, Labelling of human platelets with (^{111}In) 8-hydroxyquinoline. J. nucl. Med. 20:524, 1979.
16. Scheffel U, Tsan MF, Mitchell TG, Camargo EE, Braine H, Ezekowitz MD, Nickoloff EL, Hill-Zobel RL, Murphy EA, McIntyre PA, ^{111}Indium-labeled platelets in normal man. Kinetics, distribution and radiation dose estimations. J. nucl. Med. 23:149, 1982.
17. Hill-Zobel RL, Pyeritz RE, Scheffel N, Malpica O, Engin S, Camargo EE, Abbott M, Guilarte TR, Hill J, McIntyre PA, Murphy EA, Tsan MF, Kinetics and distribution of ^{111}In-labeled platelets in patient with homocystinuria. New Engl. J. Med. 307:781, 1982.

18. Uhlendorf BW, Conerly EB, Mudd SH, Homocystinuria: Studies in tissue culture. Pediat. Res. 7:645, 1973.

19. Poole JR, Mudd SH, Conerly EB, Edward S, Homocystinuria due to cystathionine synthase deficiency. Studies of nitrogen balance and sulfur excretion. J. clin. Invest. 55:1033, 1975.

20. Murphy EA, Francis ME, The estimation of blood platelet survival. II. The multiple-hit model. Thrombos. Diathes. haemorrh. (Stuttg.) 25:53, 1971.

21. The Panel on Diagnostic Application of Radioisotopes in Haematology. International Committee for Standardization in Haematology. Recommended methods for radioisotope platelet survival studies. Blood 50:1137, 1977.

22. Dixon WJ, Massey FJ, Introduction to statistical analysis. 2nd ed. McGraw Hill, New York, p 250, 1957.

23. Wright RR, Tono M, Pollycove M, Blood volume. Sem. nucl. Med. 5:63, 1975.

24. Nickoloff EL, The physics of left ventricular performance measurements with radioactive tracers. Ph.D. Thesis, Johns Hopk. University 1977.

25. Hill-Zobel RL, Scheffel U, McIntyre PA, Tsan MF, ^{111}In-oxine labelled rabbit platelets: In vivo distribution and sites of destruction. Blood (in press).

26. Spackman H, Stein WH, Moore S, Automatic recording apparatus for use in the chromatography of amino acids. Anal. Chem. 30:1190, 1958.

27. Guilarte TR, McIntyre PA, Radiometric-microbiological assay of vitamin-B_6: Analysis of plasma samples. J. Nutr. 111:1891, 1981.

28. Chen MF, McIntyre PA, Wagner HN Jr, A radiometric microbiological method for vitamin B_{12} assay. J. nucl. Med. 18:388, 1977.

29. Chen MF, McIntyre PA, Kertcher JA, Measurement of folates in human plasma and erythrocytes by a radiometric microbiological method. J. nucl. Med. 19:906, 1978.

30. Fowler B, Kraus J, Packman S, Rosenburg LE, Homocystinuria. Evidence for 3 distinct classes of cystathionine beta-synthase mutants in cultured fibroblasts. J. clin. Invest. 61-645, 1978.

31. Skovby F, Kraus J, Relich C, Rosenburg LE, Immunochemical studies on cultured fibroblasts from patients with homocystinuria due to cystathionine beta-synthase deficiency. Amer. J. hum. Genet. 34:73, 1982.

32. Hilden M, Brandt NJ, Nilsson IM, Schonheyder F, Investigations of coagulation and fibrinolysis in homocystinuria. Acta Med. Scand. 195:533, 1974.

33. Bolling DR, Murphy EA, The estimation of blood platelet survival. VI. Evaluation of the graphical method. Johns Hopk. Med. J. 143:25, 1978.

21 NONINVASIVE RADIOISOTOPIC TECHNIQUES FOR DETECTION OF PLATELET DEPOSITION IN MECHANICAL AND BOVINE PERICARDIAL MITRAL VALVE PROSTHESES AND IN VITRO QUANTITATION OF VISCERAL MICROEMBOLISM

M.R. DEWANJEE

INTRODUCTION

A variety of mechanical and tissue prosthetic valves are presently used in patients with diseases of cardiac valves. The major limitation of the former is the propensity for thrombus formation, embolization (1-6) and that of the latter is calcification (7-10). Although thrombotic deposition has been demonstrated in the damaged perivalvular cardiac tissue and on the prosthetic sewing ring by light and electron microscopy, no in vivo technique has been available for the direct visualization of the process of platelet deposition and embolization after surgical implantation of the prostheses.

Labelling of autologous platelets with ^{51}Cr and ^{111}In-radionuclides and its applications in thrombosis research have been described by several investigators (11-21). With the use of ^{111}In-labelled platelets we have developed, in the dog model, a noninvasive technique of imaging platelet deposition on mitral valve prostheses. In addition, in vitro studies with the gamma counter and ionization chamber also permitted quantitation of the platelet deposition on the components of mitral valve prostheses as well as quantitation of visceral microemboli. Similar imaging studies (22,23) in the acute phase were carried out successfully in patients implanted with Dacron conduits.

Methods

Study groups and implantation of Ionescu-Shiley mitral valve prostheses in dogs. Protocol for prostheses implantation, administration of ^{111}In-labelled platelets, in vivo imaging, killing the animal, isolation of prosthesis, and quantification of platelet distribution is shown in fig 1 for the one-day study.

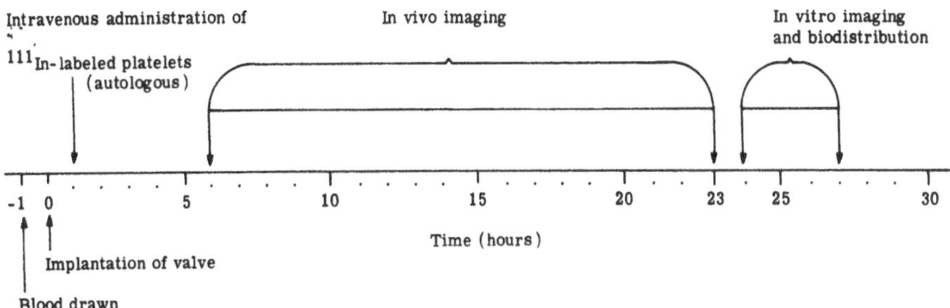

Fig. 1. Protocol (one-day study) of prostheses implantation, administration of ^{111}In-labelled platelets, in vivo imaging and sacrifice, isolation of prosthesis, in vitro imaging and biodistribution at 25 hours after tracer administration.

33 mongrel dogs, in 7 groups, weighing 18-26 kg, were studied as shown below:

Group I. Unoperated normal dogs. To determine the relative organ distribution of platelets in unoperated normal control dogs, 7 dogs were sacrificed 24 hours after administration of autologous ^{111}In-labelled platelets (see labelling method below).

Group II. Sham operation. 5 dogs were anesthetized with 2.5% methohexital sodium and maintained on halothane. Following the administration of succinylcholine, the chest was opened through the fourth left intercostal space. Following heparinization (300 units/kg i.v.), cardiopulmonary by-pass was instituted through cannulae in the right atrium and femoral artery. As the animal was cooled, the heart was fibrillated and a ventricular vent inserted through a stab wound at the apex of the left ventricle. Aortic cross-clamping was not used. Instead of excising the mitral valve, the valve was visualized, manipulated, and a cardiotomy sucker placed in the left atrium for approximately 20 min. At the end of this time, the atriotomy was closed with 4-0 Prolene. When the animal was warmed and air removed from the heart, the heart was defibrillated. By-pass was discontinued and blood reperfused into the animal until the pressure stabilized. Incisions were closed in a routine fashion with a single chest tube in the left chest. When the animal was awake and breathing on his own, the chest tube was removed, the animal was observed for 2-3 hours, and returned to the kennel. All animals received 1.2 million units of Bicillin before by-pass, 0.5 g calcium chloride, and 50 mEq of sodium bicarbonate during by-pass. Heparin was not reversed with protamine.

Group III. Implantation of Björk-Shiley mitral valve prostheses. 5 dogs were anesthetized with 2.5% methohexital sodium and maintained on halothane. The chest incision and cardiopulmonary by-pass procedures were performed as described in Group II dogs. The normal mitral valve was excised, and using interrupted mattress stitches, a 25 mm Björk-Shiley prosthesis was inserted. Discontinuation of cardiopulmonary by-pass and chest closure procedures were performed as described in Group II dogs.

Group IV. Implantation of Björk-Shiley mitral valve prostheses in dogs treated with platelet inhibitors. 5 dogs were treated with dipyridamole (2.5 mg/kg/day, orally), 2 days prior to operation. In addition, they received another dose of dipyridamole plus aspirin (15 mg/kg/day) 1 hour after operation. Surgery and implantation of 25 mm Björk-Shiley valves were performed as described in Group II dogs.

Group V, VI and VII. Implantation of Ionescu-Shiley mitral valve prostheses. 11 dogs were implanted with prostheses, 3 dogs in Group V, 3 dogs in Group VI, and 5 dogs in Group VII were killed at 1, 14, and 30 days post-implantation. Dogs were anesthetized with 2.5% methohexital sodium and maintained on halothane. The chest incision and cardiopulmonary by-pass procedures were performed as described in Group II dogs. The schematics of the Ionescu-Shiley bovine pericardial trileaflet valve prosthesis in the mitral valve annulus in the dog heart is shown in fig 2. The normal mitral valve was excised, and using interrupted mattress stitches, a 25 mm Ionescu-Shiley pericardial tissue prosthesis[1] was inserted. Discontinuation of cardiopulmonary by-pass and chest closure procedures were

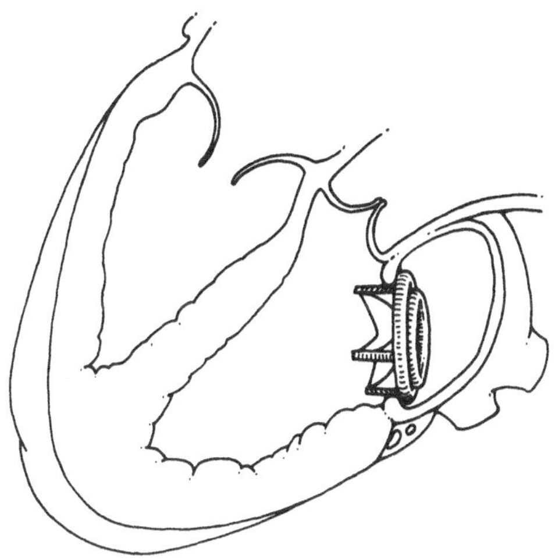

Fig. 2. Schematics of Ionescu-Shiley bovine pericardial trileaflet valve prosthesis in the annulus of mitral valve in dog heart.

performed as described in Group II dogs.

Platelet labelling with ^{111}In-(tropolone)$_3$ and in vivo imaging with a gamma camera. The labelling of the autologous platelets was performed during surgery (dog Groups II, III, and IV, based on the method of Dewanjee et al (13,14). In brief, ^{111}In(tropolone)$_3$ was prepared from ^{111}In-chloride (Medi-Physics, Inc. Emeryville, California) by adding 25 μg of oxine in 25 μl of saline to 0.5 - 0.6 mCi (18.5 - 22.2 MBq) of ^{111}In-chloride. The ^{111}In-(tropolone)$_3$ was then mixed with 4 ml of ACD-saline solution, pH was adjusted to 6.5, and platelet labelling was performed in ACD-saline medium. Free ^{111}In-(tropolone)$_3$ was removed by washing with ACD plasma. Residual platelet aggregates were removed by centrifugation at 100 g for 5 min. The efficiency of ^{111}In-labelling of platelets was 80-95%.

About 1 hours after surgery, the dogs were injected with 300 - 400 μCi (11.1 - 14.8 MBq) of autologous ^{111}In-labelled platelets suspended in 4-6 ml of ACD-plasma solution. At 24 hours after intravenous administration, Group II dogs were anesthetized with sodium pentobarbital and were imaged with a gamma camera (Searle, Pho-Gamma V) fitted with a medium-energy parallel fine-hole collimator. The camera spectrophotometer was adjusted to cover both the 174 keV and 247-keV peak of ^{111}In-radionuclide. The distribution of ^{111}In-labelled platelets in the thorax was obtained in the left lateral position, and 50,000 counts were accumulated.

Biodistribution of ^{111}In-labelled platelets. About 24 hours after intravenous administration of ^{111}In-labelled platelets, all experimental dogs were heparinized (400 units/kg) and killed with an overdose of sodium pentobarbital. The heart, lungs, liver, spleen, kidneys, brain, blood, and tissue samples from skeletal muscle, bone, and marrow were obtained and weighed. The schematics of tissue processing and tracer quantification are shown in fig 3. Distribution of radioactivity in the organs and whole body was then determined with a dose calibrator (Capintec-CRC 5R) and an automatic gamma well counter (Beckman Gamma-8000). The microprocessor was programmed to include the 174-keV, 247-keV, and 421-keV peaks. The sum peak at 421 keV corresponded to 45 - 50% of the total counts in the 3" x 3" NaI(Tl) crystal of our gamma counter. The ionization chamber and gamma counter were calibrated with ^{111}In source from the National Bureau of Standards (Bethesda, Maryland). A conversion factor of 1.42 x 10^6 cpm per microcurie of ^{111}In was obtained.

For confirmation of the results of in vivo imaging in Group III-VII dogs, the isolated heart was washed free of blood from the cardiac chambers and imaged with the gamma camera in the orientation of the in vivo imaging. Then the valve prosthesis with the immediately adjacent tissue was removed through the surgical incision in the left atrium. About 0.9 cm wide circumferential perivalvular cardiac tissue was excised, the prosthesis was separated from the perivalvular damaged cardiac tissue, and the sewing ring was cut with a scalpel and removed from the housing. Visible platelet thrombi lying on the Teflon biomaterial on the arterial side were also isolated.

The sutures attaching the 3 leaflets with the stent were cut with a scalpel blade, and the 3 leaflets were carefully

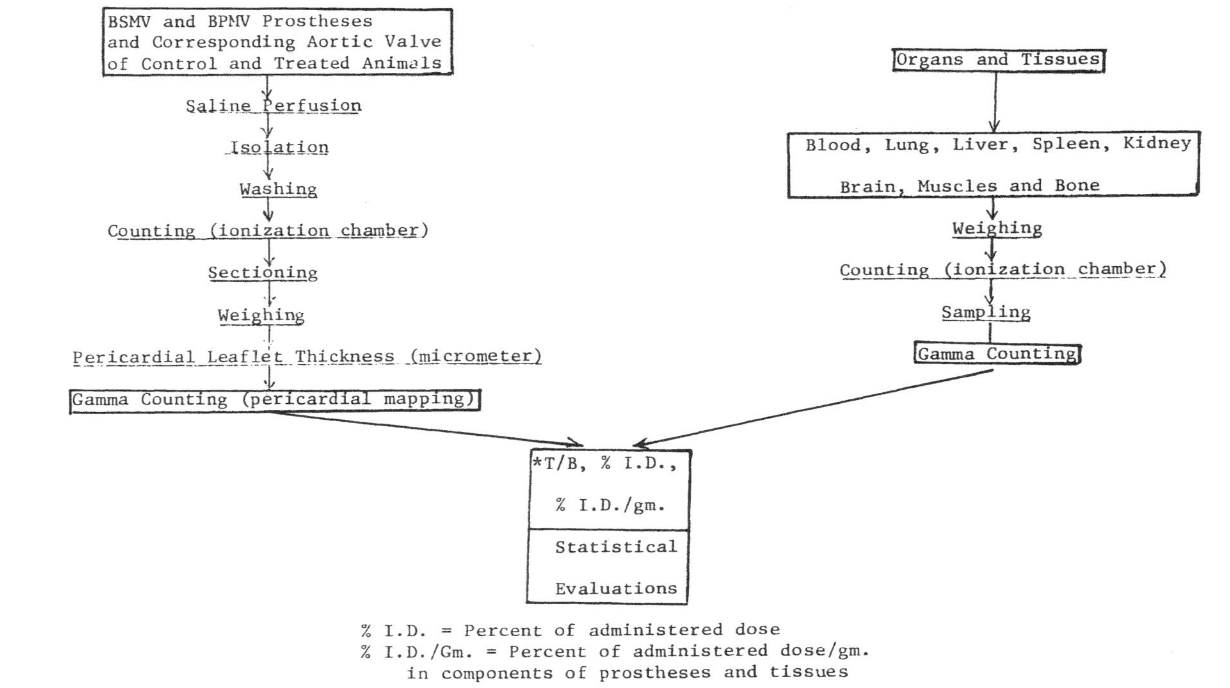

Fig. 3. Scheme of tissue processing and quantification of tracers in tissue and components of prostheses.

separated from the stainless steel stent. In addition, the leaflets of 3 normal aortic valves were harvested from aortic annulus, and these were weighed in a microbalance. The mean radioactivity of ^{111}In-labelled platelets on the 3 leaflets of valve prosthesis was compared with that of the normal aortic valve.

The radioactivity in the Teflon sewing ring, housing, the 3 leaflets or pyrolytic carbon disc, isolated platelet thrombus, perivalvular tissue, blood, brain, liver, spleen, kidneys, lung, cardiac and skeletal muscle were determined with the ionization chamber and gamma counter in all 7 groups of animals; the percentage of injected radioactivity in the viscera was then calculated. 9% and 40% of the weight of the animal was used in the calculation of blood-volume and skeletal muscle respectively. The total radioactivity in each organ was divided with decay-corrected injected ^{111}In radioactivity and percentage of injected dose was calculated for each organ. 24 hours cumulative surgical consumption of platelets was calculated by the subtraction of retained radioactivity from injected radioactivity in Group II, III, IV, and V dogs.

Quantification of visceral platelet deposition. For determination of microembolism, the mean and the standard values of radioactivity ratios were determined in the 7 groups of dogs. The renal cortex, medulla, and papilla were separated, and 4 samples of cortex, medulla, and papilla from each kidney were weighed. The radioactivity per unit weight and cortex/papilla and cortex/blood ratios were determined in all experimental dogs. For determination of microemboli in the brain, a craniotomy was performed, and brain tissue was removed and frozen for about an hour. 4 samples of gray and white matter were obtained from each dog for determination of cerebral microembolism. Similarly, samples in triplicate were obtained for determination of tissue/blood-ratio in lung, liver, spleen, cardiac, and skeletal muscle.

Platelet survival in bovine pericardial valve prosthesis-implanted dogs. 300 to 400 μCi (11.1 - 14.8 MBq) of ^{111}In-labelled autologous platelets were administered to 5 dogs (30-day study) at 10 and 21 days post-surgery. 9 blood-samples

(4ml each) were collected in preweighed heparinized tubes at 10 min, 2, 16, 24, 48, 72, 96, 120, 144, and 160 hours, and radioactivity per gram of blood was determined with a gamma counter. Platelet-survival times were calculated with a programmable calculator (Hewlett-Packard Model 97) by a least square exponential fitting program (14).

Results

^{111}In-labelled platelet imaging. The scintiphotos of the distribution of ^{111}In-labelled platelets in Group III-VII dogs taken at 24 hours after intravenous administration of radioactive platelets clearly delineated the prosthetic valve and surgically damaged tissue (figs 4-12).

For confirmation of the results of the in vivo imaging, the isolated components of the prosthetic valve were imaged in the orientation of the in vivo imaging, and this again demonstrated the site of valve implantation as the site of major platelet deposition in the thorax (figs 7A, 7B, 8A, 8B, 10A, 10B, 11A and 11B). The scintiscan and the photograph of the isolated components of the valve and the surgically damaged tissue revealed that the site of platelet deposition, as detected by imaging, was the Teflon sewing ring and the perivalvular tissue in the acute phase. In a 5-year old female patient, having surgical repair for truncus arteriosus, the Hancock conduit with porcine xenograft valve (arrows) shows uniform platelet accumulation. The optimal imaging was obtained at day 3 post-injection and day 5 post-operation.

Fig. 4. Scintiphoto of the thorax of intact dog in left anterior oblique (LAO) position 25 hours after implantation of bovine pericardial mitral valve prosthesis (BPMVP) and 24 hours after intravenous administration of ^{111}In-labelled platelets. Uptake shown by solid arrow corresponds to platelet thrombosis on suture ring and perivalvular tissue, open arrow demonstrates the site of cannulation. Upper part of liver uptake is evident in lower part of photograph. 50,000 counts were obtained in this view.

Fig. 5. Scintiphoto of the thorax of intact dog in left anterior oblique position (LAO) 7 days post-implantation of bovine pericardial mitral valve prosthesis (25 mm) and 24 hours after administration of ^{111}In-labelled autologous platelets. 50,000 counts were obtained in this view.

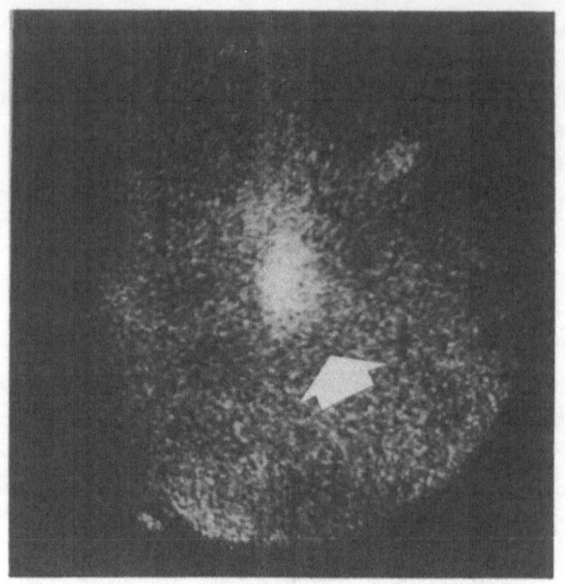

1 day

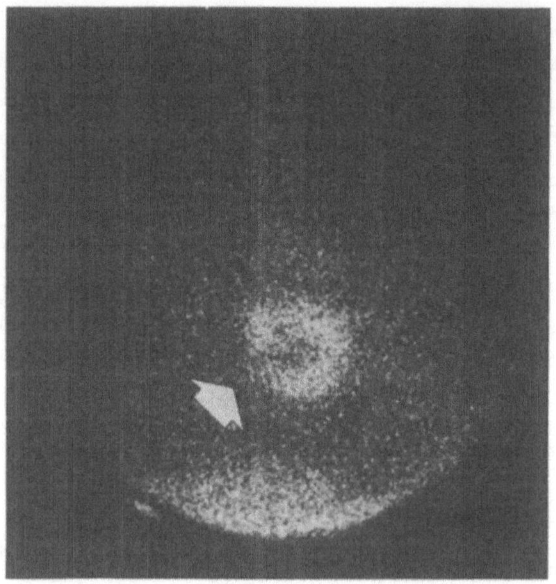

7 days

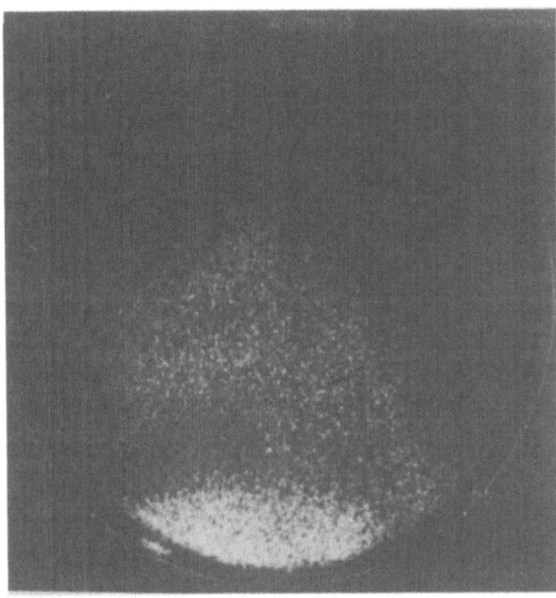

30 days

Fig. 6. Scintiphoto of thorax of a dog in LAO position 30 days post-implantation of pericardial mitral valve prosthesis (24 hours after injection). The image is almost similar to that of a normal unoperated dog).

Biodistribution of ^{111}In-labelled platelets. The biodistribution data (Tables 1 and 2) indicate that, in the Group I unoperated dogs, about 43% of the labelled platelets were in the systemic circulation, the remaining platelets being localized in decreasing order in the spleen, liver, muscle, lungs and kidneys. In the Group II sham-operated dogs, the total number of platelets in the viscera and blood was reduced because of the surgical platelet consumption. Similar reduction was also observed in the operated Group III, IV and V dogs. In comparison with the normal and sham-operated dogs, in the Group III, IV and V dogs implanted with mechanical and tissue valve prostheses, there was a significant ($p<0.01$) increase in platelet deposition in kidneys and skeletal muscle due to trapping of platelet microemboli. Since only about 30% of the total labelled platelets were in circulation, less platelets were available for pooling in the spleen and liver.

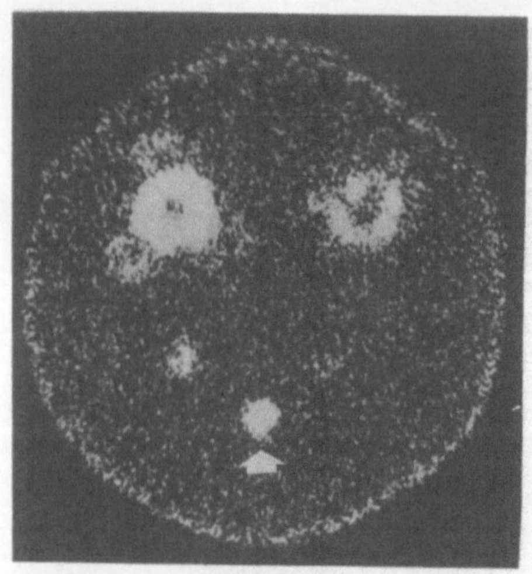

Fig. 7A:
day 1.

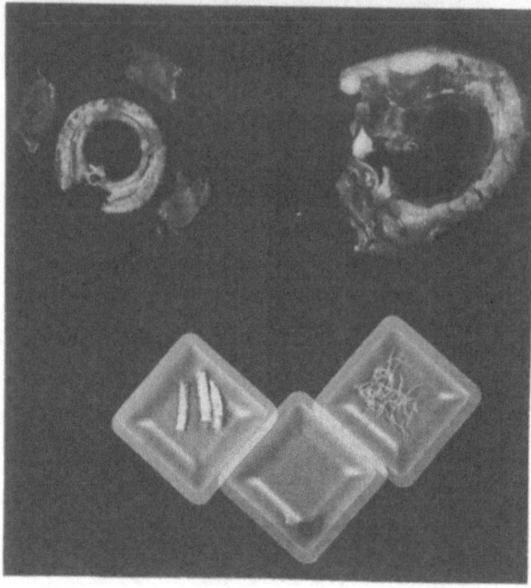

Fig. 7B:
day 1.

Fig. 7A. Scintiphoto of Teflon sewing ring with 3 leaflets around it (left), perivalvular tissue (right), stent support, thrombus on sewing (right) and Prolence suture (left to right in trays). 5000 counts were obtained in this view. The dog was implanted with 25 mm bovine pericardial mitral prosthesis (Shiley) and injected with labelled autologous platelets 1 hr post-surgery and sacrificed 25 hrs post-surgery. The sewing ring appears as the most thrombogenic material in the acute phase. 5000 counts were obtained in this view.
Fig. 7B. Photograph of sewing ring with 3 leaflets around it (left), perivalvular cardiac tissue (right) and stent support, 31.44 mg of thrombus and Prolene suture (bottom). (24 hrs post-implantation).

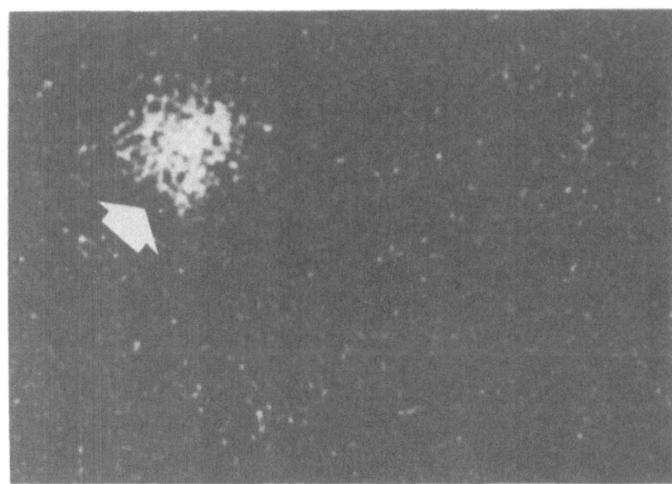

Fig. 8A.

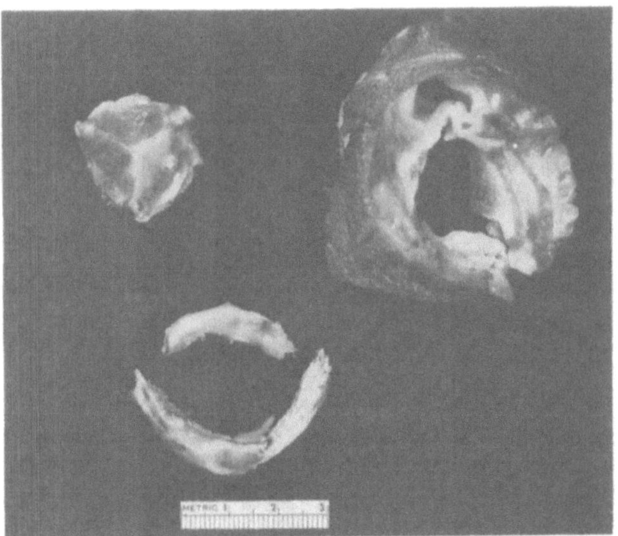

Fig. 8B.

Fig. 8A. Scintiphoto of isolated components of bovine pericardial mitral prosthesis (30 days post-implantation in dog). Note platelet deposition only on the leaflets. 5000 counrs were obtained in this view.

Fig. 8B. Photograph of isolated components of the prosthesis in the same orientation.

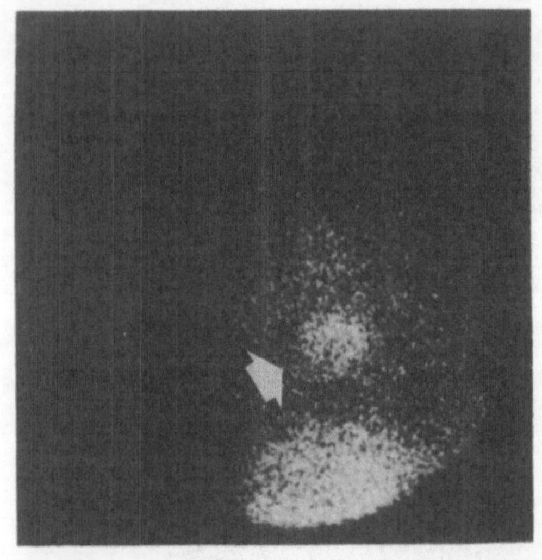

Fig. 9A:
1 day.

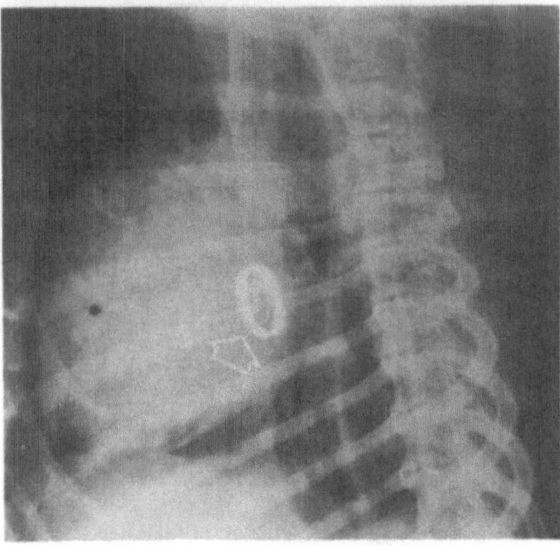

Fig. 9B.

Fig. 9A. Radiography of the 25 mm Björk-Shiley mitral valve prosthesis in dog.
Fig. 9B. Scintiphoto of the thorax of intact dog in left lateral position 25 hrs after surgery and 24 hrs after intravenous administration of ^{111}In-labelled platelets. Uptake shown by solid arrow corresponds to suture ring and perivalvular tissue. Localization of ^{111}In-labelled platelets in the upper part of the liver is also evident (lower part of photograph). 50,000 counts were obtained in this view.

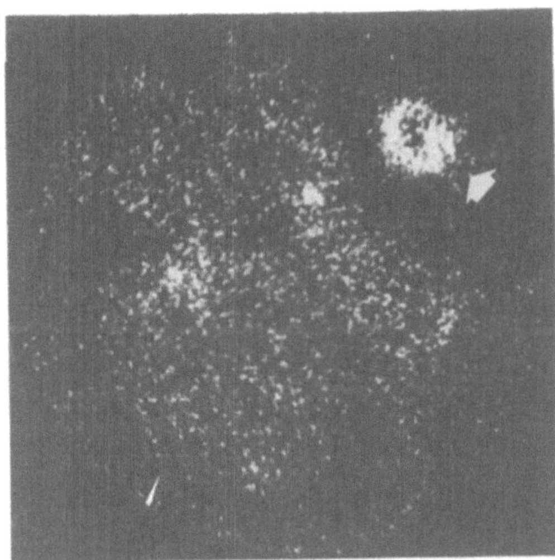

Fig. 10A:
1 day.

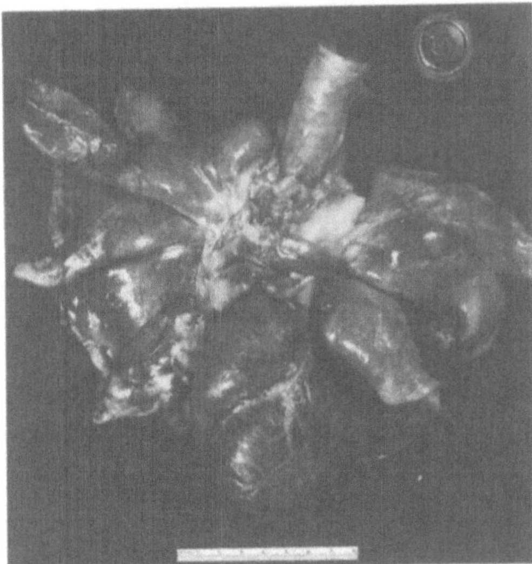

Fig. 10B:
1 day.

Fig. 10A. Scintiphoto of isolated lung and heart with Björk-Shiley prosthesis that has been separated and placed in upper right corner. 5000 counts were accumulated in this view. Solid arrow points to the site of intense platelet deposition in the prosthesis. Open arrow points to the other area of platelet deposition at the site of cannulation in the right atrium.

Fig. 10B. Scintiphoto of sewing ring (left), perivalvular tissue (right) and thrombus (bottom). Due to lack of platelet deposition in the pyrolytic carbon disc and in the stainless steel strut and housing, these components were not visible in the scintiphoto. 5000 counts were obtained in this view.

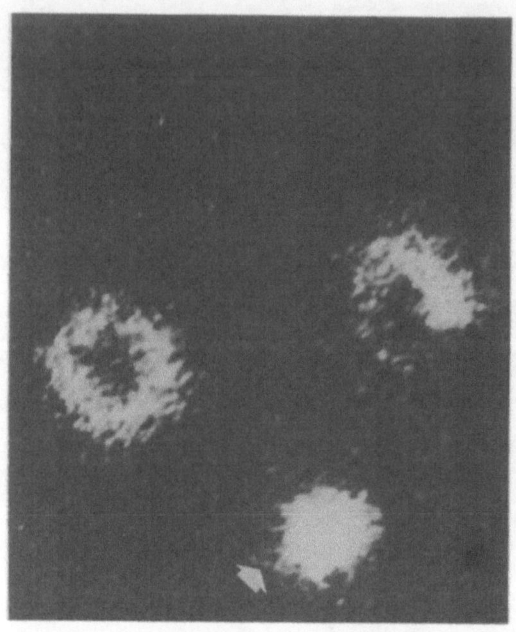

Fig. 11A. Photographs of pyrolytic carbon-coated disc in stainless steel housing (top), sewing ring (left), perivalvular tissue (right) and thrombus (bottom) were photographed in the same orientation of imaging.

Visceral platelet microemboli originating from platelet thrombi on the region of the prosthetic device are easily dispersed and are difficult to find by histopathological techniques until multiplane slices are made along the capillary network. On the other hand, comparative evaluation of the tissue/blood-ratio obtained with a tracer technique provides a simple procedure of most of the parameters important for the quantitation of microemboli in viscera.

In the spleen of the Group I and II dogs without a prosthetic valve, a major fraction of the platelet deposition is due to the normal physiological pooling of platelets. To a small extent this is true for the liver although this organ also sequesters damaged platelets. As observed in Group III, IV and V dogs with prosthetic valves, in spite of less circulat-

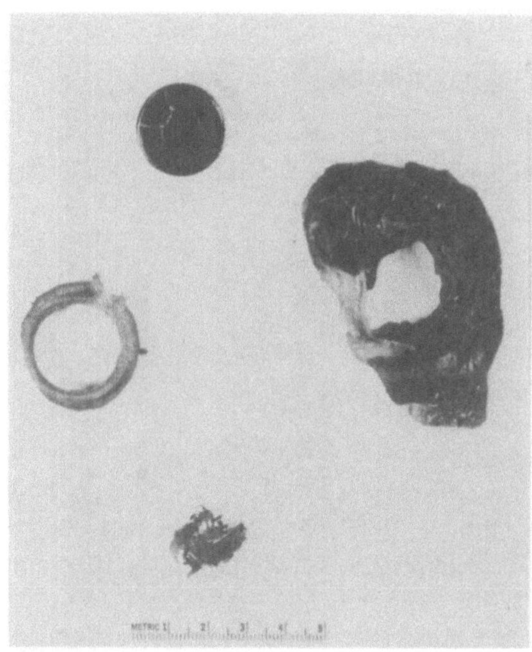

1 day

Fig. 11B. Scintiphoto of platelet deposition in the transverse slice of renal cortex. 5000 counts were accumulated in this view.

ting labelled platelets, the spleen/blood and liver/blood radioactivity ratios were high, thus indicating a combination of pooling of platelets and of entrapment of platelet microemboli. Indeed, as we have discussed in the kidney, liver, brain and in the cardiac and skeletal muscle, in Group III, IV and V dogs the absolute amount of radioactivity accumulated in these tissues was high although the organ distribution in Group VII tends toward the normal value of Group I dogs. Since these tissues normally maintain a low tissue/blood radioactivity ratio, higher level of radioactivity ratio suggests an entrapment of platelet microemboli presumably originating on the prosthetic valve. Treatment with dipyridamole aspirin caused a slight reduction of platelet thrombosis and embolization.

Due to intrinsic thrombogenicity and porosity of the sewing ring and thrombogenicity of the perivalvular damaged cardiac tissue (acute phase), the Group III, IV and V implanted

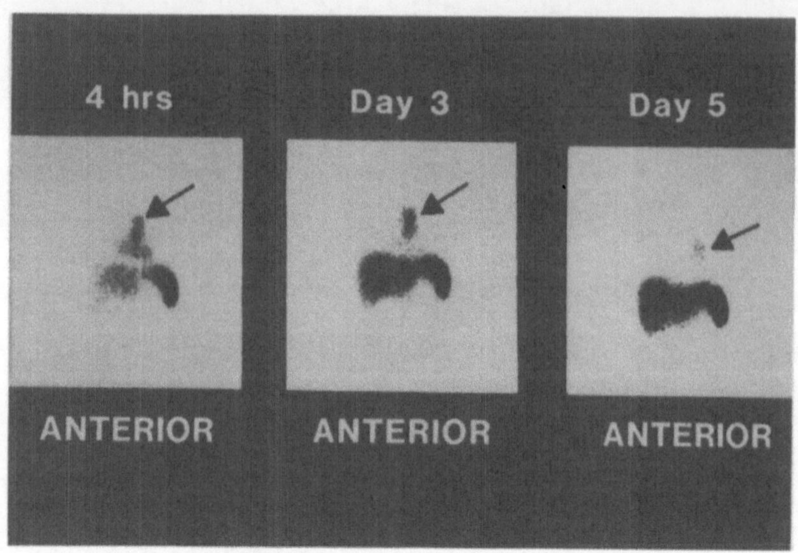

Fig. 12. Human pulmonary conduit. Montage of anterior images from 4 hrs to 5 days after injection of autologous ^{111}In-labelled platelets. Conduit (arrows) shows uniform platelet accumulation. Diminishing blood radioactivity enhances appearance of conduit.

dogs had similar platelet retention (tables 4 and 5); 0.56%, 0.20% and 0.09% of the total labelled platelets were localized in the Teflon sewing ring, thrombus on the sewing ring, and perivalvular tissue, respectively at 1, 14, and 30 days (table 5) post-implantation. Most of the visible thrombus was on the sewing ring in the atrial side, and some thrombus was also found on the perivalvular cardiac tissue between the sewing ring and the damaged cardiac tissue. Dipyridamole-aspirin treatment demonstrated a slight reduction in platelet deposition. The cannulation site in the right atrium retained about 0.1% of the total platelets.

Visceral platelet deposition. To determine the magnitude of platelet microaggregates trapped in capillary beds of internal organs and the muscular system, tissue/blood radioactivity ratios were determined. When compared with dogs of Group I and II, in the kidneys the absolute amount of ^{111}In-labelled plate-

TABLE 1. BIODISTRIBUTION (MEAN ± S.D.) OF PERCENT OF ADMINISTERED DOSE OF ^{111}IN-LABELED PLATELETS IN UNOPERATED NORMAL, SHAM-OPERATED, BJÖRK-SHILEY MITRAL VALVE PROSTHESES-IMPLANTED AND DIPYRIDAMOLE-ASPIRIN TREATED-IMPLANTED DOGS 24 HOURS AFTER INTRAVENOUS ADMINISTRATION AND 25 HOURS AFTER SURGERY

Tissue and Components of Mitral Valve Prosthesis	Normal Gr I: (n = 7)	Sham-Operated Gr II: (n = 5)	Implanted Gr III:(n = 5)	Implanted and Treated (Gr IV: (n = 5)
Liver	20.94 ± 12.38	16.53 ± 6.56	18.06 ± 2.27	18.84 ± 4.18
Spleen	32.27 ± 10.78	24.05 ± 7.17	21.52 ± 2.68	24.78 ± 6.38
Lungs	0.98 ± 0.14	1.54 ± 0.70	1.64 ± 0.44	2.45 ± 1.11
Kidneys	0.38 ± 0.15	0.95 ± 0.33	1.60 ± 0.63	1.31 ± 0.66
Skeletal muscle	2.47 ± 0.15	3.06 ± 1.39	7.93 ± 0.91	5.06 ± 3.44
Blood	42.76 ± 9.53	35.41 ± 8.58	28.66 ± 6.10	32.24 ± 4.62
Total BSMVP	---	---	0.76 ± 0.12	0.49 ± 0.18
Cumulative surgical consumption (24 hr)	---	18.2 ± 6.70	20.12 ± 7.82	14.59 ± 8.23

BSMVP: Björk-Shiley Mitral Valve Prostheses

TABLE 2. BIODISTIRBUTION (MEAN ± S.D.) OF ADMINISTERED DOSE (%) OF ^{111}IN-LABELED PLATELETS IN BOVINE PERICARDIAL MITRAL VALVE PROSTHESIS-IMPLANTED DOGS (1, 14, AND 30 DAYS POST-IMPLANTATION) 24 HOURS AFTER INTRAVENOUS ADMINISTRATION

Tissue and Mitral Valve Prosthesis	1D-Implanted Gr V: (n = 3)	14D-Implanted Gr VI: (n = 3)	30D-Implanted Gr VII: (n = 5)
Liver	19.49 ± 3.46	31.96 ± 5.01	22.36 ± 8.67
Spleen	22.56 ± 7.26	17.42 ± 6.57	28.33 ± 10.15
Lungs	1.98 ± 0.67	0.92 ± 0.47	2.70 ± 0.41
Kidneys	1.52 ± 0.51	0.64 ± 0.27	0.96 ± 0.38
Skeletal muscle	6.19 ± 0.84	4.53 ± 0.95	3.13 ± 0.79
Blood	29.89 ± 7.52	41.88 ± 14.30	43.18 ± 9.95
Total BPMVP*	0.70 ± 0.22	0.18 ± 0.09	0.04 ± .015
Cumulative post-surgical consumption (24 hr)	17.73 ± 6.96	---	---

BPMVP* Bovine Pericardial Mitral Valve Prosthesis

TABLE 3. TISSUE/BLOOD RATIO (MEAN ± S.D.) AT 24 HOURS AFTER ADMINISTRATION OF ^{111}IN-LABELED PLATELETS IN NORMAL-UNOPERATED, SHAM-OPERATED, MECHANICAL PROSTHESES (1 DAY, CONTROL AND TREATED) AND BOVINE PERICARDIAL MITRAL VALVE PROSTHESIS IMPLANTED DOGS AT 1, 14, AND 30 DAYS AFTER SURGERY

	Brain (gray) / Blood	Lung / Blood	Liver / Blood	Spleen / Blood	Cardiac Muscle / Blood	Cortex (kidney) / Blood
Normal, unoperated	0.010	0.243	1.993	11.932	0.06	0.24
Gr. I (n = 7)	±0.006	±0.062	±1.646	± 3.530	±0.02	±0.06
Sham-operated	0.012	0.406	1.526	13.181	0.05	0.41
Gr. II (n = 5)	±0.003	±0.216	±0.824	± 2.366	±0.01	±0.19
BSMVP-implanted	0.032	0.711	2.883	26.825	0.19	1.44
Gr. III (n = 5)	±0.015	±0.292	±1.244	±14.012	±0.10	±0.54
BSMVP-implanted and treated	0.015	1.322	2.542	31.475	0.23	0.93
Gr. IV (n = 5)	±0.006	±0.731	±1.101	±25.067	±0.05	±0.07
Pericardial mitral valve prosthesis	0.012	1.17	2.34	22.62	0.28	0.25
Gr. V 1 day (n = 3)	±0.011	±0.91	±1.11	± 4.92	±0.07	±0.13
Pericardial mitral valve prosthesis	0.012	0.85	2.33	17.62	0.11	0.88
Gr. VI 14 days (n = 3)	±0.011	±0.22	±1.24	± 6.57	±0.06	±0.27
Pericardial mitral valve prosthesis	.011	0.52	1.88	14.53	0.11	0.45
Gr. VII 30 days (n = 5)	± .011	±0.20	±0.93	± 5.17	±0.02	±0.15

TABLE 4. DISTRIBUTION (MEAN ± S.D.) OF PERCENT OF ADMINISTERED DOSE OF ^{111}IN-LABELED PLATELETS IN COMPONENTS OF BJÖRK-SHILEY MITRAL VALVE PROSTHESES-IMPLANTED AND DIPYRIDAMOLE-ASPIRIN TREATED-IMPLANTED DOGS 24 HOURS AFTER IMPLANTATION AND 25 HOURS AFTER SURGERY

Components	% Administered ^{111}In-Platelets Gr III: Implanted	Gr IV: Treated-Implanted
Pyrolitic carbon disc	0.0031 ± 0.0003	0.0009 ± 0.0002
Valve housing	0.0033 ± 0.0004	0.0020 ± 0.0003
Teflon sewing ring	0.30 ± 0.11	0.21 ± 0.10
Thrombus on Teflon	0.26 ± 0.04	0.20 ± 0.08
Perivalvular damaged cardiac tissue	0.19 ± 0.11	0.09 ± 0.03
Total	0.76 ± 0.12	0.49 ± 0.18

lets of Group III dogs was higher. A significantly high ($p < 0.01$) cortex/blood and cortex/papilla radioactivity ratio was obtained between Group I and the rest of the 6 groups of dogs (table 3).

The most interesting change was observed in the accumulated platelet thrombus on leaflets and sewing ring; as the sewing ring is slowly covered by fibrous ingrowth, less platelet is deposited at 1 month, and this minimal platelet deposition could not be observed by in vivo imaging (fig 6). At this period the leaflets are the most thrombogenic surface exposed to blood, although leaflet thrombogenicity at 1 month is lower than at 1 day (figs 7A, 7B, 8A and 8B) and table 3. Minor degree of calcification in the early stage could not be observed by radiography of the intact animal or isolated prostheses. Increased platelet consumption from blood-pool resulted in a decrease in platelet survival from (50 ± 10) hours in normal

TABLE 5. DISTRIBUTION OF ^{111}IN-LABELED PLATELETS IN COMPONENTS OF BOVINE PERICARDIAL MITRAL VALVE PROSTHESIS-IMPLANTED MONGREL DOGS AT 1, 14, AND 30 DAYS POST-IMPLANTATION. THE DOGS WERE SACRIFICED 24 HOURS AFTER INJECTION FOR QUANTITATION OF PLATELET-THROMBUS

Components of Prosthesis	(Mean ± S.D.) of Percent of Administered Dose (1 day, n = 3)	(14 days, n = 3)	(30 days, n = 5)
Per. Leaflets (3)	0.154 ± 0.018	0.114 ± 0.092	0.0357 ± 0.023
Teflon Sewing Ring	0.549 ± 0.154	0.044 ± 0.023	0.0020 ± .0136
Thrombus on Teflon	0.089 ± 0.057	0.022 ± 0.012	.0010 ± .0004
Perivalvular Cardiac Tissue	0.112 ± 0.019	0.018 ± 0.012	0.0012 ± .0009
$\left(\frac{\text{Per. Leaflets, CPM/mg}}{\text{Aortic Valve, CPM/mg}}\right)$	108 ± 21	57 ± 15	36 ± 30
Thrombus/Blood	545 ± 157	2.35 ± 1.66	1.34 ± 1.14

unoperated dogs to (25 ± 8) hours at 10 days and (38 ± 10) hours at 21 days post-prostheses implantation.

As the prosthesis consumes less platelets at 1 month, more platelets are in circulation although tissue/blood ratio is higher than that of normal unoperated dogs (table 3). This is also reflected in the decrease of radioactivity ratio of leaflet to that of normal aortic valve (table 5). The rate of incorporation of platelet in old thrombus also decreases significantly. The thrombus/blood ratio decreases from 545 to 2 within 2 weeks and even less (∿1) at 1 month.

Discussion

Thromboembolic events in patients with prosthetic heart valves constitute a major clinical problem. However, there is still little understanding of the clinical significance of the early and late postoperative "in situ" deposition of platelet-thrombi in prosthetic material. In addition, little is known of the incidence and magnitude of visceral microemboli following valve replacement. With the use of ^{111}In-labelled platelets, we have established a new technique for in vivo detection early postoperatively of "in situ" platelet deposition on mechanical mitral valve prostheses in the acute phase. These techniques are equally useful for tissue valve prostheses in the acute and chronic phase. We have also developed a quantitative method for the in vitro determination of platelet deposition on the components of mechanical mitral prostheses and the internal organs.

In a previous paper (16,21,22) we specifically demonstrated that ^{111}In-labelled platelets provide a sensitive marker for in vitro quantitation of platelet and platelet-thrombi deposition on the components of a mechanical mitral prosthesis (15, 16) and their reduction following administration of the platelet-inhibitor drug combination dipyridamole and aspirin. In this study we have demonstrated the shift of the site of platelet thrombus from sewing ring in the acute phase (1 day) to the pericardial leaflet in the chronic phase at 1 month. This decrease in thrombogenicity of tissue valve prosthesis is observed by in vivo imaging, in vitro quantitation of thrombus deposition, quantitative biodistribution, and estimation of microembolism by tissue/blood ratio. Although ^{51}Cr-labelled platelets were used in the past by Harker and Slichter et al (11) for the measurement of global platelet consumption, the quantitative analyses of several parameters of thrombosis and embolization were only possible with ^{111}In-labelled autologous platelets.

Dewanjee et al (20,22) developed in vivo and in vitro quantitative methods to compare levels of platelets in partially de-endothelialized vessel wall to the reference pool of circulating labelled platelets and determination of platelet/ unit area of thrombogenic surface of biomaterials. This concept was used to evaluate the effectiveness of platelet-inhibitor agents. In the past, large thrombosis in biomaterial was evaluated by tissue necrosis, (18) and microembolism was evaluated rarely by transmission electron microscopy (19). These techniques are not sensitive, are very costly, are full of artifacts, and microembolism due to disaggregation process is elusive. In vitro determination of tissue/blood determination appears most simple and sensitive and could be obtained for all organs in the animal model. We have estimated mitral valve prostheses-associated platelet thrombosis in the acute and chronic phase. This study suggests that even in tissue valve prostheses it is beneficial to use platelet-inhibitor therapy till the sewing ring develops fibrous ingrowth.

Using the methodology we have developed, we are continuing this study to evaluate other platelet-inhibitor drugs in the chronic phase. Considering the convenience of platelet labelling, administration, ease of imaging, and acceptable radiation dose, we feel that these noninvasive procedures of imaging platelet deposition could be used in patients undergoing implantation of cardiovascular prostheses and in the evaluation of platelet-inhibitor drugs following prosthetic valve replacement. Since tissue prostheses calcify in young animals, we are also evaluating the effect of a platelet-inhibitor drug, ibuprofen (Motrin), and calcification inhibitor, diphosphonate, and investigating the role of thrombosis on calcification. In addition, inhibitor drugs of thrombosis and calcification (diphosphonate) could be immobilized by cross-linking during tissue fixation with glutaraldehyde, thus reducing the degeneration of tissue prostheses.

Index terms: pericardial tissue valve prosthesis, platelet thrombosis, platelet survival imaging, visceral microembolism.

Acknowledgement

We appreciate the encouragement of Heinz W. Wahner, M.D. of Nuclear Medicine and Paul E. Zollman of Veterinary Medicine and the technical assistance of Mr. Arlan Hildestad and Mr. Sushital Chowdhury and the typing assistance of Ms. Judy Ashenmacher in preparation of the manuscript. The author is indebted to Shiley Inc. for kindly providing the mechanical and tissue valve prostheses.

REFERENCES

1. Barnhorst DA, Oxman HA, Connolly DC, Pluth JR, Danielson GK, Wallace RB, McGoon DC, Long-term follow-up of isolated replacement of the aortic and mitral valve with the Starr-Edwards prosthesis. Amer. J. Cardiol. 35:228, 1975.

2. Salomon NW, Stinson EB, Griepp RB, Shumway NE, Mitral valve replacement: long-term evaluation of prosthesis-related mortality and morbidity. Circulation 2:34, 1977.

3. Copans H, Lakier JB, Kinsley RH, Colsen PR, Fritz VU, Barlow JB, Thrombosed Björk-Shiley mitral prostheses. Circulation 61:169, 1980.

4. Moreno-Cabral RG, McNamara JJ, Mamiya RT, Brainard SC, Chung GKT, Acute thrombotic obstruction with Björk-Shiley valves. Diagnostic and surgical considerations. J. thorac. cardiovasc. Surg. 75:321, 1978.

5. Roberts WC, HAMMER WJ, Cardiac pathology after valve replacement with a tilting disc prosthesis (Björk-Shiley type): a study of 46 necropsy patients and 49 Björk-Shiley prostheses. Amer. J. Cardiol. 37:1024, 1976.

6. Friedli B, Acrichide N, Grondin P, Campeau L, Thromboembolic complications of heart-valve prostheses. Amer. Heart J. 81:702, 1971.

7. Silver MM, Pollock J, Silver MD, Williams WG, Trusler GA, Calcification in porcine xenograft valves in children. Amer. J. Cardiol. 45:685, 1980.

8. Angell WW, Angel JD, Porcine valves. Progr. cardiovasc. Dis. 23:141, 1980.

9. Barnhardt GR, Jones M, Ishihara T, Chavez AM, Rose DM, Ferrans VJ, Failure of porcine aortic and bovine pericardial prosthetic valves: An experimental investigation in young sheep. Circulation 66:150, 1981.

10. Galioto FM Jr, Midgley FM, Kapur S, Perry LW, Watson DC, Shapiro SR, Ruckman RN, Scott LP. Early failures of Ionescu-Shiley bioprosthesis after mitral valve replacement in children. J. thorac. cardiovasc. Surg. 83:306, 1982.

11. Harker LA, Slichter SJ, Studies of platelet and fibrinogen kinetics in patients with prosthetic heart valves. New Engl. J. Med. 283:1302, 1970.

12. Thakur ML, Welch MF, Joist JH, Coleman RE, Indium-111 labeled platelets: Studies on preparation and evaluation of in vitro and in vivo function. Thromb. Res. 9:345, 1976.

13. Dewanjee MK, Rao SA, Didisheim P, In-111 tropolone, a new high affinity platelet label: Preparation and evaluation of labeling parameters. J. nucl. Med. 22:981, 1981.

14. Dewanjee MK, Rao SA, Rosemark JA, Chowdhury S, Didisheim P, In-111 tropolone, a new tracer for platelet labeling. Radiology 145:149, 1982.

15. Dewanjee MK, Kaye MP, Fuster V, Noninvasive radioisotopic technique for detection of platelet deposition in mitral valve prosthesis and quantitation of cerebral renal and pulmonary microembolisms. Circulation p 8, suppl. III (abstract), 1980.

16. Dewanjee MK, Kaye MP, Fuster V, Rao SA, Noninvasive radioisotopic technique for detection of platelet deposition in mitral valve prosthesis and renal microembolism in dogs. Amer. Soc. Artif. Int. Organs 26:475, 1980.

17. Fuster V, Dewanjee MK, Kaye MP, Josa M, Metke MP, Chesebro JH, Noninvasive radioisotopic technique for detection of platelet deposition in coronary artery bypass grafts in dogs and its reduction with platelet inhibitors. Circulation 60:1508, 1979.

18. Kusserow BK, Larrow R, Nichols J, Observations concerning prosthesis-induced thromboembolic phenomena made with an in vivo embolus test system. Trans. Amer. Soc. Artif. Int. Organs 16:58, 1970.

19. Hanson SR, Harker LA, Ratner BD, Hoffman AS, In vivo evaluation of artificial surfaces with a nonhuman primate model of arterial thrombosis. J. Lab. clin. Med. 95:289, 1980.

20. Dewanjee MK, Pumphrey CW, Murphy KP, Rosemark JA, Chesebro JH, Fuster VD, Kaye MP, Evaluation of platelet-inhibitor therapy in a canine bilateral femoral graft implant model. Trans. Amer. Soc. Artif. Int. Organs 27:504, 1982.

21. Dewanjee MK, Fuster V, Rao SA, Forshaw PL, Kaye MP, Noninvasive radioisotopic technique for detection of platelet deposition in mitral valve prostheses and quantitation of visceral microembolism in dogs. Mayo Clin. Proc. (in press).

22. Agarwal KC, Wahner HW, Dewanjee MK, Fuster V, Puga FJ, Danielson GK, Chesebro JH, Feldt RH: Imaging of platelets in right-sided extracardiac conduits in humans. J. nucl. Med. 23:342, 1980.

23. Dewanjee MK, Kaye MP, Quantitation of platelet interaction with a prosthetic mitral valve in dogs. In: ^{111}Indium-labeled platelets and leucocytes. Society of Nuclear Medicine, Wahner HW, Goodwin DA (eds), Central Chapter pp 213-234, 1982.

PLATELETS, BETA-THROMBOGLOBULIN, PLATELET FACTOR 4

22 BETA-THROMBOGLOBULIN, PRESENT STATE OF THE ART

C.A. LUDLAM

The quantification of the platelet contribution to different pathophysiological conditions has always presented problems. This can now be more easily achieved following recent advances that have led to the development of new techniques. Although there are many techniques for measuring platelet behaviour in vitro e.g. aggregation, adhesion etc. It remains uncertain how such activity relates to their function in vivo. Furthermore, the necessity to quantify the platelet contribution to various disease states has become more acute with the development of antiplatelet drugs.

The measurement of platelet survival has been the reference technique for measuring platelet behaviour within the circulation, however, within the past 10 years other sensitive tests have been developed for measuring activation of both platelets and the coagulation system. Sensitive radioimmunoassays for fibrinopeptide A and fragment E have enabled the effect of trace quantities of thrombin and plasmin to be detected. Platelet activation, on the other hand, can be determined by measuring the plasma concentration of platelet granule proteins liberated as a result of their stimulation or lysis. Platelet factor 4 (PF4) and B-thromboglobulin (Btg) are two such proteins that have been extensively investigated in the past decade both in healthy subjects and in patients with a broad spectrum of different disorders 1-6.

Platelets possess three principle types of storage granules. Dense bodies contain mainly low molecular weight chemicals e.g. Ca++, ATP: lysosomes storing a variety of hydrolases, and α-granules harbouring several interesting proteins including Btg, PF4, thrombospondin and fibrinogen. Some of these e.g. Btg, appear to be unique to platelets, whereas others may be found associated with other cell types. As well as being present in mast cells (McLaren et al) (7), PF4 is liberated from α-granules into the plasma from which it in turn becomes associated with vascular endothelial cells (8).

It was the antiheparin activity of platelets, originally termed platelet factor 4 (9), that enabled it to be isolated and characterized. It is now clear, however, that this protein does not contribute significantly to the heparin neutralizing activity of platelet poor plasma which is due to other acute phase reactant proteins, e.g. α_1 acid glycoprotein and fibrinogen. The primary amino acid sequence of PF4 is known and the lysine-rich C-terminal residues are presumably responsible for its heparin neutralizing activity (10). Within platelet α-granules it is bound to a proteoglycan carrier and once released it associates with a wide variety of plasma glycoproteins. Btg has a primary amino acid structure very similar to PF4 (although it possesses relatively little anti-heparin activity), presumably because both have evolved from a common ancestral protein (11). Evidence has been presented to demonstrate that Btg is derived from another protein termed "low affinity PF4" following proteolysis of a quadrapeptide from its N terminus and this latter protein may well be derived intern from platelet basic protein following the release of a polypeptide (12). PF4 is reported to have anti-collagenase activity and to be chemotactic for neutrophils and monocytes (10), whereas Btg's function remains unknown; the suggestion that it inhibits PGI_2 synthesis by endothelial cells (13) remains unconfirmed (14).

Sensitive radioimmunoassays have been set up for many of the α-granule proteins. When the first assay for Btg was developed it rapidly became apparent that its plasma level was critically dependant upon the technique used to prepare the plasma (4). A method was devised to inhibit the release reaction in vitro by cooling the blood anticoagulated with EDTA, and by the addition of two antiplatelet agents PGE_I and theophylline. These act synergistically to increase the cAMP concentration within the cell Other investigators have devised other anticoagulant/antiplatelet cocktails e.g. EDTA, cAMP, PGE_I (15), citrate, theophylline, adenosine (16), EDTA/citrate, adenosine, PEG_I (17) and ACD, aspirin, PGE_I (18). All these different collection procedures result in similar plasma Btg levels and it therefore seems likely that these may represent the true circulating level in vivo. It is interesting to note that these different cocktails all contain two antiplatelet agents: several studies indicate that if blood is collected in the presence of only a single antiplatelet agent Btg/PF4 levels are usually higher and therefore do not reflect the true basal circulating concentration (19,20).

Although some platelet "dust" (21) may remain in the plasma following centrifugation and contribute to the apparent plasma Btg level, studies by Dawes et al (8) have demonstrated that the plasma level is very similar to that in amniotic fluid with which it may be in equilibrium. When radiolabelled Btg is injected into the circulation it disappears with a half time of approximately 100 min whereas PF4 is cleared very rapidly from the circulation and its half-life is therefore difficult to measure.

In healthy individuals the normal plasma concentration Btg is 20-50 ng/ml and for PF4 ⩽-5 ng/ml, and it appears to be remarkably constant within each person. There is a positive correlation between the plasma Btg and PF4 levels. The plasma Btg level does, however, rise with age particularly over 50 years (4,22). There is a reciprocal relationship between the plasma Btg or PF4 level and platelet lifespan, i.e. high plasma Btg/PF4 are associated with shorter platelet survival (4). Although in many clinical situations Btg and PF4 may parallel each other there are two important instances when the relative concentrations of these two proteins diverge. In renal failure plasma Btg rises together with creatinine whereas PF4 appears independent of renal function (1,2,3,4,23,24). As Btg has a molecular weight of approximately 36,000 it is probably filtered by the glomerulus and reabsorbed by tubular cells; its plasma concentration parallels that of β_2 microglobulin, a protein also filtered and reabsorbed by the kidney (25). Pf4 is only raised in renal failure if there is platelet activation e.g. acute glomerulonephritis, whereas in patients with chronic renal insufficiency the PF4 level is normal. The second major differrence between Btg and PF4 is that after the injection of heparin a very large increase in plasma PF4 level is observed probably due to the removal of PF4 from the surface of endothelial cells whereas there is no change in the Btg concentration. This observation is obviously important to take into account if patients with thromboembolism are being treated with heparin when the blood-sample is collected (8).

Both plasma and urinary concentrations of Btg and PF4 have been measured in a variety of clinical conditions in which platelets may be important. Venous and arterial thromboembolism are associated with platelet activation and aggregation within the circulation. Venous thrombosis is associated with elevated plasma and urinary Btg concentrations (3,26,27). In patients presenting with symptoms or signs suggestive of a deep venous thrombosis (DVT), elevated urinary Btg concentrations are more specific for the presence of a thrombus than an increased plasma concentration. Immediately post-operative there is a marked increase in urinary Btg in all patients which fall to within the normal range in 2-3 days. In those who develop a DVT a rise in Btg is observed and the increase in urinary concentrates appears more specific and sensitive for the presence of thrombosis than an increase in the plasma level. These promising results, especially for urinary measurements, suggest that this could be a fruitful area for future research in the field of thrombus detection.

Arterial insufficiency either in the form of transient ischaemic attacks, angina, strokes or myocardial infarction result in elevated Btg and PF4 plasma concentrations. When patients admitted to a coronary care unit are studied many have elevated concentrations of platelet proteins; increased levels are however observed in individuals in whom the chest pain is due to non-myocardial causes. In these patients the mechanism by which Btg becomes elevated is unclear. During the first few days levels of platelet proteins fall before rising in the second week possibly due to the formation of intracardiac thrombi or DVT. Chronic coronary artery insufficiency is associated with elevated PF4 levels but these do not fall following coronary artery bypass grafting (15,28,29,30).

If it were possible to identify more accurately which patients with rheumatic heart disease and prosthetic cardiac valves were at high risk of a thromboembolic episode this would be a major clinical advance. To this end measurements of Btg and PF4 have been made in these conditions and increased levels observed imply that there is chronic activation of the circulating platelets. The results from one small study suggest that high levels may be predictive for future clinically detectable embolic events (3,31,32).

Platelets may be important in the pathogenesis of the vascular complications of diabetes mellitus and to investigate further their possible roles plasma Btg and PF4 levels have been measured and related to both metabolic control and the presence of complications. Btg and PF4 do not appear to be related to the degree of chronic metabolic control as assessed by blood-glucose estimations or HbA_{ic} levels (33,34). Newly diagnosed diabetes with hyperglycaemia however, have raised levels which fall as the blood-glucose is brought under control (35). The presence of major vascular complications is associated with elevated platelet proteins; some reports demonstrate that patients with microvascular complications have levels similar to patients without demonstrable complications. This may, to some extent, be related to the method for collecting and preparing the plasma (vide supra) or else different patient selection (36,37). All studies agree that in the presence of renal failure due to diabetic nephropathy the plasma Btg rises sharply.

Platelet proteins have been studied in patients with both congenital and acquired primarily haematological disorders. The May-Hegglin anomaly and Bernard-Soulier syndrome are both associated with giant platelets and high platelet Btg content but this probably only reflects the increased platelet volume containing more α-granules (38). Deficiencies of Btg/PF4 have been observed in patients with α-storage pool disorder and the grey-platelet syndrome (39). Patients with acquired platelet disorders have also been studied. Aplastic anaemia is associated with very low plasma Btg levels (1,2,3,4). Patients with idiopathic thrombocytopenic purpura have concentrations within the normal range: when platelet destruction is intravascular however, as in thrombotic thrombocytopenic purpura, Btg levels are markedly raised (40). Myeloproliferative disorders are associated not only with raised platelet counts but in many individuals platelet dysfunction can be demonstrated. In patients with polycythaemia rubre vera, chronic myeloid leukaemia and essential thrombocythaemia the plasma Btg concentration is proportional to the whole blood-platelet count (1,2,3,4,41,42). Furthermore alterations in the platelet counts are reflected in corresponding changes in Btg. Recent studies suggest that the platelets have a partial storage pool disorder which could either arise as a result of defective megakaryocyte synthesis or be acquired within the circulation (43). The measurement of plasma and urinary Btg/PF4 levels has provided one more tool for the assessment of platelet function in vivo. Not only may they reflect platelet activation but they may have great potential for measuring the inhibitory effects of antiplatelet drugs.

REFERENCES

1. Ludlam CA, Anderton JL, Platelet B-thromboglobulin: Platelet function testing. Day HJ, Holmsen H, Zucker MB (eds), U.S. Dept. of Health, Education and Welfare. Publ. Hlth Serv. Nat. Inst. Health, pp 267-293, 1976.

2. Ludlam CA, Cash JD, Studies on the liberation of B-thromboglobulin from human platelets in vitro. Brit. J. Haemat. 33:239, 1976.

3. Ludlam CA, Moore S, Bolton AE, Pepper DS, Cash JD, The release of a platelet specific protein measured by a radioimmunoassay. Thromb. Res. 6:543, 1975.

4. Ludlam CA, Evidence for the platelet specificity of B-thromboglobulin and studies on its plasma concentration in health individuals. Brit. J. Haemat. 41:271, 1979.

5. Kaplan KL, B-thromboglobulin. Progress in Haemostasis and Thrombosis 5. pp 153-178, 1980.

6. Zahavi J, Kakkar VV, B-thromboglobulin: A specific marker of in-vivo platelet release reaction. Thrombos. Haemost. 44:23, 1980.

7. McLaren KM, Holloway L, Pepper DS, Human platelet factor 4 and tissue mast cells. Thromb. Res. 19:293, 1980.

8. Dawes J, Smith RC, Pepper DS, The release, distribution and clearance of human B-thromboglobulin and platelet factor 4. Thromb. Res. 12:851, 1978.

9. Conley LC, Hartman RC, Lalley JS, The relationship of heparin activity to platelet concentration. Proc. Soc. for Exp. Biol. and Med. 69:284, 1948.

10. Deuel TF, Senior RM, Chang D, Griffin GL, Heinrikson RL, Kaiser ET, Platelet factor 4 is chemotactic for neutrophils and monocytes. Proc. Nat. Acad. Sci. USA 78:4584, 1981.

11. Begg GS, Pepper DS, Chesterman CN, Morgan FJ, Complete covalent structure of human B-thromboglobulin. Amer. Chem. Soc. 17:1739, 1978.

12. Niewiarowski S, Walz DA, James P, Rucinski B, Kueppers F, Identification and separation of secreted platelet proteins by isoelectric focusing. Evidence that low-affinity platelet factor 4 is converted to B-thromboglobulin by limited proteolysis. Blood 55:453, 1980.

13. Hope W, Martin TJ, Chesterman CN, Morgan FJ, Human B-thromboglobulin inhibits PGI_2 production and binds to a specific site in bovine aortic endothelial cells. Nature 282:210, 1979.

14. Ager A, Gordon JL, Influence of human B-thromboglobulin on prostaglandin production by pig aortic endothelial cells in culture. Thromb. Res. 24:95, 1981.

15. Levine SP, Lindenfield J, Ellis JB, Raymond NM, Krentz LS, Increased plasma concentrations of platelet factor 4 in coronary artery disease. Circulation 64:626, 1981.

16. Kaplan KL, Noseel HL, Drillings M, Leszink G, Radioimmunoassay of PF4 and B-thromboglobulin: Development and application to studies of platelet release in relation to fibrinopeptide A generation. Brit. J. Haemat. 39:129, 1978.

17. Handin RI, McDonough M, Lesch M, Elevation of PF4 in acute myocardial function: Measurement by radioimmunoassay. J. Lab. clin. Med. 91:340, 1978.

18. Files JC, Malpass TW, Yee EK, Ritchie JL, Harker LA, Studies of human platelet α-granule release in vivo. Blood 58:607, 1981.

19. Franchi F, Canciani MT, Mannuci PM, The B-thromboglobulin test. Thrombos. Haemost. 44:107, 1980.

20. Randi ML, Fabris F, Casonato A, Girolami A, The effect of anticoagulant mixtures on Btg and PF4 levels. Thrombos. Haemost. 46:569, 1981.

21. Wolf P, The nature and significance of platelet products in human plasma. Brit. J. Haemat. 13:269, 1967.

22. Dewar HA, Marshall T, Weightman D, Prakash V, Boon PJ, B-thromboglobulin in antecubital vein blood: The influence of age, sex and blood-group. Thrombos. Haemost. 42:1159, 1979.

23. Van Hulsteijn H, Van Es A, Bertina R, Briët E, Plasma B-thromboglobulin and platelet factor 4 in renal failure. Thromb. Res. 24:175, 1981.

24. Andrassy K, Deppermann D, Ritz E, Koderisch J, Seelig H, Different effects of renal failure on B-thromboglobulin and high affinity platelet factor 4 (HA-PF4) concentrations. Thromb.Res. 18:469, 1980.

25. Depperman D, Andrassy K, Seelig H, Ritz E, Post D, Beta-thromboglobulin is elevated in renal failure without thrombosis. Thromb. Res. 17:63, 1980.

26. Bolton AE, Cooke ED, Lekhwani CP, Bowcock SA, Urinary B-thromboglobulin levels as a diagnostic marker for postoperative deep vein thrombosis. Thromb. Res. 19:249, 1980.

27. De Boer AC, Han P, Turpie AGG, Butt R, Zielinsky A, Genton E, Plasma and urine B-thromboglobulin concentration in patients with deep vein thrombosis. Blood 58:693, 1981.

28. Kutti J, Safai-Kutti S, Svardsudd K, Swedberg K, Wadenvik H, Plasma levels of platelet factor 4 in patients admitted to a coronary care unit. Scand. J. Haemat. 26:235, 1981.

29. Sobel M, Salzman EW, Davies GC, Handin RI, Sweeney J, Ploetz J, Kurland G, Circulating platelet products in unstable angina pectoris. Circulation 63:300, 1981.

30. Rasi V, Ikkala E, Torstila I, Plasma B-thromboglobulin in acute myocardial infarction. Thromb. Res. 25:203, 1982.

31. Pumphrey CW, Dawes J, Elevation of plasma B-thromboglobulin in patients with prosthetic cardiac valves. Thromb. Res. 22:147, 1981.

32. Cella G, Schivazappa L, Casonato A, Molaro LG, Girolami A, Westwick J, Lane DA, Kakkar VV, In vivo platelet release reaction in patients with heart valve prosthesis. Haemostasis 9:263, 1980.

33. Matthews JH, O'Connor JF, Hearnshaw JR, Wood JK, B-thromboglobulin and glycosylated haemoglobin in diabetes mellitus. Scand. J. Haemat. 23:421, 1979.

34. Betteridge DJ, Zahavi J, Jones NAG, Shine B, Kakkar VV, Galton DJ, Platelet function in diabetes mellitus in relationship to complications

glycosylated haemoglobin and serum lipoproteins. Eur. J. Clin. Invest. 11:273, 1981.

35. Preston FE, Marcola BH, Ward JD, Porter NR, Timperley WR, Elevated B-thromboglobulin levels and circulating platelet aggregates in diabetic microangiopathy. Lancet 1:238, 1981.

36. Borsey DQ, Dawes J, Fraser DM, Prowse CV, Elton RA, Clark BF, B-thromboglobulin in diabetes mellitus. Diabetologia 18:353, 1980.

37. Elving LD, Casparie AF, Miedema K, Russchen CJ, Plasma B-thromboglobulin in diabetics with and without microangiopathic complications. Diabetologia 21:160, 1981.

38. Fabris F, Casonato A, Randi ML, Girolami A, Plasma and platelet B-thromboglobulin levels in patients with May-Hegglin anomaly. Haemosthasis 9:126, 1980.

39. Levy-Toledano S, Caen JP, Breton-Gorius J, Rendu F, Cywiner-Golenzer C, Dupuy E, Legrand Y, Maclouf J, Gray platelet syndrome: α granula deficiency. J. Lab. clin. Med. 98:831, 1981.

40. Han P, Turpie AGG, Genton E, Plasma B-thromboglobulin: Differentiation between intravascular and extravascular platelet destruction. Blood 54:1192, 1979.

41. Boughton BJ, Corbett WEN, Ginsburg AD, Myeloproliferative disorders: A paradox of in vivo and in vitro platelet function. J. clin. Path. 30:228, 1977.

42. Cortelazzo S, Viero P, Barbui T, Platelet activation in myeloproliferative disorders. Thrombos. Haemost. 45:211, 1981.

43. Pareti FI, Gugliotta L, Mannucci L, Guarini A, Mannucci PM, Biochemical and metabolic aspects of platelet dysfunction in chronic myeloproliferative disorders. Thrombos. Haemost. 47:84, 1982.

23 BETA-THROMBOGLOBULIN AND PLATELET FACTOR 4 IN POLYCYTHEMIA AND THROMBOCYTHEMIA

Y. NAJEAN, O. POIRIER

INTRODUCTION

As already has been discussed elsewhere in this volume, the clinical significance of excessive values of βTG and PF-4 still remain a matter for discussion. Although they were suggested seven years ago (1), the potential application of these assays remains controversial. In spite of positive conclusions, from a statistical point of view, a detailed analysis of the published reports shows a low predictive value in terms of sentitivity of the tests; thus, there is no difference between myocardial infarct and simple coronary artery disease (2,3), no difference between dying and surviving patients (4), a low statistical difference of the marker values as a function of the severity of the arterial disease in diabetics (5,6). Thus Files (4) was able to conclude that this assay "does not identify individuals with stable chronic atherosclerotic vascular disease and not provide a means for identifying patients at risk".

Polycythemic patients are a high risk group for vascular accidents: age, vascular antecedents, hyperviscosity related to excessive hematocrit during relapses, increase of the platelet count are favoring factors. We have been able to study 191 patients in a an attempt to clarify the following points:

- the value of simultaneous assay of βTG and PF-4;
- the relationship between these factors and age and platelet count;
- the relationship between these factors and the vascular status, as it can be estimated from the clinical study (thromboembolic antecedents);
- finally, during follow-up, the relationship of these factors to the occurence of a new thromboembolic accident and with

Table 1. Reproducibility of the βTG and PF-4 values in polycythemic patients, with similar values of the platelet counts at successive determinations

	Platelet count at the successive assays	Similar results (difference <30%)	Different results (>30%)
βTG	$<400.10^9/1$	25	12
	$>400.10^9/1$	17	3
PF-4	$<400.10^9/1$	22	15
	$>400.10^9/1$	8	12

Table 2. Correlation between βTG and PF-4

Platelet count	$<250.10^9/1$	250 - 400	400 - 500	>550
Correlation coefficient (r)	0.67 (37 cases)	0.58 (36 cases)	0.49 (21 cases)	0.44 (22 cases)

Table 3a. Difference between β TG and PF-4, according to the platelet count at the time of dosage, and to the presence of arterial vascular antecedents

	Platelet count (10^3/cmm)	No arterial antecedent (116 cases)		Arterial antecedent (75 cases)		Statistical significance (F test)
β TG	100 - 245	(37)	51,3 ± 23,6	(25)	74,0 ± 31,5	0,01 > P > 0,001
	250 - 395	(36)	67,3 ± 26,1	(25)	133,8 ± 52,8	P < 0,001
	400 - 545	(21)	128,5 ± 45,7	(12)	141,8 ± 59,0	N S
	⩾ 550	(22)	152,5 ± 40,4	(13)	173,2 ± 37,3	N S
PF-4	100 - 245	(37)	15,6 ± 11,1	(25)	26,3 ± 26,7	0,02 > P > 0,01
	250 - 395	(36)	24,7 ± 10,5	(25)	46,4 ± 46,0	0,01 > P > 0,005
	400 - 545	(21)	43,7 ± 25,7	(12)	43,8 ± 21,4	N S
	⩾ 550	(22)	45,8 ± 27,7	(13)	55,0 ± 37,1	N S

the prescription of anti-aggregating drugs.

βTG (Amersham, U.K.) and PF-4 (Abbott Laboratories, Diagnosis, Division, Chicago, U.S.A.) were assayed in the same plasma sample, taken by the same physician, in the same laboratory, with the same material and at the same time (between 10 am and 1 pm) for all cases.

Reproducibility of the results

As shown in table 1, βTG and PF-4 assays give reproducible results at consecutive dosages, more than one year of delay in most the cases, when the platelet counts remain similar. It can however be noted that βTG reproducibility is better than that of PF-4 ($p<0.02$). Hematocrit changes do not interfere with changes of platelet marker values.

Correlation between βTG and PF-4

As already proven in physiological situations, βTG and PF-4 are closely correlated, with a mean βTG/PF-4 ratio of 3.5. The correlation coefficient is given in table 2. It can however be noted that, when platelet count is high (table 2) or when vascular antecedents are observed (table 3a and b), the correlation is lower than in normal situations, with higher increase of βTG than of PF-4.

As previously noted, simultaneous assay of PF-4 and βTG is justified (7,8,9,1). Urinary excretion of PF-4 is indeed greater than that of βTG and in cases of renal insufficiency the relative retention of βTG renders its assay uninterpretable (10). On another hand, the circulating life span of PF-4 is much shorter than of βTG, which makes its in vivo increase lower. In the case of in vitro release of the markers, a parallel increase may imply a technical error in sampling. Kaplan and Owen (11) clearly stated that "studies in which only one of the proteins has been measured ... are difficult to interpret".

Correlation between platelet markers and the platelet count

In the whole group the correlation coefficient was found to be highly significant: $r = 0.54$ for βTG and 0.45 for PF-4.

Table 3b. Ratio βTG - PF-4 in patients with or without thromboembolic antecedents

	Patients with platelet count $>500.10^9/L$	Patients with platelet count $<500.10^9/1$ with βTG > 50 ng/ml	Patients with platelet count $<500.10^9/1$ with βTG < 50 ng/ml
Arterial antecedents	5.04 ± 3.21	4.64 ± 2.39	4.66 ± 3.58
Absence of arterial antecedents	3.17 ± 1.50	3.83 ± 2.20	3.41 ± 1.36
	F = 4.35 (1.25)	F = 3.01 (1.97)	F = 1.31 ± 1.18)
	$p < 0.05$	$0.1 > p > 0.05$	N S

Table 4. βTG and PF-4 values in 116 cases without thromboembolic antecedent, as a function of the platelet count (116 cases)

platelet count	$100 - 250.10^9/1$	250 - 400	400 - 500	⩾ 550
βTG (ng/ml)	51.3 ± 23.6	67.3 ± 26.1	128.5 ± 45.7	152.5 ± 40.4
PF-4 (ng/ml)	15.6 ± 11.1	24.7 ± 10.9	43.7 ± 25.9	45.8 ± 27.7

Detailed results, for the patients without arterial antecedents, are given on table 4. Repetivite assays do confirm these results. 42 from the 57 cases twice tested in absence of significant change of the platelet count showed similar results: 8 of the 10 cases tested before and after relapse with clear increase of the platelet count demonstrated similar increase of markers; in 19 cases studied before and after 32 P-induced remission, 16 exhibited a parallel decrease of both the platelet markers.

The present results confirm previous data (4,9,12,13). Their importance, from a clinical point of view, rests in that the "normality" obliged us to take into consideration the current platelet count; any improvement or worsening also must be interpreted in function of the platelet concentration.

The ratio βTG vs PF-4 is higher in patients with thromboembolic antecedents, even if the statistical significance is low (table 3b). This fact, again, gives importance to the simultaneous assay of both the factors.

Correlation of βTG and PF-4 with patient's age

Multiparametric analysis shows that, at similar platelet count and when arterial antecedents are taken into consideration, it remains a weak correlation between the marker levels and age: $r = 0.29$ for βTG and 0.28 for PF-4 ($p < 0.02$).

Correlation between βTG and PF-4, and antecedent of thromboembolic events

Precise clinical data were obtained in all the cases included in the present study. Cerebral vascular accident was noted in 19 cases, myocardial infarct in 18, leg arthritis in 26, and several consecutive accidents in 12. When the platelet count is considered statistically significant difference is observed between the patients with, or without, thromboembolic antecedents (table 3b). Once again, the difference is more important for βTG than for PF-4.

From these data, sensitivity (i.e. the ratio of cases with values in excess of one s.d. from the mean expected value to the number of cases with thromboembolic antecedent) is 0.70 for βTG

Table 5. βTG and PF-4 values observed in 11 patients who experienced thromboembolic accident in the 12 months following these assays

	Patient's age	Accident	Platelet count 10^3 at the time of marker's assay	βTG (into brackets expected value)	PF-4	ratio βTG/PF-4
1.	57	phlebitis	170	56 (51)	5 (16)	11.1
2.	69	angina	750	120 (152)	26 (46)	4.7
3.	55	phlebitis	250	56 (51)	15 (16)	3.7
4.	55	phlebitis	450	144 (128)	20 (44)	7.2
5.	67	stroke	450	94 (128)	16 (44)	5.8
6.	75	phlebitis	700	73 (152)	13 (46)	5.7
7.	26	retro-placental hemorrhage	860	176 (152)	29 (46)	6.1
8.	73	leg arteritis	120	72 (51)	8 (16)	9.0
9.	81	phlebitis	1200	150 (162)	40 (46)	3.8
10.	75	phlebitis	275	26 (67)	10 (25)	2.6
11.	51	myocardial infarct	126	24 (51)	8 (16)	3.0
						m = 5.7

Table 6. βTG and PF-4 values in patients treated by anti-aggregating agents

	31 patients treated by aspirine + dipyridamol		14 patients tested before and after ticlopidine therapy		
	results below the expected value	results higher the expected value	drop	similar result	increase
βTG	14	17	4	6	4
PF-4	16	15	5	7	2

and 0.53 for PF-4. But a low specificity of both these biological tests impedes correct clinical analysis.

Occurence of a vascular accident after platelet marker assays (table 5)

All the patients have been followed and the risk factors eliminated as much as possible (hematocrit maintained below 50% and if possible platelet count below $600.10^{9}/1$. Nevertheless, 11 cases had a vascular accident in the year following the platelet markers assay. If there is no clear excess of the markers value, the observed ratio βTG/PF-4 is higher than that observed in the whole group of patients (5.7 vs 3.5).

Correlation between platelet marker values and anti-aggregation therapy

No prospective analysis of anti-aggregating therapy has been done by using the in vitro platelet marker assays. Such a study however would be useful, since the clinical usefulness of anti-aggregating drugs remains a matter of controversy. In polycythemia, preliminary results of aspirine + dipyridamol in phlebotomized patients do not seem improve the prognosis, in spite of a hemorrhagic toxicity (Polycythemia Vera Study Group; non-published results of protocol 05).

We have compared the observed values of βTG and PF-4 in 31

cases treated by aspirine + dipyridamole with than expected; no statistical difference was observed. 14 cases have been tested before and after ticlopidine therapy; 4 only demonstrated evident decrease of the βTG and/or PF-4 levels (table 6). So the value of these assays for estimating the clinical interest of anti-aggregating therapy still remains to prove. A prospective protoco is presently running.

Conclusion

In spite of a large number of assays, no definitive conclusion can be drawn. We only can conclude that simultaneous assay of both the markers is necessary, that platelet count and age are to be taken into consideration for clinical interpretation, and that a statistically valid correlation does exist between the marker levels and thromboembolic antecedents.

However, the two useful informations, i.e. the predictive value of these tests, and their interest for demonstrating in vivo usefulness of anti-aggregating drugs, still remain not answered. We can hope from prospective studies an answer to these questions, since the practical interest of the platelet markers is obviously not to verify the platelet count and the vascular antecedents, but to help to forecast the future and to choose a possible preventive treatment.

REFERENCES

1. Rucinski B, Niewarowski S, James P, Walze DA, Budyski AZ, Antiheparin proteins secreted by human platelets. Purification, characterization and radio-immuno-assay. Blood 58:47, 1979.
2. Wadenvik H, Erikson KA, Safai S, Swedberg K, Kutti J, Plasma concentration of platelet factor 4 in acute myocardial infarction. Scand. J. Haemat. 26:369, 1981.
3. White GC, Marouf AA, Platelet factor 4 levels in patients with coronary artery disease. J. Lab. clin. Med. 97:369, 1981.
4. Files JC, Malpasse TW, Yee EK, Ritchie JL, Harker LA, Studies of human platelet-granule in vivo. Blood 58:607, 1981.
5. De Boer AC, Butt R, Turpie AGG, Genton E, The use of the evacuated blood collection tube in the determination of plasma beta-thromboglobulin. Thromb.Res. 20:693, 1980.
6. Levine PH, Fisher M, Fullerton AL, Duffy CP, Hoogasian JJ, Human platelet 4: Application in cerebral vascular disease. Amer. J. Hemat. 10:375, 1981.
7. Niewarowski S, Walz DA, James P, Rucinski R, Kueppers F, Identification and separation of secreted platelet proteins by iso-electric focusing. Blood 55:450, 1980.
8. Kutti J, Safai-Kutti S, Saroulis GC, Good RA, Plasma levels beta-thromboglobulin and platelet factor 4 in relation to the venous platelet concentration. Acta haemat. 64:1, 1980.
9. Lokiec F, Najean Y, Intérêt clinique du dosage radio-immunologique de la beta-thromboglobuline et du facteur plaquettaire 4. Nouv. Press Méd. 9:2833, 1980.
10. Dawes J, Smith RC, Pepper DC, The release distribution and clearance of human factor 4 and beta-thromboglobulin. Thromb. Res. 12:851, 1978.
11. Kaplan KL, Owen J, Plasma levels of beta-thromboglobulin: an platelet factor 4 as indices of platelet activation in vivo. Blood 57:199, 1981.
12. Chesterman CN, MacCready JR, Doyle JD, Morgan FJ, Plasma levels of platelet factor 4 measured by radio immuno-assay. Brit. J. Haemat. 40:489, 1978.
13. Ludlam CA, Evidence for the platelet specificity of beta-thromboglobulin and studies on its plasma concentration in healthy individuals. Brit. J. Haemat. 41:271, 1979.

24 BETA-THROMBOGLOBULIN, PLATELET FACTOR 4 AND CORONARY HEART DISEASE

E. PELISSIER, M. BAILLET, C. TZINCOCA, E. TERRIER

INTRODUCTION

The role of platelets in coronary heart disease and atherosclerosis is the subject of many contradictory publications, in which both the type of platelet tests performed and the delay between the clinical onset of the disease and the time of the tests widely differ.

The in vivo platelet activation can be measured, in plasma, by assaying 2 specific platelet proteins released from the α-granules, β-thromboglobulin (B.TG) and platelet factor 4 (PF4). These 2 proteins have been found either increased or normal during myocardial infarction or exercise-tolerance tests (1,2,3). It seemed therefore interesting to study, in 126 patients, the levels of B.TG and PF4, comparatively with the importance of the clinical symptoms, the electrocardiographic modifications and the extent of coronary lesions, identified by angiography or anatomically during surgery for coronary by-pass. The simultaneous assay of both proteins allowed a more accurate interpretation of abnormal results.

Patients and methods

In 126 patients suffering from severe coronary heart disease (116 men, 10 women; mean age 54, range 31-75 years), assays were performed 2 to 5 days before coronary artery by-pass grafting. B.TG and PF4 were assayed by radioimmuno-assay (RIA) (Amersham kit for B.TG, Abbott kit for PF4).

Blood-samples were placed in melting ice immediately after sampling and centrifuged within the following 30 min. Statistical analysis of the mean results was performed using the Student t test.

All values above the mean ± 2SD for the controls, determined from a series of 62 normal subjects (29 men and 33 women, aged between 18 and 50 years: 24.2 ± 9.9 ng/ml for B.TG and 4.3 ± 2.0 ng/ml for PF4 were considered as abnormal. Pathological results were thus above 44.0 ng/ml for B.TG and above 8.3 ng/ml for PF4.

Results

The B.TG and PF4 levels varied in the same way for all the patients (correlation coefficient r = 0.81) (fig 1). There was linear regression according to the following equation: PF4 = 0.29 (B.TG) - 1.69. The PF4 level was increased every time the B.TG level was above 44 ng/ml, except in one case (B.TG 51 ng/ml, PF4 7 ng/ml). But the PF4 level was proportionally more increased than the B.TG level in 6 patients, 3 of whom were treated with sub-cutaneous calcium heparinate or intra-venous heparin.

The mean levels of B.TG and PF4 were higher than the mean control values. B.TG was above 44 ng/ml in 55 cases (43 percent of patients).

B.TG patients: 43.5 ± 17.9 ng/ml* Controls: 24.2 ± 9.9 ng/ml*
PF4 patients: 11.2 ± 6.8 ng/ml** Controls: 4.3 ± 2.0 ng/ml**

* $P < 0.001$
** $P < 0.001$

B.TG and PF4 levels varied according to clinical symptoms. The mean levels for both proteins were higher in the group of patients with unstable angina pectoris or threat syndrome ($P < 0.001$) than in the group of patients with stable chronic angina. In the most severely ill patients, B.TG levels exceeded the threshold value of 44 ng/ml 27 times (67 percent) whereas in stable chronic angina, the threshold was exceeded in only 12 cases (26 percent).

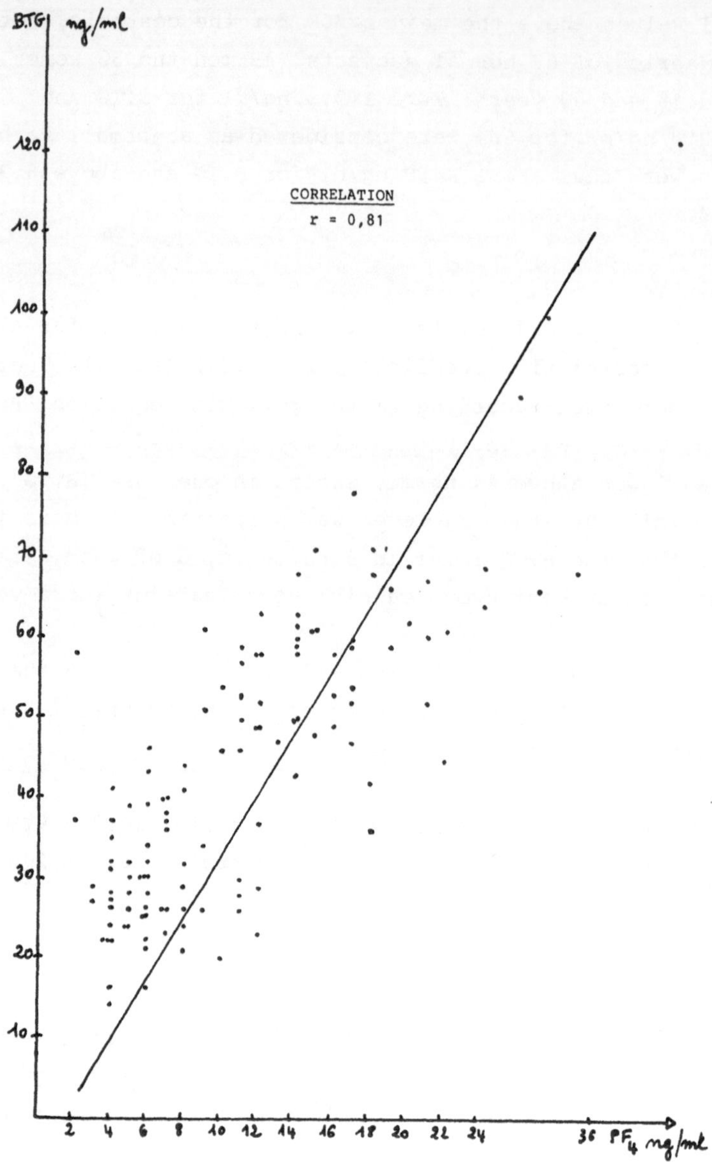

Fig. 1.

	B.TG ng/ml	PF4 ng/ml
AORTIC VALVULOPATHY		
Without angina pectoris n=28	34.6 ± 12.7	7.8 ± 4.3
Stable angina pectoris n=46	36.9 ± 15.1	9.0 ± 4.8
Unstable angina pectoris n=40	51.8 ± 18.3	14.7 ± 7.7

B.TG and PF4 levels varied with the type of lesion detected by electrocardiography.

	B.TG ng/ml	PF4 ng/ml
ISCHEMIA AND/OR NECROSIS		
Absence n=34	32.9 ± 12.3*	7.2 ± 3.8**
Presence n=61	51.1 ± 20.4*	12.7 ± 7.0**

* P <0.001
** P <0.001

The B.TG levels were above 44 ng/ml in 37 patients with necrosis and/or ischemia (60 per cent), instead of 5 patients in the first group (15 per cent).

B.TG and PF4 levels also increased with the number of stenosed vessels detected by coronary arteriography. 8/27 patients (30 per cent) had B.TG levels above 44 ng/ml when only one vessel is affected, against 23/36 (63 per cent) when 3-4 vessels are abnormal.

	1 vessel (n=27)	2 vessels (n=61)	3-4 vessels (n=36)
B.TG ng/ml	38.4 ± 23.0*	41.9 ± 16.7	49.5 ± 15.7*
PF4 ng/ml	9.6 ± 6.7+	10.3 ± 6.2	13.6 ± 6.0**

* 0.02 < P> 0.01
** 0.02 < P> 0.01

B.TG and PF4 levels were higher when the number of coronary artery grafts increased. The difference was highly significant between one graft, on the one hand, and 3-4 grafts on the other. The same difference was found when the patients with B.TG levels above 44 ng/ml were compared: one graft: 9/38 patients (24 per cent), 3-4 grafts: 17/24 patients (71 per cent).

	1 graft n= 38	2 grafts n= 64	3 grafts n= 24
B.TG ng/ml	37.3 ± 14.3*	40.7 ± 16.0	53.0 ± 14.4*
PF4 ng/ml	7.5 ± 4.8**	10.8 ± 5.9	19.1 ± 5.3**

* P 0.001

** P 0.001

Patients treated with calcium heparinate had higher B.TG and PF4 levels than patients without anticoagulant therapy, but the difference was only slightly significant for B.TG (0.10 <P> 0.05), and not significant for PF4.

There was no significant difference between the 3 evenly distributed age groups: less than 50 years, 50 to 55 years. The number of subjects over 60 was too small to allow interpretation.

No correlation was found between B.TG and PF4 levels and platelet number in whole blood.

Discussion

The simultaneous assay of B.TG and HA-PF4 revealed a positive correlation between these 2 parameters with a regression coefficient of r= 0.81, which has also been found by Lokiec et al (4). For these authors, B.TG and HA-PF4 are a measure of the same physiological function, as they are released in the same way from the α-granules, and increase in parallel in identical pathological circumstances. Nevertheless their simultaneous assay on the same blood sample has been recommended (5) to interpret abnormal results: the artificial in vitro release determines a decrease in the B.TG/PF4 ratio, comparatively to controls. Thus, in our series of 126 patients, PF4 was relatively higher than B.TG in 6 cases: the hypothesis that PF4 was released after sampling cannot be excluded in 3 of them who were not under anticoagulation by heparin.

In unstable angina and threat syndrome, B.TG and PF4 levels were found higher than in aortic valvular disease without angina, or in stable angina. Neri Serneri et al (6) also found an increase in B.TG essentially in the active forms of coronary heart disease. For Smitherman et al (7), the B.TG level is abnormal in 59 per cent of patients with unstable angina (result close to our own: 67 per cent, defined by criteria similar to those used to diagnose unstable angina and threat syndrome).

A positive correlation was also found with the electrocardiographic signs of post-infarction myocardial ischemia and/or necrosis: 37/61 patients had a B.TG level above 44 ng/ml (i.e. 60 per cent). These results seem, at first glance, to be in contradiction with those of Rasi et al (8) who showed a normal B.TG level 4 to 6 months after myocardial infarction. However, the ECG results were not mentioned during the period of observation. Similarly, Stratton et al (3) and Mathis et al (2) concluded that there was no positive correlation between B.TG and PF4 and signs of ischemia induced by the exercise test (depression or downsloping of the S-T segment). But these results are in contradiction with those of Green (1), who had earlier described an increase of more than 50 per cent in the PF4 level in subjects with a positive exercise test. In our series of patients, ECG signs of myocardial ischemia, when they exist, are present in the resting state, and are always associated with signs of necrosis which reveal a past, more or less patent, infarction.

The correlation between B.TG - PF4 and the number of narrowed vessels revealed by coronary arteriography, may be biased by the possible severity of an isolated abnormality trunk of the left coronary artery and by the usual under-estimation of the lesions revealed by the technique (9). The number of by-passes performed during surgery therefore seems to be a better criterium when at least, the left coronary artery stenosis is corrected by 2 different grafts. The positive correlation between B.TG and PF4 and number of by-passes is highly significant in our series and tends to show that the release of these 2 proteins, and therefore platelet activation, is proportional to the extent of coronary lesions. Platelet activation, whether cause or consequence of the lesions (7) can lead by the prostaglandin pathway to the synthesis of thromboxane A2, generally considered as a possible mediator for coronary artery spasm (10). This hypothesis on the role of platelets in myocardial ischemia has led to an increasing interest in anti-aggregant substances, some of which (11) seem to decrease the mortality and morbidity of myocardial infarction.

In conclusion, the B.TG and PF4 immuno-assays could be a means of detecting the patients with increased platelet reactivity who might benefit from treatment with anti-aggregant substances (12).

REFERENCES

1. Green LH, Seroppian E, Handin RI, Platelet activation during exercise-induced myocardial ischemia. New Engl. J. Med. 302:193, 1980.

2. Mathis PC, Wohl H, Wallach SR, Engler RL, Lack of release of platelet factor 4 during exercise-induced myocardial ischemia. New Engl. J. Med. 304:1275, 1981.

3. Stratton JR, Malpass TW, Ritchie JL, Pfeifer MA, Harker LA, Studies of platelet factor 4 and B. thromboglobulin release during exercise: Lack of relationship to myocardial ischemia. Circulation 66:33, 1982.

4. Lokiec F, Najean Y, Intérêt clinique du dosage radio-immunologique de la B. thromboglobuline et du facteur plaquettaire 4. Nouv. Presse Méd. 9:2833, 1980.

5. Kaplan KL, Owen J, Plasma levels of B. thromboglobulin and platelet factor 4 as indices of platelet activation in vivo. Blood 57:199, 1981.

6. Neri Serneri GG, Gensini GF, Abbate R, Mugnaini C, Laureano R, Conte A, Increased fibrinopeptide A (FPA) plasma levels and thromboxane A2 (TxA2) production by platelets in patients with ischaemic heart disease (IHD). Circulation 58:II Abstr. nr. 350, 1978.

7. Smitherman TC, Milam M, Wood J, Willerson JT, Frenkel EP, Elevated B. thromboglobulin in peripheral venous blood of patients with acute myocardial ischemia: direct evidence for enhanced platelet reactivity in vivo. Amer. J. Cardiol. 48:395, 1981.

8. Rasi V, Ikkala E, Torstila I, Plasma B. thromboglobulin in acute myocardial infarction. Thromb. Res. 25:203, 1982.

9. Ganz W, Editorial: Coronary spasm in myocardial function: Fact or fiction? Circulation 63-487, 1981.

10. Lewy RI, Smith JB, Silver MJ, Saia J, Walinsky P, Wiener L, Detection of thromboxane B_2 in peripheral blood of patients with Prinsmetal's angina. Prostaglandins and Medicine 5:243, 1979.

11. The anturane reinfarction trial: Reevaluation of outcome. New Engl. J. Med. 306:1005, 1982.

12. Salem HH, Koutts J, Firkin BG, Circulating platelet aggregates in ischaemic heart disease and their correlation to platelet life span. Thromb. Res. 17:707, 1980.

25 BETA-THROMBOGLOBULIN RELEASE AND THROMBOXANE SYNTHESIS IN DIABETIC PLATELETS: EFFECT OF GLYCEMIC CONTROL AND RETINOPATHY

P.J. GUILLAUSSEAU, E. DUPUY, J. MACLOUF, A. WARNET, J. LUBETZKI

INTRODUCTION

An increased tendency to microvascular and atherosclerotic lesions is well known in diabetes mellitus patients. Platelet hyperactivity has been reported by several investigators (1,2,3,4). The factors responsible for this hyperaggregability are still a matter of discussion, though plasmatic factors and intrinsic platelet abnormalities have been described (1,2).

Plasma and platelet β-TG levels, β-TG release induced by thrombin and Calcium Ionophore A 23187 and TX synthesis of platelets stimulated by thrombin have been studied in 2 groups of diabetics and compared with respect to sex and age matched controls.

Patients and methods

Subjects: 3 groups of subjects have been studied: 12 type I (insulin-dependent) diabetics (IDD) of recent onset without any complication (RO) (age: 26 ± 6 years, 8 men and 4 women, diabetes duration: several days - 1 year), 6 type I diabetics with proliferative retinopathy (PR) (age: 28.8 ± 2.3 years, 3 men, 3 women, diabetes duration 12 - 15 years) and 12 sex and age matched normal volunteers as control group (age: 33 ± 10 years, 8 men, 4 women).

Metabolic studies: the 12 recent onset type I diabetics were studied before and after 15 days of strict metabolic control (insulin 3 injections daily) as in patients in the metabolic department. Metabolic parameters are described in table 1. Blood sugar was determined by enzymatic method on plasma, total HbA_1 by the method of Kynoch and Lehman (5).

Table 1. Metabolic parameters

	Before	After	p
Fasting blood sugar (mM)	11.3 ± 1.5	6.9 ± 0.9	<0.025
Post prandial blood sugar (mM)	15.6 ± 1.4	10.4 ± 1.6	<0.025
Hb A1 (N= 6 ± 1.6) (%)	12.3 ± 0.5	10.5 ± 0.6	<0.025

Methods: plasma β-thromboglobulin (BTG) was assayed by radioimmunoassay (RIA) according to Ludlam and Cash (6) using the Amersham kit (Amersham Ltd), France). Platelets were isolated from plasma by metrizamide gradient as described by Levy-Toledano et al (7). Total BTG platelet content was measured by RIA tritonated platelets (1% Triton X100) (SIGMA). Thromboxane A_2 was evaluated by RIA of its stable metabolite thromboxane B_2 (TXB_2) using an iodinated tracer as described elsewhere (8). Isolated platelets were stimulated either by bovine thrombin (Hoffman La Roche) at 0.025, 0.1 and 0.25 U/ml final concentrations or by calcium ionophores A 23187 (Calbiochem) at 0.125 and 0.25 final concentrations. The release reaction was blocked after 2 min by 0.1 M EDTA (SIGMA) in ice. After centrifugation (10.000 g - 15 sec) the supernatant was frozen and kept at - 20°C until analysis.

All results are expressed as mean ± SEM ($\bar{m}$ ± SEM). Paired and unpaired Wilcoxon tests and the paired student t-test were used for statistical analysis.

Results

Plasma BTG levels: a significant increase in plasma BTG levels was observed in diabetics, specially in patients with proliferative retinopathy (fig 1). In diabetics without complications (DO) no difference was observed before and after metabolic control (fig 2).

Total BTG platelet content: no difference was observed in diabetics compared to control subjects, in diabetics with proliferative retinopathy compared to diabetics without vascular complication (fig 3) and in diabetics before and after metabolic

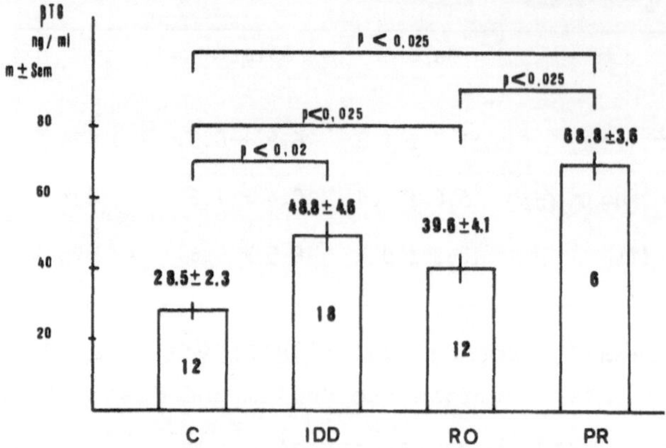

Fig. 1. Plasma BTG levels in diabetics.

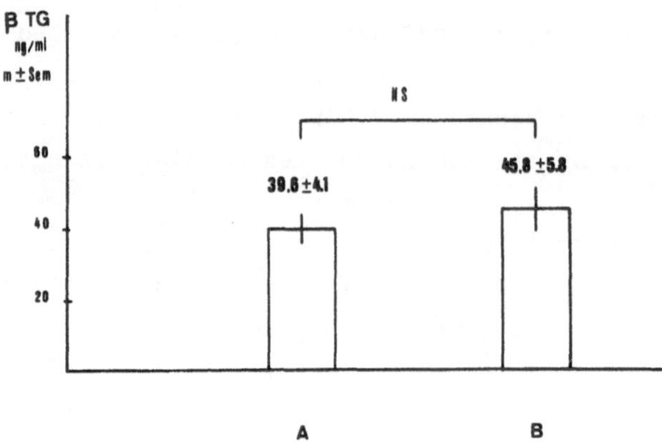

Fig. 2. Plasma BTG levels in diabetics without microangiopathy.

improvement (fig 4).

Thrombin induced BTG release: an enhanced BTG release was only observed with low thrombin concentration (0.025 U/ml) in diabetics compared to control, without any difference between patients with or without complications (fig 5) and after equilibrium (fig 6). At higher thrombin concentrations (0.1 U/ml) (fig 7) and (0.25 U/ml) (fig 8) no difference between diabetics and control was observed.

Calcium ionophore A 23187 induced BTG release: at concentra-

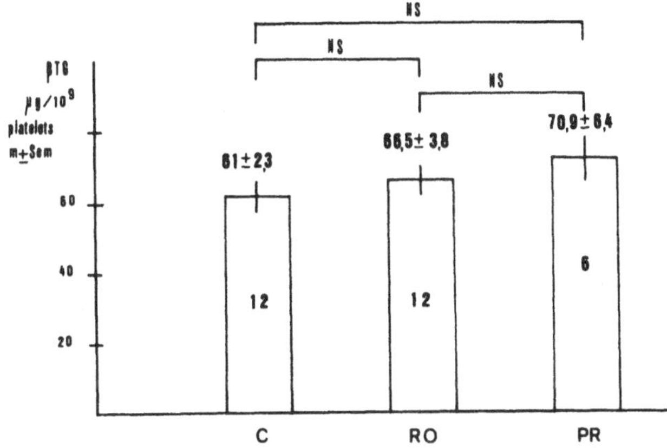

Fig. 3. Total BTG platelet content in diabetics without angiopathy (RO), with proliferative retinopathy (PR).

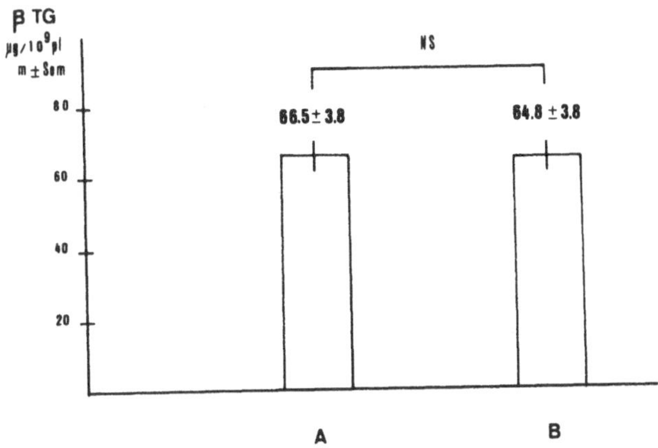

Fig. 4. Total BTG platelet content in diabetics (RO) before (A) and after (B) equilibrium.

tions of 0.125 uM and 0.25 uM of ionophore A 23187, BTG release was parallel in diabetics with and without microangiopathy and in controls (fig 9,10).

With the highest concentration of ionophore (0.05 μM) an increased BTG release was noticed in diabetics without complications. After metabolic control, the release of BTG returned to normal values (fig 11).

Thrombin induced TXB_2 synthesis: As for BTG release enhanced TXB_2 synthesis was only observed with low thrombin concentration

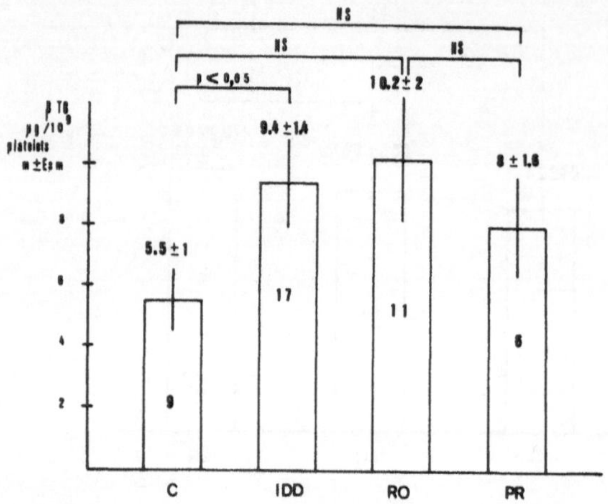

Fig. 5. Thrombin (0.025 U/ml) induced BTG release in diabetics.

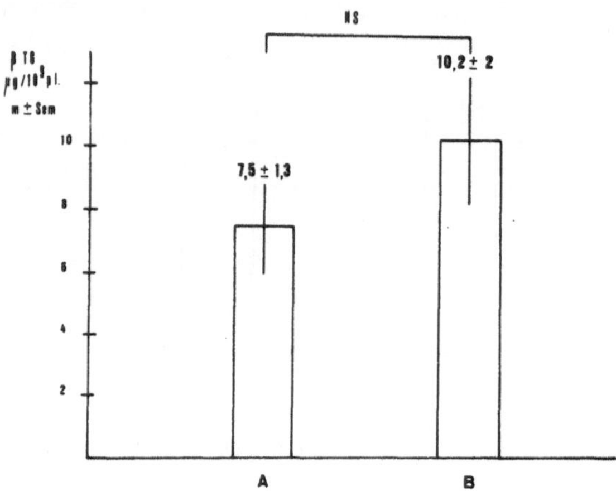

Fig. 6. Thrombin (0.025 U/ml) induced BTG release in RO before (A) and after (B) glycemic control.

(0.025 U/ml) (fig 12) without modification after glycemic control (fig 13) and without difference between diabetics with and without microangiopathy.

Discussion

As previously described by other groups (9-15) increased plasma BTG levels, reflected as in vivo platelet hyperactivity,

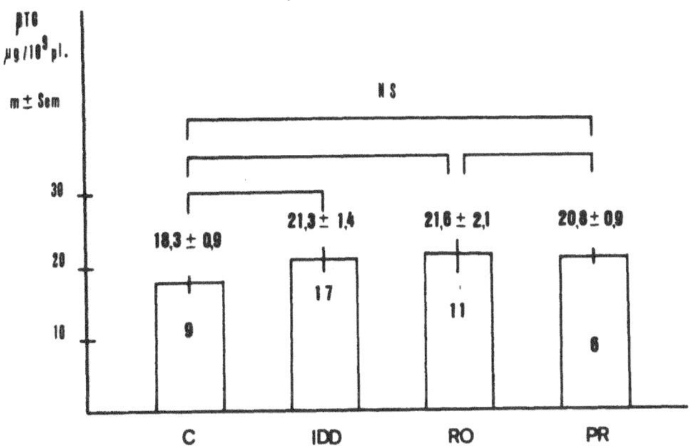

Fig. 7. Thrombin (0.1 U/ml) induced BTG release in diabetics compared to control.

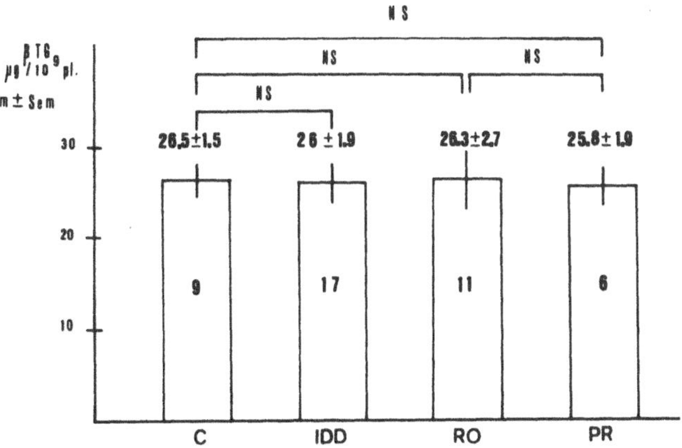

Fig. 8. Thrombin (0.25 U/ml) induced BTG release in diabetics compared to control.

was observed in diabetics mainly in diabetics with vascular complications but without influence of glycemic control.

These abnormalities are not related to a modification in total platelet BTG which is comparable in diabetics and controls, but to a platelet hyperactivity and low thrombin concentration without influence of short term glycemic control. Artificial pancreas realizing perfect euglycemia (16) is probably needed

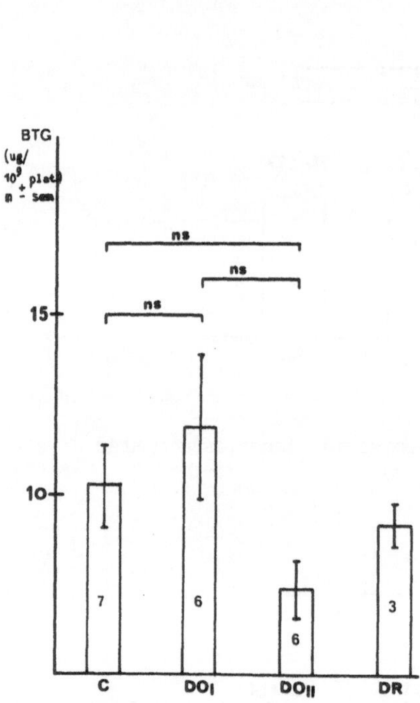

Fig. 9. Calcium Ionophore (0.125 uM) induced BTG release in diabetics without complications before (DOI) and after (DOII) equilibrium and in diabetics with proliferative retinopathy (DR).

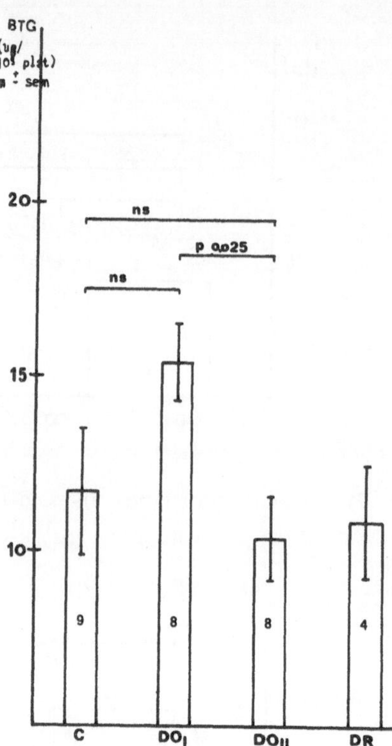

Fig. 10. Calcium Ionophore (0.25 uM) induced BTG release in diabetics without angiopathy before (DOI) and after (DOII) equilibrium and in diabetics with proliferative retinopathy (DR).

to reverse platelet disorders. Enhanced TXA_2 synthesis is associated to increase BTG release with the same thrombin concentration in diabetics compared to controls without any influence of retinal state nor metabolic control.

Previous observations have reported similar results after platelet stimulation by thrombin (17) ADP (18) or collagen (17) in which the metabolism of endogenous arachidonic acid is involved. TXA_2 synthesis derived from exogenous arachidonic acid seems to be normal (17). An alteration in the platelet membrane phospholipids could be suggested. This disorder may not be specific of platelets since increased adhesion of diabetic erythrocytes to normal cultured endothelial cells

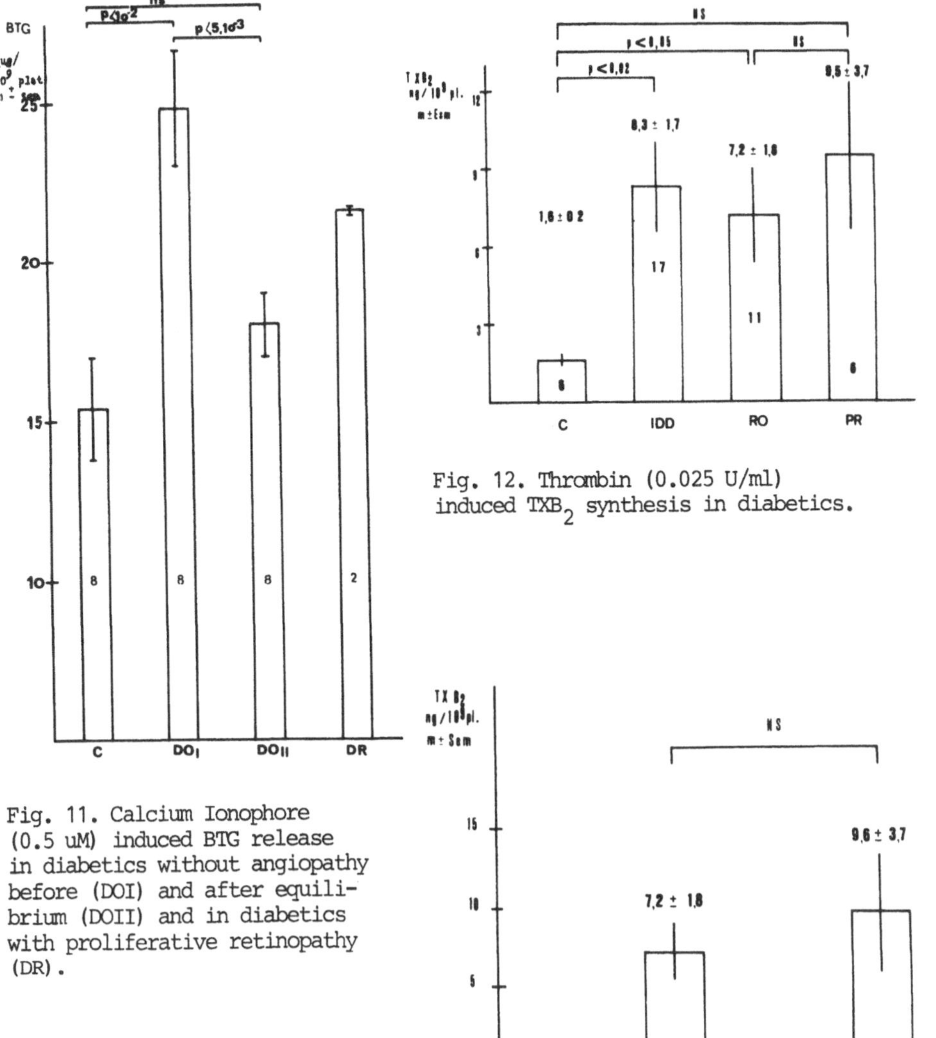

Fig. 11. Calcium Ionophore (0.5 uM) induced BTG release in diabetics without angiopathy before (DOI) and after equilibrium (DOII) and in diabetics with proliferative retinopathy (DR).

Fig. 12. Thrombin (0.025 U/ml) induced TXB_2 synthesis in diabetics.

Fig. 13. Thrombin (0.025 U/ml) induced TXB_2 synthesis in diabetics without angiopathy before (A) and after (B) equilibrium.

has been demonstrated (19).

Since decreased production of prostacyclin has been observed in diabetic vessels (20-21) an imbalance between platelet and vascular arachidonic acid metabolism could be implicated. Morever, exogenous prostacyclin inhibitory effect is diminished in diabetic platelets (22-26).

Calcium Ionophores activate platelets without aggregation via calcium fluxes (27). In this study, Ionophore-induced BTG release is enhanced in diabetics compared to controls with return to normalization after metabolic improvement.

Platelet hyperactivity associated with increased plasma BTG levels, enhanced thrombin-induced BTG release and TXA_2 synthesis are observed at the onset of diabetes without microangiopathy. The abnormalities seem to be marked in proliferative retinopathy, suggesting that the development of angiopathy is itself aggravated by the progression of vascular lesions.

REFERENCES

1. Bern MM, Platelet function in diabetes mellitus. Diabetes 27:342, 1978.
2. Colwell JA, Halushka PV, Platelet function in diabetes mellitus. Brit. J. Haemat. 44:521, 1980.
3. Dupuy E, Guillausseau PJ, Gaudeul P, Kartalis G, Wild AM, Pastureau A, Soria C, Malbec D, Duprey J, Lubetzki J, Caen J, Fonctions plaquettaires des diabétiques ayant une angiopathie. Nouv. Presse Méd. 8:3123, 1978.
4. Lecrubier C, Scarabin PY, Grauso F, Samama M, Platelet aggregation related to age in diabetes mellitus. Haemostasis 9:43, 1980.
5. Kynoch PAM, Lehmann H, Rapid estimation (2½ hours) of glycosylated haemoglobin for routine purposes. Lancet 2:16, 1977.
6. Ludlam CA, Cash JD, Studies on the liberation of B-thromboglobulin from human platelets in vitro. Brit. J. Haemat. 33:239, 1976.
7. Levy Toledano S, Bredoux R, Rendu F, Jeanneau C, Savariau E, Dassin E, Isolement et fonctions des plaquettes. Nouv. Rev. franc. Hémat. 16:367, 1976.
8. Maclouf J, Pradel M, Pradelles P, Dray F, ^{125}I derivatives of prostaglandins. A novel approach in prostaglandin analysis by radioimmunoassay. Biochem. biophys. Acta 431:139, 1976.
9. Betteridge DJ, Zahavi J, Jones NAG, Shine B, Kakkar VV, Galion DJ, Platelet function in diabetes mellitus in relationship to complications, glycosylated haemoglobin and serum lipoprotein. Eur. J. Clin. Invest. 11:273, 1981.
10. Borsey D, Dawes J, Fraser DM, Prowse CV, Elton RA, Clarke BF, Plasma thromboglobulin in diabetes mellitus. Diabetologica 18:353, 1980.
11. Burrows AW, Bêta thromboglobulin in diabetes: relationship with blood glucose and fibrinopeptide A. Horm. Metab. Res. 11:22, (suppl), 1981.
12. Elving LD, Casparie AF, Miedema F, Russchen CJ, Plasma bêta-thromboglobulin in diabetes with and without microangiopathy complications. Diabetologica 21:160, 1981.
13. Paulsen EP, McLung NM, Sabio H, Some characterization of spontaneous platelet aggregation in young insulin-dependent diabetic subjects. Horm. Metab. Res. 11:15, (suppl), 1981.
14. Rasi V, Ikkala E, Hekali R, Myllyla G, Factors affecting plasma B-thromboglobulin in diabetes mellitus. Med. et Biol. 58:369, 1980.
15. Schernthaner G, Sinzinger H, Silberbauer K, Freyler H, Muhlauser I, Kaliman J, Vascular prostacyclin. Platelet sensitivity to prostaglandins and platelet specific proteins in diabetes mellitus. Horm. Metab. Res. 11:33, (suppl), 1981.
16. Voisin P, Kolopp M, Rouselle P, Gaillard S, Pointel JP, Stoltz JF, Debry G, Drouin P, Influence du contrôle métabolique sur la viscosité sanguine et l'activité plaquettaire chez les diabétiques insulino-dépendants. Nouv. Rev. franc. Hémat. 24:187, 1982.
17. Lagarde M, Burtin M, Berciaud P, Blanc M, Velardo B, Dechavanne M, Increase of platelet thromboxane A_2 formation and of its plasmatic half life in diabetes mellitus. Thromb. Res. 19:823, 1980.

18. Ziboh VA, Marota H, Lord J, Cagle DW, Lucky W, Increased biosynthesis of thromboxane A_2 by diabetic platelets. Eur. J. Clin. Invest. 9:223, 1979.

19. Wautier JL, Paton RC, Wautier MP, Pintigny D, Abadie E, Passa P, Caen JP, Increased adhesion of erythrocytes to endothelial cells in diabetes mellitus and its relation to vascular complications. New Engl. J. Med. 305:237, 1981.

20. Silberbauer K, Schernthaner G, Sinzinger H, Piza-Katzer H, Winter M, Decreased vascular prostacyclin in juvenile-onset diabetes. New Engl. J. Med. 300:366, 1979.

21. Johnson M, Harrison HE, Raftery AT, Elder JB, Vascular prostacyclin may be reduced in diabetes in man. Lancet 1:325, 1979.

22. Betteridge DJ, Eltakir KEH, Reckless JPD, WILLIAMS KI, Diminised sensity of platelets from diabetic subjects to prostacyclin. Diabetologica 19:258 (abstract) 1980.

23. Garcia-Conde, Amado JA, Merino J, Benet I, Prostaglandins and platelet function in diabetes. Thrombos. Haemost. 42:335 (abstract) 1979.

24. Johnson M, Harrison HE, Platelet abnormalities in experimental diabetes. Thrombos. Haemost. 42:333 (abstract) 1979.

25. Lagarde M, Berciaud P, Burtin M, Dechavanne M, Refractoriness of diabetic platelets to inhibitory prostaglandins. Prostaglandins 7:341, 1981.

26. Preston FE, Greaves M, Leach E, Jackson CA, Boulton AJM, Ward JD, Reduced platelet sensitivity to prostacyclin in diabetes mellitus. Diabetologica 23:193 (abstract) 1982.

27. Levy-Toledano S, Maclouf J, Bryon P, Savariau E, Hardisty R, Caen JP, Human platelet activation in the absence of aggregation a calcium dependent phenomenon independent of thromboxane formation. Blood 59:1078, 1982.

26 HEMORHEOLOGY AND PLATELET ACTIVATION: THEORETICAL AND EXPERIMENTAL ASPECTS

Ph. VOISIN, A. LARCAN, J.F. STOLTZ

INTRODUCTION

Rheological and biophysical processes of aggregation or platelet adhesion can be diagramatically divided in 3 more or less simultaneous phases (1):

a) Transport of cells towards the vascular wall or towards other cells.

b) Activation phase: cell activation is achieved by aggregating agents released by platelets or other blood-cells (mainly erythrocytes). This primarily biochemical phase may also be related to flow and rheological parameters (rheological activation).

c) Adhesion, aggregation phase and platelet deposits: from a kinetic point of view, there is no doubt that the slowest process determines the overall rate of the whole process.

Theoretical aspects

Transport stage: in order for the platelets to perform their physiological function, there must be a mechanism that carries them to the vessel wall. But in undesirable situations such as thrombogenesis, this mechanism can be considered as one of the initiating factors.

In the absence of flow, the platelets undergo only Brownian translational rotational motion, the former having a diffusion coefficient $D = KT/6\eta\ b$ where K is the Boltzmann constant (1.38×10^{-16} erg/degree) T the absolute temperature, η the plasma viscosity and b the radius of the equivalent platelet sphere. At 37°C, $D = 1.7 \times 10^{-9}$ cm/s.

Thus, in a time Δt, the random walk due to Brownian translational diffusion of a platelet is given by $D = \overline{\Delta\chi}^2/2\Delta t$. This result is a mean distance of only 0.6 μ m/s from its starting point (2,3). This is a small distance compared to the mean distance of about 30 μm between platelets at a normal cell concentration. Alternatively, the frequency of two-body collisions between cells due to Brownian translational diffusion is given by $f_\partial = 16\,\Pi \eta b D$ ($f_\partial = 2.7 \times 10^{-3}$ per platelet per sec).

However, this mechanism does not take into account the complex interactions which occur in blood. In normal blood, about 40% of volume is occupied by red blood-cells and in such a concentrated suspension the collisions between the cells become the governing factor. If one notes that each platelet is surrounded by an average of 20 erythrocytes, it becomes understandable that the collisions of platelets with red blood cells lead to an increase in the diffusion coefficient.

Friedman and Leonard (4) found this coefficient to be about $10^{-7}cm^2/s$ and Turitto et al (10) found values between 0.5 and $2.5 \times 10^{-7}cm^2/s$ depending on the shear rate. It appears that the mechanism of platelet transport does not follow a simple diffusion process but depends on the diffusion mechanism which is supplemented by the presence of red blood-cells (5,6,7,8,9). An analysis of the whole process leads to the introduction of an effective diffusion coefficient (Deff $\neq \dot{\gamma}^{2/3}$ H). A convective diffusion analysis is given for the enhancement of platelet transport induced by red cells spinning into blood-flow (7,8,10).

Activation phase: Blood-platelets are known to aggregate in response to numerous stimuli, including ADP, arachidonic acid, collagen and thrombin, to which they may be exposed in vivo. The platelets probably possess membrane receptors for these stimuli. When these agents interact with their receptors, intracytoplasmic calcium mobilization, actomyosin activation and platelet aggregation occur.

Platelet aggregation requires extracellular calcium, energy and contact between the cells. During the aggregation the platelets secrete their granule content and form PGG_2 and TXA_2 from their arachidonic acid. The aggregation induced by the primary stimulus will, by means of a synergic effect, be increased by the secreted ADP. Although the molecular phases leading to platelet activation are now fully recognized, the participation of rheological factors has still not been clearly determined. However the rheological factors may intervene during this phase via two mechanisms:

- the direct shear activation of platelets (11,12,13). In this case, it is a direct stimulation under the action of applied stresses of the aggregating metabolic pathways.
- the release of aggregating substances from other cells (i.e. each human erythrocyte contains about 10^8 molecules of ADP. If disruption occurs these molecules are released and the ATP may be rapidly converted to ADP yielding up to about 10^{15} molecules of ADP per erythrocyte (14).

Moreover,it is well known that red cells subjected to shear stress,release ADP which aggregates platelets. It is for this reason that in a recent work, Aursnes (15) show a lower threshold concentration for ADP induced platelet aggregation and underlined the hypothesis that ADP from red cells is important in thrombogenesis and should therefore be reappraised.

Adhesion and aggregation: The importance of rheological factors is underlined by the experiments carried out by Begent and Born (16) who studied the dimensions of platelet thrombi growing in venules after stimulation by ADP (iontophoretic application in venules of hamster cheek pouch) and has shown that the height to length ratio is constant for a given flow rate, but is inversely proportional to it (increased from 0.0 to 4.4 mm/s declined above 0.4 mm, no aggregation above 2.5 mm/s). Various experimental cell deposits in arterial branches were studied with models. During the first minutes, a slow growth of cell deposits occurs and the concentration of particles per unit surface area of the wall is proportional to V_2 (velocity perpendicular to the wall); after few minutes platelets are oriented with pseudopodia, parallel to the stream lines. In vivo there is slight but definite direct relationship between rate or RBC velocity and the time required to initiate an adherent platelet aggregate. Rosenblum and El Sabban (17) have failed to show a biphasic relation and found a linear relationship between the time required to produce aggregation and the velocity (or shear rate). The velocities were greater than 0.4 (2 to 13 mm/s) and arteriolar diameters smaller than 40 to 70 µm observed by Begent (16).

Experimental aspects of platelet activation

In our experiments we have studied the platelet activation in the course of various experimental rheological circumstances in using β-thromboglobulin, specific platelet protein which is secreted in plasma during release re-action and which can be considered as an index of platelet activation (18).

Material and methods.

Experimentation: Samples of total blood or platelet rich plasma (PRP) were introduced into a coaxial cylinder viscometer (Couette type) which was able to measure shear rates ranging from 0 to 20 000 s^{-1}. The equipment was carefully siliconized before each experiment and the exposure time was standardized at 5 min.

Collection of blood: Blood was obtained by clear venepuncture in fasting healthy volunteers who had taken no drugs for at least a week, from an antecubital vein without a tourniquet. The samples were collected on 3.8% sodium citrate 9:1 (v/v) and kept at room temperature. An aliquot part of blood was centrifuged at 150 g for 15 min at 20°C in order to obtain PRP.

Total blood or PRP were inserted in the viscometer (about 3 ml) and sheared at different shear stresses or left without motion for a control sample. Then, samples were collected into ice-bath cooled tubes containing EDTA and theophylline. The tubes were centrifuged for 30 min at 2 500 g, at 4°C, and 0.5 ml of PPP carefully removed from the middle layer of supernatant, for a duplicate assay. The rest of supernatant was used immediately for the determination of lactate - dehydrogenase activity or hemolysis measurement.

β-Thromboglobulin assay: After proper plasma dilution, β-TG levels were determined by radioimmunoassay using a commercially - available kit (Amersham-International, Versailles France). As the β-TG plasma level increases progressively in non-sheared samples, the value of a simultaneous

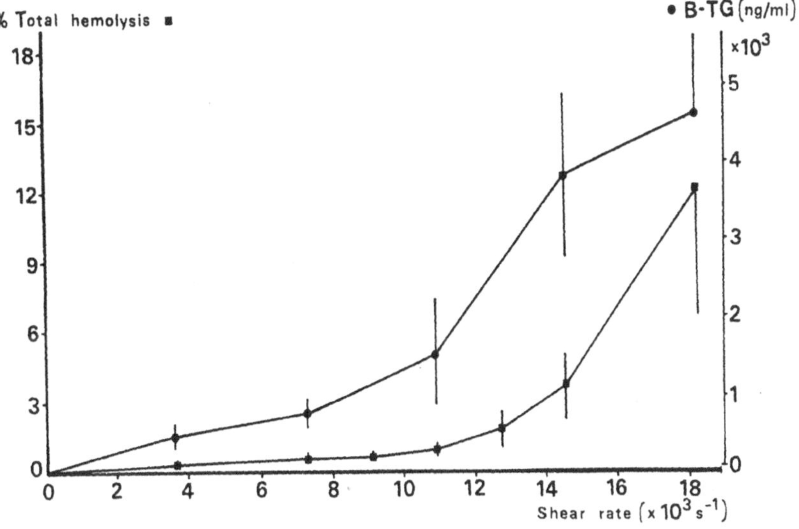

Fig. 1. Percentage of total hemolysis and plasma β-TG levels in samples of whole blood stressed at different shear rates (M ± SD).

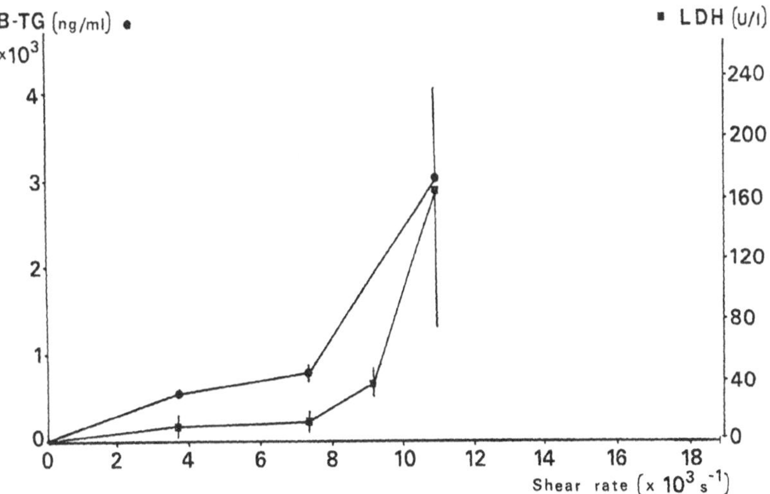

Fig. 2. Plasma LDH activity and β-TG levels in samples of PRP stressed at different shear rates (M ± SD).

control was subtracted from every result of sheared samples.

Lactate-dehydrogenase activity: The enzyme activity was measured in PPP with Boerhinger-Mannheim GmbH test, according to the method described by Wroblewski and Ladue (19). The results were given in IU/l after subtraction of the activity measured in a non-sheared plasma.

Hemolysis measurement: 100µl of plasma were diluted with 5 ml of Isoton (Coultronics SA) and OD was read at 460 and 540 nm in a Perkin Elmer 55 spectrophotometer (Coleman Instruments). The results were given in percentage of total hemolysis, obtained in mixing 5 drops of Zap'Oglobine (Coultronics SA) with 3 ml of the same blood and in taking an aliquot of 100 µl to dilute it.

Results: Hemolysis was undetectable in control samples which remained for 5 min in viscometer at the beginning and at the end of each experimental series. Besides, no difference in LDH activity was observed between these samples and total blood or PRP at room temperature.

In whole sheared blood, hemolysis remained lower than 1% up to 11 000 s^{-1}. Beyond it increased rapidly to reach on average 12% at 18 000 s^{-1}.

Lactate-dehydrogenase activity which was measured simultaneously, revealed an important increase from 10 000 s^{-1}. Nevertheless it remained closely connected with hemolysis as seen by the correlation coefficient between these 2 parameters ($r = 0.96$; $p < 0.001$).

As index of platelet activation, β-TG plasma level enhanced progressively up to 11 000 s^{-1} independently from all other factors. Then the release curve rose perceptibly in connection to haemolysis (fig 1).

PRP samples could only be sheared lower than 11 000 s^{-1}. Then the increase of plasma LDH activity and β-thromboglobulin level (fig 2) remained slow up to 7 000 s^{-1}, but rose very rapidly beyond. Moreover there was a significant correlation between these 2 parameters ($r = 0.77$; $p < 0.05$).

Discussion

The effect of shear field on the release phenomena and on platelet synthesis have been little studied. However, recent works (12,20-28) have shown in particular that:

- Low shear stresses (50 to 100 dyn/cm^2) resulted in the liberation of small amounts of ADP, ATP and serotonin.
- Shear stress of 100 to 200 dyn/cm^2 caused a decrease in serotonin uptake rates and a progressive loss of platelets due to platelet aggregation. These observations were associated with a progressive release from platelet of β-thromboglobulin and formation of malondialdehyde. As concerns platelet aggregation, the work of Klose et al (29) shows that the spontaneous aggregation and the aggregation induced by ADP were functions of the shear rate and the contact duration. On the other hand, it seems that platelets are less aggregable after exposure during 5 min to a shear field.
- For stresses above 200 dyn/cm^2 a progressive loss of lactate dehydrogenase can be observed indicating platelet damage.

Finally a rising pressure enhances the PF_4 release evoked by turbulence in stirred samples (30).

A comparison between these works and our experiments is difficult because the methods and mode of expression of results are different. However, we confirmed an irreversible trauma of red blood-cells with release of hemoglobin, ADP and cytoplasmic components. Moreover, the continuous plasma β-TG increase from the lowest shear rates, suggested a platelet activation in whole blood, apparently connected with the shear stress. But the importance and simultaneous increase of hemolysis, LDH activity and β-TG levels provide evidence that there is also participation in platelet activation of substances released by sheared RBC.

In PRP, the LDH activity remains very inferior to that in whole blood, when β-TG levels were the same as in blood. It confirms that at low shear rates platelet aggregation and granule secretion mainly occur. The cellular lysis would intervene only at the highest shear rates and might be of mechanical origin. These results are also similar to those published by other authors for the same time of shear stress exposure.

Our preliminary study is obviously incomplete and will have to be confirmed by more detailed observations. In particular it does not allow us to specify the relationship between the microrheological properties of platelets and the role of molecular microviscosity in the phenomena (31), We would also like to study the probable relationship between the membrane structure (ionized groups, microtubules, lipid composition) and this parameter.

REFERENCES

1. Stoltz JF, Voisin Ph, Thrombotic processes and shear activation of platelets: Pharmacological approaches. Clin. Hemorh. (in press).

2. Goldsmith TH, Blood flow and thrombosis. Thrombos. Diathes. haemorrh. Stuttg. 32:35, 1974.

3. Yu SK, Goldsmith HL, Some rheological aspects of platelet thrombosis platelet drugs and thrombosis. (Hirsh J, Karger S (eds), 1975.

4. Friedman LI, Leonard EE, Platelet adhesion to artificial surfaces: consequences of flow, exposure time, blood condition and surface nature. Fed. Proc. 30:1641, 1971.

5. Baumgartner HR, Haudenschild LA, Adhesion of platelets to subendothelium. Ann. N.Y. Acad. Sci. 201:22, 1972.

6. Baumgartner HR, Muggli R, Tschopp TB, Turitto VT, Platelet adhesion, release and aggregation in flowing blood: effects of surface properties and platelet function. Thrombos. Haemost. 35:124, 1976.

7. Baumgartner HR, Platelet and fibrin deposition on subendothelium: opposite dependence on blood shear rate. In: Thrombosis and Haemostasis. VIth Intern. Congr. on thrombosis and haemostasis, Philadelphia 1977. p 38, 1977.

8. Antonini G, Guiffari G, Quemada D, Effect du mouvement induit des hématies sur le transport plaquettaire. Biorheology 12:133, 1975.

9. Dosne AM, Michel H, Merville C, Drouet L, Bodevin E, Caen JP, Interactions des plaquettes avec le sous-endothékium artériel. Groupe français d'étude sur l'hémostase et la thrombose, Toulouse mars 1976. Nouv. Rev. franc. Hémat. 16:273, 1976.

10. Turitto VT, Baumgartner HR, Platelet interaction with subendothelium in flowing rabbit blood: Effect of blood shear rate. Microvasc. Res. 17:38, 1979.

11. Born GVR, Richardson PD, Activation time of blood platelets. J. Membrane Biol. 57:87, 1980.

12. Schmidt-Schonbein H, Rieger H, Platelet activation by shear forces: On the influence of flow conditions and platelet properties on platelet behaviour. Proc. of the Vth Intern. Congr. on Thromboembolism. Coccheri S (ed). Quaderni della coagulazione, Bologna, pp 104-111, 1978.

13. Voisin Ph, Larcan A, Stoltz JF, Activation rhéologique des plaquettes sanguines: Etude prélininaire. J. Mal. Vasc. (in press).

14. Williams AR, The induction of intravascular thrombi in vivo by means of localized hydrodynamic shear stresses. Basic aspects of blood trauma pp 63-73, 1979.

15. Aursnes I, Gjesdal K, Abildgoard U, Platelet aggregation induced by ADP from unsheared erythrocytes at physiological Ca^{++} concentration. Brit. J. Haemat. 47:149, 1981.

16. Begent N, Born GVR, Growth rate in vivo of platelet thrombi produced by iontophoresis of ADP as a function of mean blood flow velocity. Nature 227:926, 1970.

17. Rosenblum WI, El Sabban FC, Influence of shear rate on platelet aggregation in cerebral microvessels. Microvasc. Res. 23:311, 1982.

18. Zahavi J, Kakkar VV, B-Thromboglobulin: A specific marker of in vivo platelet release reaction. Thrombos. Haemost. 44:23, 1980.

19. Wroblewski F, Ladue JS, Lactic deshydrogenase activity in blood. Proc. Soc. exp. Biol. Med. 90:210, 1955.

20. Anderson GH, Hellums JD, Moake J, Alfrey CP, Platelet response to shear stress: Changes in serotonin uptake, serotonin release and ADP induced aggregation. Thromb. Res. 13:1039, 1978.

21. Anderson GH, Hellums JD, Moake J, Alfrey CP, Platelet lysis and aggregation in shear fields. Blood cells 4:499, 1978.

22. Colantuoni G, Hellums JD, Moake JL, Alfrey CP, The response of human platelets to shear stress at short exposure time. Trans. Amer. Soc. Artif. Organs 23:626, 1977.

23. Sutera SP, Flow induced trauma to blood cells. Circ. Res. 41:2, 1977.

24. Schmidt-Schonbein H, Richardson P, Born GVR, Rieger H, Forst R, Rothing-Winkel I, Rheology of thrombotic processes occuring in flow: The interaction of erythrocytes and thrombocytes. 3rd Intern. Congr. of Biorheology, abstr. nr. 168, La Jolla, 1978.

25. Schmidt-Schonbein H, Born GVR, Richardson PD, Cusak N, Rieger H, Forst R, Rothing-Winkel I, Lasberg P, Wehmeyer A, Rheology of thrombotic processes in flow: The interaction of erythrocytes and thrombocytes subjected to high flow forces. Biorheology 18:415, 1981.

26. Dewitz TS, Martin RR, Solis RT, Hellums JD, McIntyre LV, Microaggregate formation in whole blood exposed to shear stress. Microvasc. Res. 26:263, 1978.

27. McIntyre LV, Kuntamukkula MS, Moake JL, Petersen DM, The use of rheological techniques to evaluate platelet function. Alterations caused by drug therapy. In: Biorheology, Huang CH, Copley AL (eds), AICHE Symposium Series, 182:74, 1978.

28. Stevens DE, Joist JH, Sutera SP, Role of platelet-prostaglandin synthesis in shear induced platelet alterations. Blood 56:753, 1980.

29. Klose HJ, Rieger H, Schmidt-Schonbein H. A rheological method for the quantification of platelet aggregation (PA) in vitro and its kinetics under defined conditions. Thromb. Res. 7:261, 1975.

30. Torsellini A, Maggi L, Guidi G, Lombardi V, Modifications of platelet function induced by variation of hydrostatic pressure in an experimental model. 1st Conference on hemostasis and thrombosis, abstr.nr. 77, Florence, 1977.

31. Nathan G, Fleisher A, Dvilansky A, Livne A, Parola AH, Membrane dynamic alterations associated with activation of human platelets by thrombin. Biochimica biophys. Acta 598:417, 1980.

GRANULOCYTES

27 ^{111}IN-LEUKOCYTE SCINTIGRAPHY IN THE DIAGNOSIS OF VASCULAR GRAFT INFECTION

E.A. VAN ROYEN, M.H. RÖVEKAMP, R.J.A.M. VAN DONGEN, J.B. VAN DER SCHOOT, M.R. HARDEMAN

INTRODUCTION

Infection at the site of a vascular graft is a serious complication in vascular surgery especially when synthetic materials have been used (1). Prosthetic grafts are widely employed in aorto-iliac, aorto-femoral and femoro-popliteal bypasses. X-ray investigation, angiography, ultrasound and computer tomography are of limited value in the diagnosis of graft infection (2,3,4). Delay in diagnosis and treatment of this complication results in a high morbidity and mortality. Some reports are available on the use of ^{67}Ga-citrate scintigraphy (3), however its accumulation in normal intestinal structures is a serious drawback. We investigated the effectiveness of ^{111}In-leukocytes scintigraphy in the diagnosis of vascular graft infection. The possible accumulation of labelled leukocytes was assessed both subjectively by visual interpretation and quantitatively by computer evaluation.

Methods

Patients: A control group consisted of 13 patients who were submitted to ^{111}In-leukocyte scintigraphy for other reasons and had no arterial graft.

Group 1 included 18 scintigrams performed in 17 patients, 10 to 30 days after aorto-iliac grafting, with an uneventful post-operative course.

Group 2 consisted of 12 scintigrams in 10 patients with non-infectious complications after vascular surgery (e.g. intra-abdominal bleeding, groin or wound hematomas, wound healing disturbances).

Group 3 included 24 scintigrams in 19 patients with early (e.g. within 3 months after surgery) infectious complications of

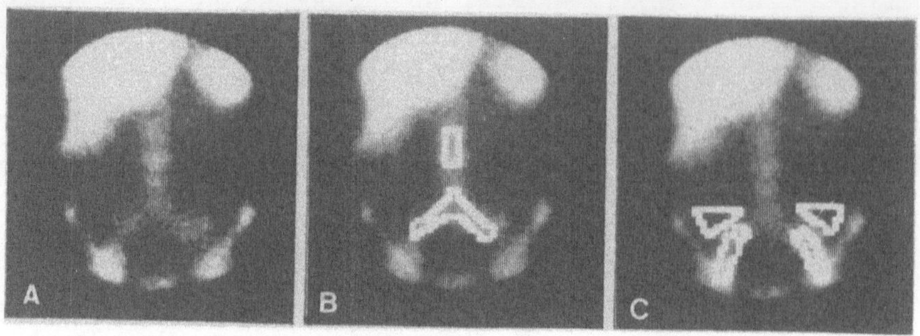

Fig. 1. a) Normal scan. b) Regions of interest: proximal aorta, graft area. c) Regions of interest: ileo femoral arteries, left and right iliac fossae.

Table 1. ^{111}In-leukocyte uptake

	control group units SEM	group 1 units SEM	significance (Wilcoxon)
graft	28.6 ± 2.6	33.6 ± 2.9	n.s.
aorta	35.1 ± 3.4	40.9 ± 3.4	n.s.
L ileofemoral artery	24.6 ± 2.3	33.0 ± 2.7	$p<0.01$
R ileofemoral artery	24.5 ± 2.4	33.7 ± 3.1	$p<0.025$
graft/aorta ratio	0.83± 0.02	0.81± 0.02	n.s.
L/R ileofemoral ratio	1.02± 0.02	0.98± 0.02	n.s.

aorto-iliac, aorto-femoral, femoro-popliteal or thoracic-aortic reconstruction.

Group 4 included 21 scintigrams in 18 patients presenting with possible late vascular graft infection (i.e. after 3 months after surgery.

^{111}In-leukocyte scintigraphy

Leukocytes were isolated and labelled with ^{111}In-oxinate as described elsewhere. The administered dose was 300-500 µCi. Scintigrams were performed on a LFOV gamma camera linked to a Gamma II computer employing both 173 and 247 KeV photopeaks, 20-24 hours after reinjection of the labelled suspension. Both anterior and lateral views were taken for a 10 min period. Analogue images were assessed by 2 observers as to ^{111}In-activity above the graft region or focal accumulation elsewhere. Quantitative ^{111}In-uptake

Table 2. Sensitivity and specificity

	group 1	group 2	group 3	group 4	total
true positive	-	-	6	13	19
true negative	17	7	13	7	44
false positive	1	4	3	1	9
false negative	-	1	2	-	3
accuracy 84%					
specificity 83%					
sensitivity 86%					

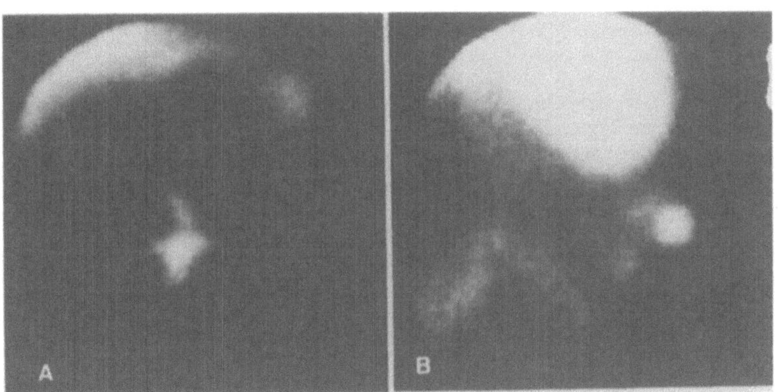

Fig. 2. Wound infection. a) Anterior view. b) Right lateral view: anterior localization of activity.

was measured by marking regions of interest on the video image around proximal aorta, bifurcation c.q. graft area, L and R ileofemoral arteries and L and R iliac fossa (fig 1). The amount of activity within these regions was calculated in units (counts/pixel/100 μCi/10 min after correction for physical decay). Useful parameters were provided by calculating a graft/aorta ratio and L/R ratio's for ileofemoral arteries and iliac fossae.

Results

The results obtained in the control group without vascular surgery and group 1, (10-30 days after uncomplicated vascular surgery) are given in table 1. In the latter group ^{111}In-uptake

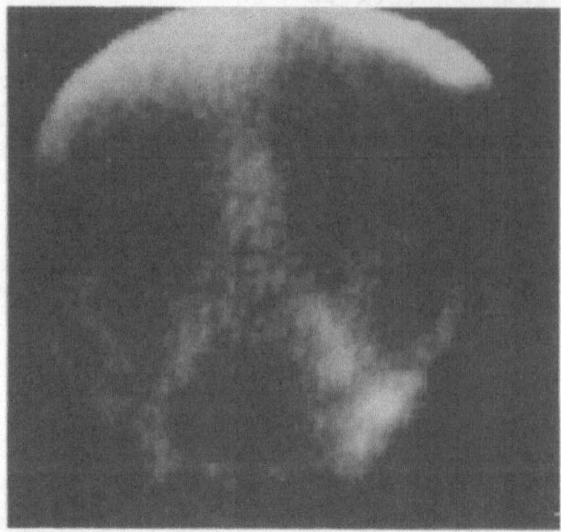

Fig. 3. Infected aorto-femoral graft 8 months post-operative. Clinical presentation: groin abscess. Scintigraphy: focal activity in the left groin and along the left iliac artery. Surgery: infected left limb of the prosthesis.

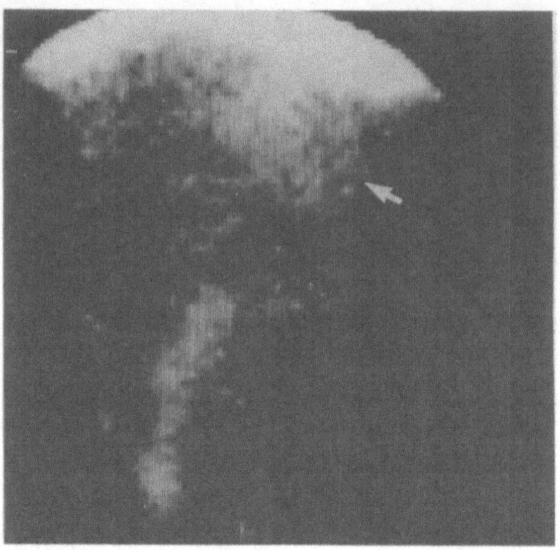

Fig. 4. Infected aorto-iliac graft 12 months post-operative. Clinical symptom: GI bleeding. Scintigraphy: focal activity proximal, extending in the bowel (arrow) and distal at the right iliac artery. Surgery: aorto-duodenal fistula involving the proximal anastomosis and an infected right limb.

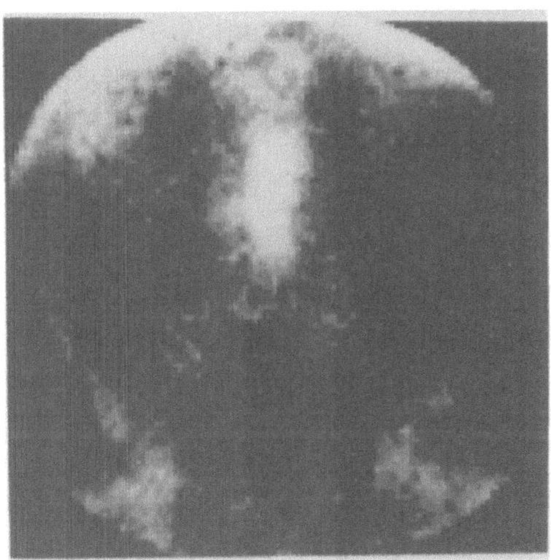

Fig. 5. Infected aorta-iliac graft 7 months after implantation. Clinical symptom: septicaemia. Scintigraphy: focal activity at the proximal anastomosis. Surgery: aorto-duodenal fistula.

values tended to be somewhat higher above the various regions. Significance was only reached above the L and R ileofemoral arteries. In group 2, representing non-infectious complications, abnormal activity was found in 4 out of 12 scintigrams. These foci were located at the aorta-iliac regions and at the site of groin hematoma. Quantitative values i.e. the L/R ratio of fossa iliaca and iliac arteries were above the normal range (>2 s.d.) in these patients. Therefore, they have been classified as false positive. One patient was qualified false negative in which graft infection developed 5 months after the scintigram. The final results are given in table 2. Follow-up during 10-28 months after surgery revealed no graft infection in these patients.

Group 3 Early infection (n=24)

Superficial wound infection overlying the graft was detected in 2 cases. Graft activity itself showed to be abnormal on the lateral view (fig 2). Abnormal ^{111}In-leukocyte accumulation at the graft was found in 9 cases. Increased graft/aorta ratio's (1.07-1.86 and abnormal L/R ratio's were found. Re-operation or drainage procedures confirmed infection in 6 of them, while in 3 no infection could be proved. Follow-up of the negative scans (15 cases) revealed infection in 2 of them. The final results are given in table 2.

Group 4 Late infection (n=21)

Abnormal ^{111}In-leukocyte activity was found in 14 cases. Reoperation or drainage procedures confirmed infection in 13 of them One scintigram proved to be false positive. No false negative scintigrams were recorded during a follow-up of 4-21 months. Table 2 demonstrates the results.

Discussion

^{111}In-leukocyte scintigraphy proved to be a valuable tool in the search of vascular graft infection. The procedure is easy to perform even in critically ill patients. One 10 min view of the abdomen is often sufficient to establish or to reject the diagnosi of graft infection. In uncomplicated vascular surgery, almost no activity is found in abdominal structures apart from liver and spleen. This competes favourable to ^{67}Ga-scintigraphy. Quantitative evaluation of the scintigram revealed some slight increase activity only at the site of the operation likely related to norma wound healing (5). Computer measurements of the amount of ^{111}In-activity proved to be helpful as to the decision whether or not infection was present. False positive results were mostly observed in case of intra-abdominal and retroperitoneal hematomas, possibly resulting in an inflammatory response.

Three results were considered being false negative. In one patient with sepsis and an occluded graft, an infection was demonstrated at operation shortly after the scintigram was made. The 2 others, however, presented with infection, 5 months later. It is questionable if one could expect the scintigram to be positive that period before clear infection developed. The sensitivity and specificity calculated from our results are high. In comparison tc other procedures ^{111}In-leukocyte scintigraphy offers a reliable non-invasive technique in the diagnosis of vascular graft infectic

REFERENCES

1. Szilagyi DE, Smith RF, Elliot JP, Vrandecic MP, Infection in arterial reconstruction with synthetic grafts. Ann. Surg. 176:321, 1972.

2. Becker RM, Blundell PE, Infected aortic bifurcation grafts: experience with fourteen patients. Surgery 80:544, 1976.

3. Simpson AJ, Astin JK, Peck MR, Diagnosis of an abdominal graft abscess by combined ultrasonography and scintigraphy. Clin. Nucl. Med. 4:338, 1979.

4. Haaga JR, Baldwin GN, Reich NE, Bevin E et al, CT Detection of infected synthetic grafts: preliminary report of a new sign. Amer. J. Roentgenol. 131:317, 1978.

5. Sauvage LR, Berger K, Barros D'Sa AAB et al, Dacron arterial prostheses. In: Graft materials in vascular surgery. Dardick H (ed), Medical Books Symposia Specialist, Miami Florida, pp 153, 1978.

28 DIAGNOSIS OF INTRA ABDOMINAL INFLAMMATORY PROCESSES WITH ^{111}IN-LABELLED LEUCOCYTES

M.H. RÖVEKAMP, W.H. BRUMMELKAMP, J.B. VAN DER SCHOOT, S.Chr.C. REINDERS FOLMER, E.A. VAN ROYEN

INTRODUCTION

The diagnosis of occult inflammatory processes is one of the most challenging tasks in clinical practice. An accurate and speed diagnosis is important for early and adequate treatment (1-3). To this end, the search has been going on for some time for newer, more reliable methods. ^{67}Ga-citrate scintigraphy has been successfully used, but it has its limitations (4-6). Ultrasonography and computed tomography have proved their clinical usefulness in the detection and location of abdominal and retroperitoneal abscesses. However, both methods do have specific limitations as well (7-13).

In the search for a more specific scintigraphic technique aimed at overcoming the disadvantages of ^{67}Ga-citrate, the use of labelled leucocytes has been advocated in the diagnosis of inflamm tory lesions (14). A comparative study performed by McAfee and Thakur revealed ^{111}In-oxinate as the most efficient labelling agen for this purpose (15,16). This report includes the results we obtained over a 2½ year period by use of this method in patients suspected of intra-abdominal, retroperitoneal or pelvic inflammatory processes.

Method

Leucocytes were isolated as previously described (17,18) and labelled with a commercial preparation of ^{111}In-oxinate. The dose administered was about 350 μCi. Scintigrams were performed 20 to 2 hours after administration of the labelled cells. If indicated, an additional Tc^{99m}-Sn colloid liver and spleen scintigram was made and computer-assisted subtraction was performed.

Patients

A total of 225 examinations were performed in 184 patients, of these,165 patients (73%) were in a postoperative phase. Most patients had symptoms suggesting an occult inflammatory process varying from mild clinical signs to severe sepsis. In some patients, there was reason for scintigraphy due to a previously diagnosed intrahepatic or intrasplenic lesion, the origin of which had to be determined.

In 50 patients in this series, in addition to the ^{111}In leucocyte scan, ultrasonography and/or computed tomography were also performed, within a two-week period. The results obtained by means of these three modalities with these patients were evaluated in a retrospective study.

Results

On all 225 scintigrams, the previously described normal distribution in liver, spleen and bone marrow was observed. No activity was observed in the kidneys. A slight colonic uptake, without evident pathology, was observed on nine(4%) of the scintigrams. On 141 scintigrams, an abnormal accumulation of activity was observed; 89 of those could be subjected to a surgical follow-up. An inflammatory process was confirmed in 82 of these 89 positive scintigrams (table 1). Localization of focal activity agreed with the findings at surgery (fig. 1-4). The other seven scintigrams had to be classified as false positive. The final diagnosed lesions in these patients are given in Table 2.

52 Scintigrams were subjected to a clinical non-surgical follow-up. Of these 41 scintigrams were classified as true positive and 11 had to be considered as false positive (table 1). The final diagnosed lesions in these patients are given in table 2.

On 84 scintigrams, no abnormal focal activity was observed, beside the normal distribution of activity. 21 Scintigrams were subjected to a surgical follow-up. A localized inflammation was demonstrated on 10 occasions, these scintigrams were subsequently classified as false negative. The final diagnosis of these patients are listed in table 3. In the other 11 cases, no inflammation could be demonstrated. The remaining 63 scintigrams were subjected to a

Table 1. Results (n = 225)

	confirmed at operation, needle aspiration, or autotopsy			
true positive	123	82	accuracy	87%
true negative	73	11		
false positive	18	7	specificity	80%
false negative	11	10	sensitivity	92%

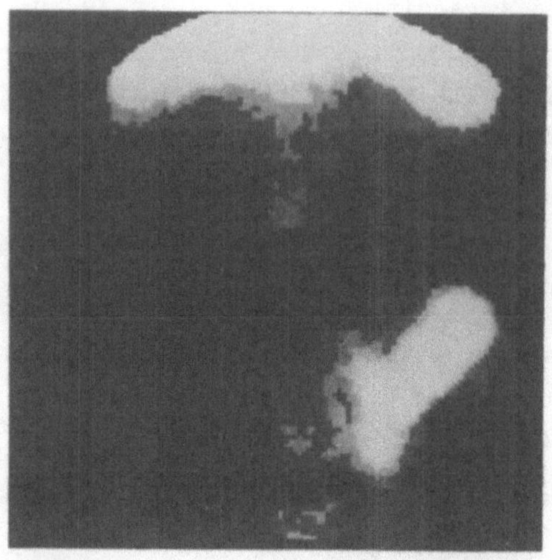

Fig. 1. Paracolic/rectal absces

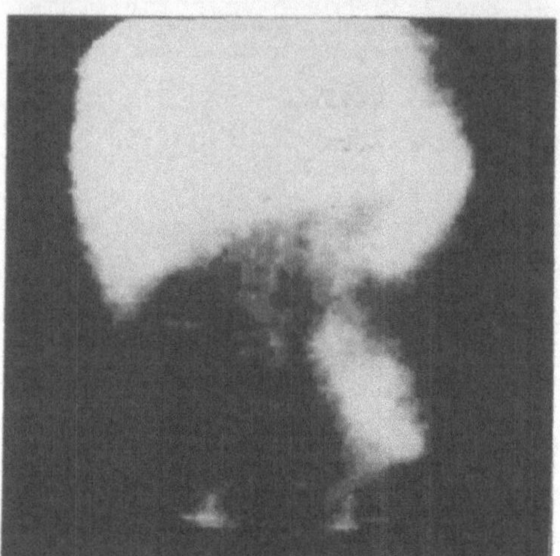

Fig. 2. Left subphrenic abscess after splenectomy with extension into the left retrocolic space.

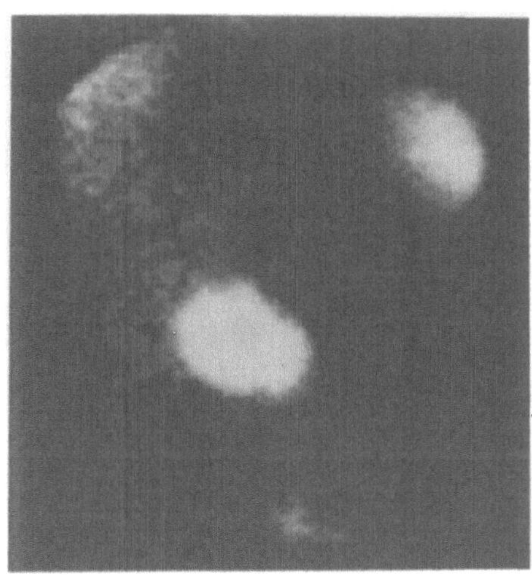

Fig. 3. Gallbladder empyema.

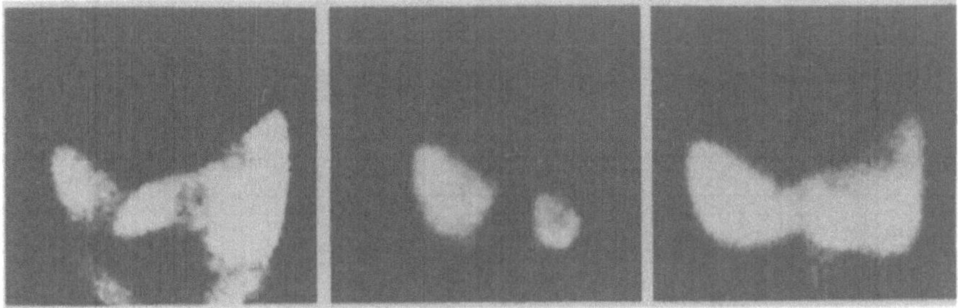

Fig. 4. Subtraction scintigram of an intrahepatic abscess. a. Indium-111 leucocytes. b. Subtraction of liver area. c. Technetium-99m-Sn-colloid.

Table 2. False-positive results.

final diagnosed lesion	scans	confirmed at operation needle aspiration, or autopsy
intra-hepatic metastases/tumour	4	3
liver-hilus metastases	1	
gallbladder carcinoma	1	1
bile fistula	1	1
retroperitoneal haematoma	1	
colitis	1	
colostomy	1	1
wound/drain site	2	
left subphrenic haematoma after splenectomy	2	
kidney transplant rejection	1	1
none	3	
	18	7

Table 3. False-negative results.

final diagnosed lesion	scans	confirmed at operatio or needle aspiration
right lower quadrant mass after appendectomy	1	
small abscess with ileo-cutaneous fistula	1	1
small infected haematoma	2	2
infected liver cyst	2	2
splenic abscess (typhoid)	1	1
presacral abscess (Crohn's disease)	1	1
chronic ileo-coecal inflammation (Crohn's disease)	1	1
cholangitis	1	1
infected intramedullary nail (femur shaft)	1	1
	11	10

Table 4. Results obtained in 45 patient with leucocyte scintigraphy and ultra-sonography.

	leucocyte scintigraphy	ultrasonography
true positive	22	19
true negative	20	17
false positive	2	5
false negative	1	4
accuracy	93%	80%

clinical non-surgical follow-up. The clinical course after 62 scintigrams proceeded without further development of clear signs c localized inflammation, so that these scintigrams were considered to be negative. In one patient, the scan was classified as false negative (table 3). Table 4 lists the results obtained in the 45 patients in whom leucocyte scintigraphy as well as ultrasonography was performed. The accuracies obtained were leucocyte scintigraphy 93% and ultrasonography 80%. Computed tomography as well as leucocyte scintigraphy was performed in an additional five patients, and in 11 of the above mentioned 45, all three medalities were used. This series of 16 computed tomographic studies was not further analyzed, because of the small number in comparison to the other series of 45 investigations.

Discussion

The overall results as listed in table 1 were 123 true-positive and 74 true-negative scans, accounting for an accuracy of 87,5%. 18 False-positive and 10 false-negative results account for respectively a 92% sensitivity and an 80% specificity. The occurence of false results could be related to several factors: (a) the labelled cell suspension, (b) the lesion, and (c) the scintigraphic technique. Concerning the false negative results; (a) a sufficient number and proper functioning of the labelled cells is essential. The viability of the cells was clearly demonstrated by their migration into inflammatory lesions. (b) The degree, nature and duration of the inflammatory response at the site of the lesion is important. A lesion with a low cellular response or with a cellular response with a scarce infiltration of P.M.N. leucocytes will probably accumulate too less ^{111}In activity to be detected. The presence of a dense fibrous wall around the lesion, as may be found in liver and spleen, will also prevent sufficient migration of leucocytes, resulting in a negative scintigraphy. The false-negative results observed in this series, could be related, in most cases, to these factors (table 3). (c) Lesions next to, or within, organs or structures normally accumulating activity can be difficult to detect. In case of liver and spleen, the subtraction technique provided a useful additional means in the detection of upper-abdominal lesions.

Concerning false-positive results; (a) Contamination of the cell preparation with other cells, especially platelets, probably causes accumulation of activity at other non-inflammatory sites. (b) False-positive scintigrams may be the result of leucocyte accumulation in non-infectious lesions. Most of the false-positive scans in this series were based on leucocyte accumulation as an aspecific cellular response brought about by various lesions (table 2). (c) Some pitfalls in the scintigraphic technique, especially encountered when the ^{111}In leucocyte Tc^{99m}-Sn colloid subtraction is used in diagnosing upper-abdominal processes, can cause false-positive results.

In the series of 45 patient in whom both leucocyte scintigraphy and ultrasonography were performed, more false results were observed with ultrasonography, resulting in a lower accuracy. Others report a similar diagnostic accuracy in comparison with these two modalities.

For the differential diagnosis between the inflammatory or non-inflammatory origin of lesions localized by ultrasound or computed tomography, a complementary use of these three modalities were found to be very useful by us and by others. In the search for occult inflammatory processes, the possibility of whole body imaging is an advantage of the ^{111}In leucocyte scintigram, compared with ultrasonography and computed tomography.

Conclusions

In this series of 225 ^{111}In leucocyte scintigrams this method was found to be a reliable diagnostic means in the search for occult abdominal inflammatory processes. An accurate localization of lesions was observed. Performing ^{111}In leucocyte scintigraphy, in combination with ultrasonography or computed tomography, was found to be useful in defining a possible inflammatory origin of localized lesions diagnosed with the latter two modalities.

Summary

Over a 2½ year period, 225 scintigrams with ^{111}In-oxinate labelled leucocytes were performed in 184 patients suspected of an intra-abdominal, retroperitoneal or pelvic inflammatory process. In patients suspected of an upper abdominal process, an ^{111}In leucocyte Tc^{99m}-Sn colloid subtraction was performed, in order to eliminate the normal liver and spleen uptake. 123 Scintigrams were considered true positive and 73 true negative. A diagnostic accuracy of 87% was calculated. With 18 false-positive scans an 80%-specificity and with 11 false-negative a 92% sensitivity were obtained. False-negative results in the majority of the scintigrams were based on leucocyte accumulations, due to aspecific cellular inflammatory reactions. False-negative results were mainly related to intra-hepatic, intra-splenic or older lesions. In 50 patients, ultra sonography and/or computed tomography was also performed. A higher diagnostic accuracy was observed with leucocyte scintigraphy compared to ultrasonography.

REFERENCES

1. Altemeier WA, Culbertson WF, Fullen WD et al, Intra-abdominal abscesses. Amer. J. Surg. 125:70, 1973.
2. Sherman NJ, Davis JR, Jesseph JE, Subphrenic abscesses, a continuing hazard. Amer. J. Surg. 117:117, 1969.
3. Altemeier WA, Alexander JW, Retroperitoneal abscesses. Arch. Surg. 83:512, 1961.
4. Caffee HH, Watts G, Mena I, Gallium-67 citrate scanning in the diagnosis of intra-abdominal abscesses. Amer. J. Surg. 133:665, 1977.
5. Moinuddin M, Rockett JF, Gallium imaging in inflammatory diseases. Clin. Nucl. Med. 1:271,1976.
6. Forgacs P, Wahner HW, Keys Th F, Gallium scanning for the detection of abdominal abscesses. Amer. J. Med. 65:949, 1978.
7. Halber MD, Daffner RH, Morgan CL et al, Intra-abdominal abscess: Current concepts in radiologic evaluation. Amer. J. Roentgenol. 133:9, 1979.
8. Maklad NF, Brouce D, Doust BD, Ultrasonic diagnosis of post-operative intra-abdominal abscess. Radiology 113:417, 1974.
9. Doust BD, Quiroz F, Stewart JM, Ultrasonic distinction of abscesses from other intra-abdominal fluid collections. Radiology 125:213, 1977.
10. Jensen F, Pedersen JF, The value of ultrasonic scanning in the diagnosis of intra-abdominal abscesses and hematomas. Surg. Gynec. Obstet. 139:326, 1974.
11. Koehler PR, Knochel JQ, Computed tomography in the evaluation of abdominal abscesses. Amer. J. Surg. 140:675, 1980.
12. Haaga JR, Alfidi RJ, Havrilla Th R et al, CT detection and aspiration of abdominal abscesses. Amer. J. Roentgenol. 128: 465, 1977.
13. Wolverson MK, Jagannadharao B, Sundaram M et al, CT as a primary diagnostic method in evaluating intra-abdominal abscesses. Amer. J. Roentgenol. 133:1089, 1979.
14. Thakur ML, Coleman RE, Welch MJ, Indium-111-labeled leukocytes for the localization of abscesses: preparation, analysis, tissue distribution, and comparison with Gallium-67 citrate in dogs. J. Lab. clin. Med. 89:217, 1977.
15. McAfee JG, Thakur ML, Survey of radioactive agents for in vitro labelling of phagocytic leukocytes. I. Soluble agents. J. nucl. Med. 17:480, 1976.
16. McAfee JG, Thakur ML, Survey of radioactive agents for in vitro labelling of phagocytic leukocytes. II. Particles. J. nucl. Med. 17:488, 1976.
17. Rövekamp MH, Hardeman MR, Van der Schoot JB et al, ^{111}Indium-labelled leucocyte scintigraphy in the diagnosis of inflammatory disease, first results. Brit. J. Surg. 68:150, 1981.
18. Rövekamp MH, Indium-111 labelled leucocyte scintigraphy in the diagnosis of inflammatory disease: a clinical study. Ph D Thesis 1982, pp 17-37.

29 ^{111}IN-AUTOLOGOUS LEUCOCYTES IN THE DIAGNOSIS AND MANAGEMENT OF INFLAMMATORY BOWEL DISEASE

S.H. SAVERYMUTTU, A.M. PETERS, H.J.F. HODGSON, V.S. CHADWICK, J.P. LAVENDER

INTRODUCTION

^{111}In-labelled autologous leucocytes are now established as an accurate method for the localization of intra abdominal abscesses (1-3). This technique has also been applied with success to other conditions with an inflammatory component (4). Active inflammatory bowel disease appears ideally suited for investigation by this technique as histologically it is characterized by leucocyte infiltration of the bowel wall and a leucocyte rich faecal exudate. In preliminary studies we (5) and others (6) showed that inflamed bowel could be imaged with ^{111}In-labelled leucocytes. Labelled cel from inflamed gut, unlike those within abscesses are rapidly excreted into the bowel lumen and counting of faecal radioactivity permits a quantitative assessment of leucocyte excretion. Since the granulocyte is the dominant type in active inflammatory bowel disease we have used a pure granulocyte separation in addition to the conventional mixed leucocytes preparation. The aim of this prospective study was to assess the value of ^{111}In-labelled leucocytes in localizing inflamed bowel and to study the relationship between disease activity and labelled leucocyte excretion. Control studies were performed in patients with the irritable bowel syndro and with a variety of non inflammatory bowel disorders such as gut carcinoma.

Methods

Leucocyte labelling and scanning. Mixed leucocyte preparations were labelled using ^{111}In-acetylacetonate (7) and pure granulocyte preparations labelled with ^{111}In-tropolonate (8). Gamma camera abdominal scans were performed between 40 min and 5 hours after reinjection of the labelled cells and also at 24 hours. A four day faecal collection was commenced immediately after the administration of the labelled cells in daily aliquots and the total ^{111}In content measured.

Patients studied. A total of 142 studies were performed in 115 patients. The diagnoses and cell preparation used are shown in table 1.

Table 1. Diagnosis and cell preparation used

Diseases	Mixed leucocytes	Pure granulocytes
Crohn's disease	22	32
Ulcerative colitis	8	31
Irritable bowel syndrome	11	14
Non inflammatory bowel disorders	14	12

All patients had routine biochemistry and haematology checked at the time of the study. Patients with Crohn's disease and ulcerative colitis completed a chart for calculation of the Crohn's disease activity index (CDAI) (9). For both groups of patients a disease activity score was calculated from the charts using the coefficients derived for Crohn's disease. In the ulcerative colitis patients in order to avoid confusing nomenclature it is referred to as the ulcerative colitis activity index (UCDAI). Two patients with ulcerative colitis had an active peripheral arthritis at the time of the study.

Results

Scanning. Abdominal scans in patients with the irritable bowel syndrome or noninflammatory bowel conditions showed in all cases activity confined to the liver, spleen and bone marrow with no evidence of bowel localization (fig. 1). Fig. 2. illustrates an early scan (at 40 min) in a patient with distal ileal Crohn's disease showing abnormal localization in the right iliac fossa corresponding to the site of disease shown on the barium follow through. An abdominal scan performed 15 hours afterwards (fig.3) shows activity now in the colon representing labelled cells

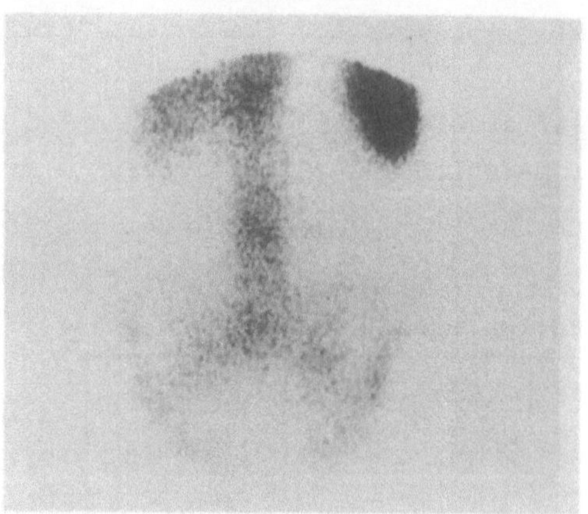

Fig. 1. Abdominal scan in a patient with the irritable bowel syndrome showing a normal distribution of activity.

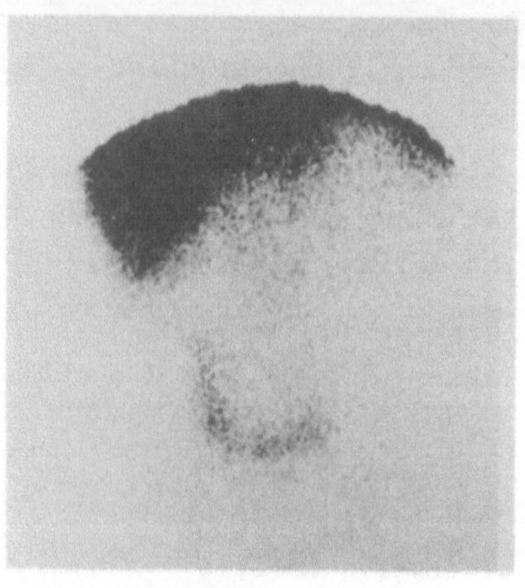

Fig. 2. Abdominal scan at 40 min Crohn's disease affecting the distal ileum.

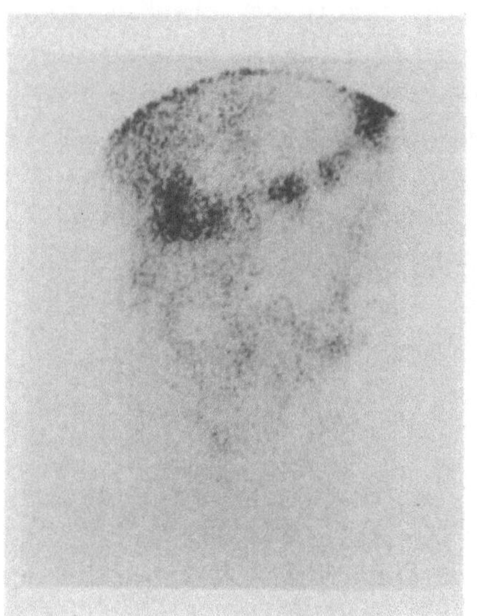

Fig. 3. Abdominal scan at 15 hours in patient in fig. 2, showing distal transit of labelled leucocytes.

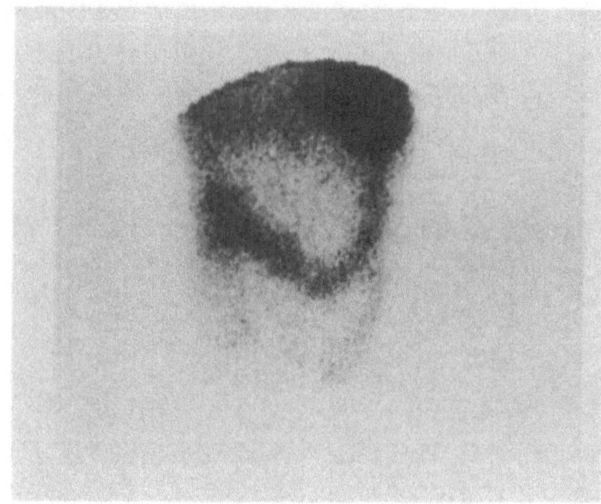

Fig. 4. Abdominal scan at 3 hours in a patient with ulcerative colitis involving the whole large bowel.

Tabel 2. Agreement of disease extent assessed on scan with radiology

	Small bowel disease	Large bowel disease
Mixed leucocytes	33%	80%
Pure granulocytes	63%	85%

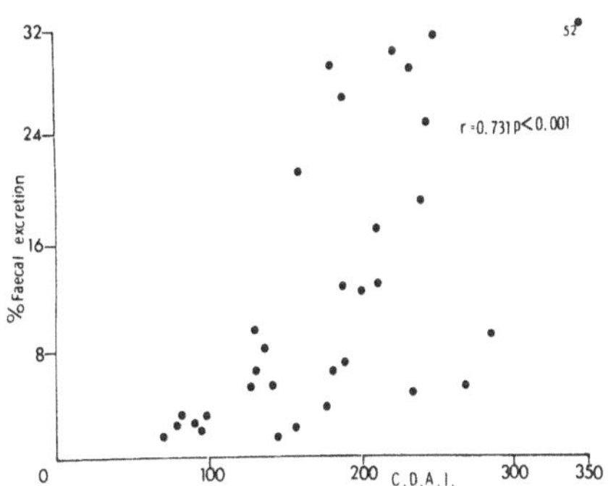

Fig. 5. Faecal ^{111}In-excretion vs CDAI in patients with Crohn's disease receiving pure granylocytes.

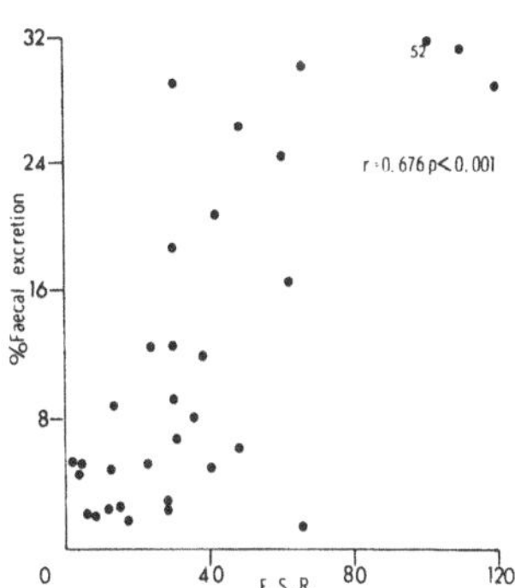

Fig. 6. Faecal ^{111}In vs ESR in patients with Crohn's disease receiving pure granulocytes.

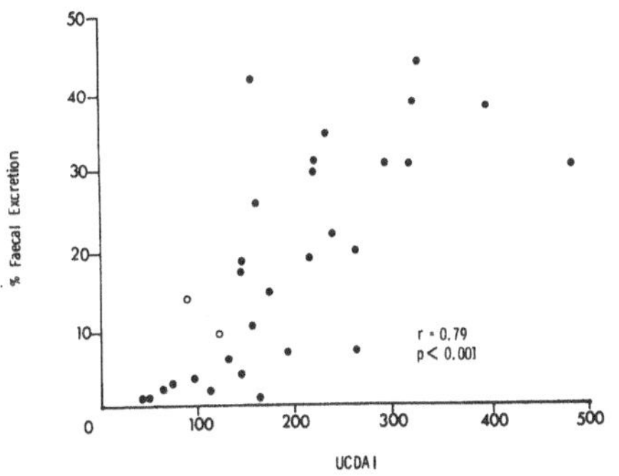

Fig. 7. ^{111}In-excretion vs UCDAI in patients with ulcerative colitis receiving pure granulocytes. °Indicates patients with active peripheral arthritis.

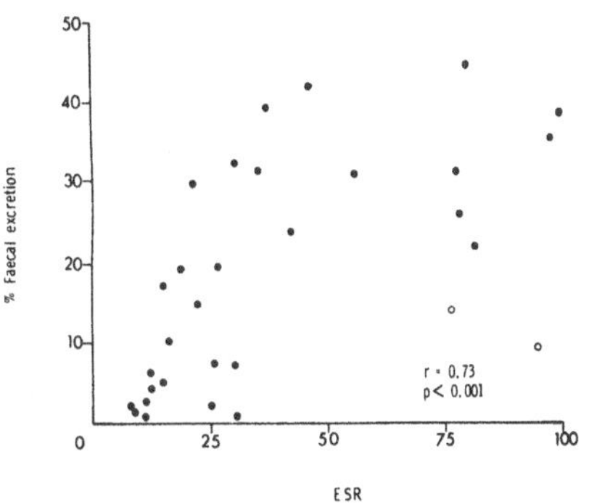

Fig. 8. Faecal ^{111}In-excretion vs ESR in patients with ulcerative colitis receiving pure granulocytes. °Indicates patients with active peripheral arthritis.

entering the bowel lumen and undergoing interluminal bowel transit with the faecal stream. An example of a scan in a patient with ulcerative colitis is shown in fig. 4 demonstrating activity outlining the large bowel. Later scans also showed distal intraluminal transit of the labelled cells. Table 2 summerizes the relationship between disease extent assessed by scan and radiology and the cell preparation used.

Faecal leucocyte excretion

a) Mixed leucocyte studies. The range of faecal leucocyte excretion in patients with the irritable bowel syndrome or noninflammatory bowel disease was 0.1 to 1% (mean 0.4% ± SD 0.31) of the injected dose. In the 30 studies in patients with ulcerative colitis and Crohn's disease, faecal excretion ranged from 0.3% to 11%. Higher levels of excretion were found in patients with the more active disease.

b) Pure granulocyte studies. The range for faecal leucocyte excretion in 14 patients with the irritable bowel syndrome receiving pure granulocyte preparation was 0.2 - 1.6% (mean 0.53 ± SD 0.42). In 32 studies in patients with Crohn's disease using granulocyte preparation, faecal ^{111}In were higher than the mixed leucocyte preparation ranging from 1.1% - 52%. There were significant correlations between faecal granulocyte excretion and CDAI (r= 0.7 $p<0.001$) (fig. 5) and with ESR (r= 0.68 $p<0.001$) (fig. 6). In studies in patients with ulcerative colitis using pure granulocyte preparation there were similar correlations between faecal granulocyte excretion and UCDAI (r= 0.79 $p<0.001$) (fig. 7) and with ESR (r= 0.73 $p<0.001$((fig. 8). The advantage of the specificity of faecal granulocyte excretion for bowel inflammation can be seen in the two patients with an active peripheral arthritis complicating ulcerative colitis with disproportionately high ESR estimatic for the degree of activity.

Discussion

This study demonstrates that ^{111}In-labelled leucocytes can be used to obtain gamma camera images of inflamed bowel in both ulcerative colitis and Crohn's disease. Positive scans are specific for inflammation as no false positive results were observed in the irritable bowel syndrome or noninflammatory bowel disorders. Pure granulocytes were superior to mixed leucocytes in producing clearer bowel images and better agreement with radiology for judging the extent of diseased bowel. The poorer quality of the small bowel image compared to the large bowel image is due to a combination of factors including background bone marrow activity, small bowel movement during the scanning period and overlapping small bowel loops.

The technique of ^{111}In-leucocyte scanning offers several advantages over the alternative approach using ^{67}Ga-citrate. ^{67}Ga-citrate is normally excreted into the bowel thus having the potential to produce false positive bowel images in normal subjects (10). Furthermore ^{67}Ga-citrate scanning has been shown to have limited value in localizing inflamed bowel in Crohn's disease (11).

Quantitation of faecal ^{111}In-leucocyte excretion is a new method of assessing inflammatory activity in both Crohn's disease and ulcerative colitis. Although pure granulocyte separation and labelling involves additional expertise, the use of such a preparation offers several advantages over the conventional mixed leucocyte preparation. A smaller radiation dose may be given and the possible damaging effects on lymphocytes are avoided. Faecal granulocyte excretion showed a highly significant correlation with both clinical and laboratory assessment of disease activity.

^{111}In-labelled autologous leucocytes provides a novel approach to the problem of imaging and assessing inflammatory bowel disease. In the single procedure, gamma scanning permits a noninvasive assessment of distribution while faecal counting allows an objective estimation of inflammatory activity. These properties should lead to the widespread use of this technique in the clinical management of inflammatory bowel disease.

REFERENCES

1. Thakur ML, Lavender JP, Arnot RN, Silvester DJ, Segal AW, Indium-111-labelled autologous leucocytes in man. J. nucl. Med. 1977, 18:1014, 1977.

2. Coleman RE, Black RE, Welch DM, Maxwell JG, Indium-111-labelled leucocytes in the evaluation of suspected abdominal abscesses. Amer. J. Surg. 139:99, 1980.

3. Knocker JQ, Koehler PR, Lee TC, Welch DM, Diagnosis of abdonimal abscesses with computer tomography, ultrasound and ^{111}In-leucocyte scan. Radiology 137:425, 1980.

4. Davies RA, Thakur ML, Berger HJ, Wackers F, Gottschalk A, Zaret B, In-111-labelled autologous leucocytes for imaging the inflammatory response to acute myocardial infarction. J. nucl. Med. 21:89, 1980.

5. Saverymuttu SH, Peters AM, Lavender JP, Hodgson HJH, Chadwick VS, Imaging disease bowel with Indium-111-labelled leucocytes. Brit. J. Radiol. 54:707, 1981.

6. Segal AW, Ensell J, Munro JA, Sarner M, Indium^{111} tagged leucocytes in the diagnosis of inflammatory bowel disease. Lancet 2:230, 1981.

7. Sinn H, Silvester DJ, Simplified cell labelling with Indium-111-acetylacetone. Brit. J. Radiol. 52:758, 1979.

8. Danpure HJ, Osman SO, Brady F, The labelling of blood cells in plasma with ^{111}In-tropolonate. Brit. J. Radiol. 55:247, 1982.

9. Best WR, Becktel JM, Singleton JW, Kern F, Development of the Crohn's disease activity index. Gastroenterology 79:439, 1976.

10. Hopkins GB, Kan M, Mende CW, Early ^{67}Gallium scintigraphy for the localisation of abdominal abscesses. J. nucl. Med. 16:990, 1975.

11. Rheingold OJ, Tedesco FJ, Block FE, Mac Donald DA, Midle AG, Gallium-67 citrate scintiscanning in active inflammatory bowel disease. Dig. Dis. Sci. 24:363, 1979.

30 DIAGNOSIS OF ORTHOPEDIC PROSTHESES INFECTION WITH ^{111}IN-LABELLED LEUCOCYTES

M.H. RÖVEKAMP, E.A. VAN ROYEN, S.CHR.C. REINDERS FOLMER, E.L.F.B. RAAYMAKERS

INTRODUCTION

The major concern after partial or total prosthetic hip replacement still lies in differentiating between failure resulting from septic or aseptic loosening (1). A definitive diagnostic answer, in the pre-operative phase, to the question septic or aseptic is most important for the final management and outcome for the patient. The various parameters and diagnostic methods currently being used too often result in an unreliable answer to that question (2). Infection after hip surgery can present itself early post-operative (within the first 12 weeks after surgery); delayed post-operative (sign occurring up to one year after surgery) and late post-operative (more than one year after surgery) (3). Late post-operative accounts for approximately 50% of all infections.

In the diagnosis of loosening arthroplasties, scintigraphy with Tc^{99m}-diphosphonate and ^{67}Ga-citrate has been used and considered helpful by some authors (4-7).

Scintigraphy with ^{111}In-oxinate labelled leucocytes has been recently demonstrated to be a useful and more specific test than ^{67}Ga-citrate in diagnosing occult inflammatory processes (8,9). A diagnostic accuracy of 80-90% was obtained in several series with intra-abdominal, retro-peritoneal inflammatory lesions and vascular graft infection (10-16). Others reported the diagnosis of endocarditis, (17), acute osteomyelitis, septic arthritis, etc. (18). In this study, the value of the ^{111}In-oxinate leucocyte scintigraphy as a diagnostic means in the differentiation between septic or non-septic loosening of hip arthroplasties has been evaluated.

Methods

Leucocytes were isolated and labelled with ^{111}In-oxinate as described earlier (14,15). Scintigrams were performed 20-24 hours after injection of 350 μCi of labelled cells. Anterior views were taken of both hip joints, symmetrically, enabling left and right comparison to be made. In 9 patients, the results of the ^{111}In-leucocyte scans were compared with the findings on a Tc^{99m}-diphosphonate scan, in order to correlate areas of increased activity, indicating bone formation, with areas of increased ^{111}In-leucocyte activity.

Patients

32 Scintigrams were performed in 31 patients after hip surgery Operations performed were: 14 total hip replacements; 12 femoral head replacements; 4 screw fixations for femoral neck fracture; and 1 osteotomy with internal fixation. 15 Patients in whom 16 scintigrams were performed, were suspected of an early infection, 9 patients (9 scintigrams) of a delayed infection, and 7 patients (7 scintigrams) of a late infection. All patients presented symptoms suggestive of infection and/or loosening of the prosthesis. 19 Scintigrams were followed by an operation, 2 by a puncture and 11 by conservative management. The average clinical follow-up after scintigraphy was 9 months, with a minimum of 2 months and a maximum of 2½ year.

Results

Of the 32 scintigrams performed, 13 demonstrated distinct abnormal accumulation of activity at the site of the hip joint or proximal femur; 7 showed abnormal activity, but less marked than the former 13 scintigrams. No abnormal accumulation of activity was observed on 12 scintigrams. Scans were considered to be true positive only, when the clinical diagnosis of an "infected hip" was supported by positive bacterial growths.

Positive scintigrams showing a distinct abnormal accumulation of activity: 8 patients with positive scintigrams were re-operated and aspiration was performed in 2 patients. 4 Scans were classifie as true positive and 6 scans were considered to be false positive (table 1) (fig 1-4). 3 Positive scintigrams in 3 patients were

Table 1. Results

		confirmed at operation or needle aspiration		
true positive	6	5	accuracy	50%
true negative	9	3		
false positive	14	10	specificity	40%
false negative	3	3	sensitivity	70%
	32	21		

Table 2. Results in relation to the lengths of postoperative periods

	early(<3 months)	delayed (3 months-1 year)	late(>1 year)
true positive	3	1	2
true negative	7	1	1
false positive	5	6	3
false negative	1	1	1
	16	9	7

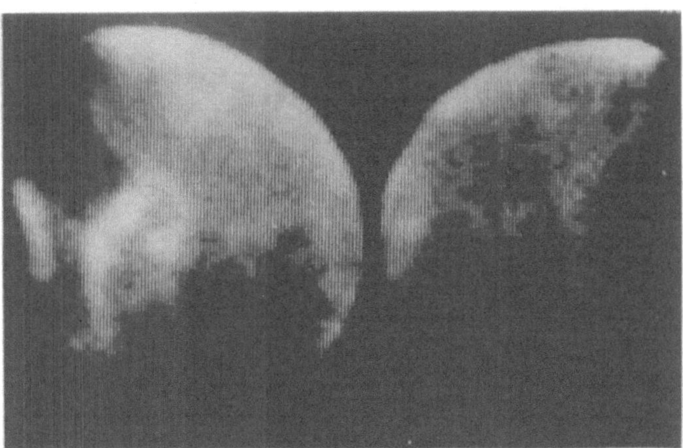

Fig. 1. a) Right early post-operative wound and deep infection after femoral head replacement. b) Left hip: normal.

Table 3. Clinical diagnosis

scan	distinct accumulation of activity	minor accumulation of activity	no abnormal activity
infected			
deep infection/purulent	3		2
septic loosening/low - grade infection	2		1
femoral head necrosis/ infected		1	
non-infected			
non-septic loosening	2	1	3
non septic loosening + destructed acetabulum	2	2	
femoral head necrosis/ non-infected		1	
apecific inflammatory response/culture negative	2		
non clinical signs	2	2	6

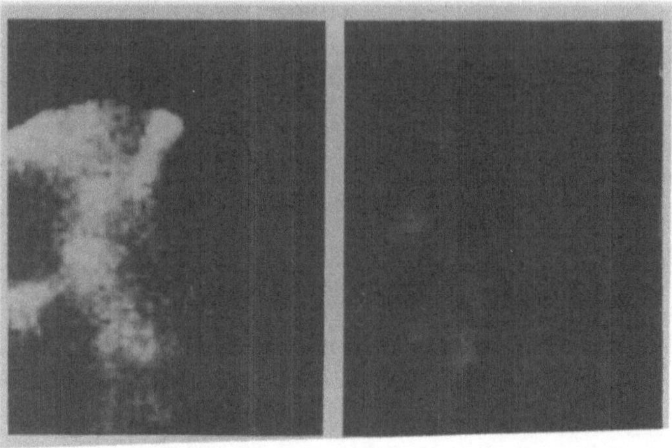

Fig. 2. Late post-operative deep infection. a) Right hip: ^{111}In-leucocytes. b) Left hip: Tc^{99m}-diphosphonate.

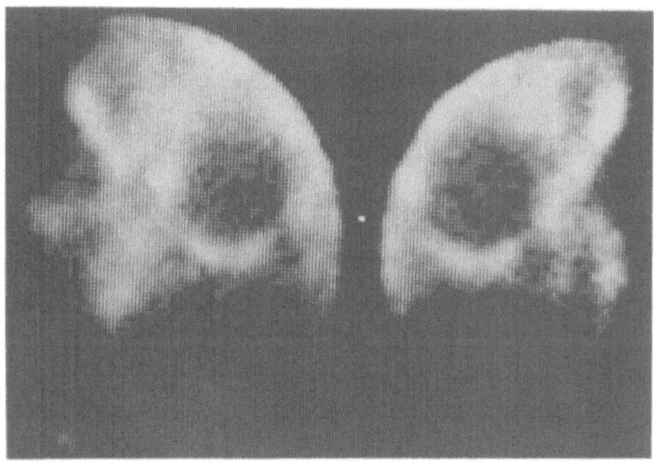

Fig. 3. a) Right hip: delayed post-operative lowgrade infection of a total hip replacement. b) Left hip: normal.

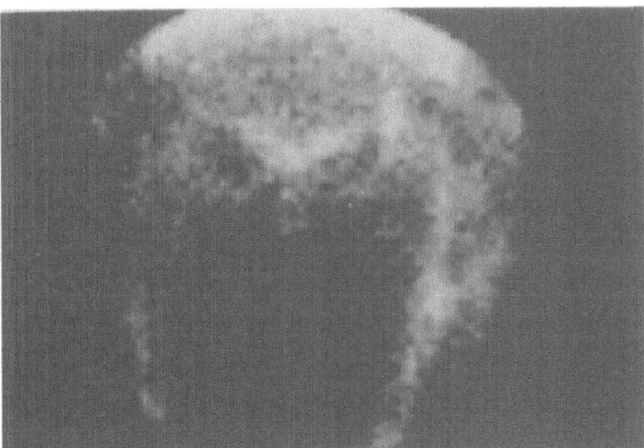

Fig. 4. Right hip: normal. Left hip: false positive scan of an early mechanical loosening due to perforation of the femur shaft.

subjected to clinical non-surgical follow-up. In 2 patients clinical symptoms subsided without evidence of infection, these scans being classified as false positive (table 1). In the other patient, clinical symptoms were highly suspect for a low-grade infection. This scan was considered as true positive.

Positive scintigrams showing only a minor abnormal accumulation of activity: 5 of these were followed by re-operation. One scan was considered true positive and 4 as false positive (table 1). In 2 other patients, re-operation was not performed, both were scanned within 3 months after operation, clinical signs slowly returned to normal in these patients. These scans were classified as false positive (table 1).

Negative scintigrams: No focal activity could be observed at the site of the arthroplasty on 12 scintigrams. 5 of these scans were followed by re-operation and 1 by aspiration. Clear evidence of infection was found in 2 patients. In another patient, the histological appearance was typical for a low-grade infection, these 3 scans were classified as false negative (table 1). The other 3 scans were true negative (table 1). 6 Scans were not followed by a surgical procedure. The clinical follow-up revealed no further development of signs of infection. These scans were considered as true negative (table 1).

Table 2 shows the results in relation to the lengths of post-operative periods.

Discussion

In this series of ^{111}In-labelled leucocyte scanning of infections after arthroplasty and other operations on the hip joints varying results with a low diagnostic accuracy were obtained (table 1). We assume, that the unpredictable different local reactions to arthroplasty, which, in a later phase, do not differ markedly whether an infection is present or not, 19 are the predominant causative factors for the observed high number of false results. Table 3 demonstrates that the same clinical entity causes either accumulation of activity or not, in both infected or non-infected conditions.

Conclusion

Although leucocyte scintigraphy has been shown to be of use in demonstrating inflammatory and infectious processes in various localizations, it turned out to be of limited value in the pathology of hip arthroplasties. This seems mainly to be inherent in the peculiarities of complications of prostheses, especially in the delayed and late manifestations.

Summary

In this study the value of ^{111}In-oxinate leucocyte scintigraphy as a diagnostic means in differentiation between septic or non-septic complications after hip surgery has been evaluated. 32 Scintigrams were performed in 31 patients, with different types of operations performed and in 3 different time intervals postoperatively.

The overall accuracy obtained was 50%, the specificity 40% and sensitivity 70%. This low diagnostic accuracy seemed mainly to be inherent in the peculiarities of complications observed after arthroplasties.

REFERENCES

1. Hunter GA, Welsh RP, Cameron HU et al, The results of revision of total hip arthroplasty. J. Bone Jt. Surg. 61-B: 419, 1979.

2. Gelman MI, Coleman RE, Stevens PM et al, Radiography, radionuclide imaging, and arthrography in the evaluation of total hip and knee replacement. Radiology 128:677, 1978.

3. Eftekhar NS, Principles of total hip arthroplasy. The C.V. Mosby Comp. Saint Louis pp 552-593, 1978.

4. Pearlman AW, The painful hip prosthesis: Value of nuclear imaging in the diagnosis of late complications. Clin. Nucl. Med. 5:133, 1980.

5. Weiss PE, Mall JC, Hoffer PB et al, ^{99m}Tc-Methylene diphosphonate bone imaging in the evaluation of total hip prostheses. Radiology 133:727, 1979.

6. Williamson BRJ, McLaughin RE, Wang GJ et al, Radionuclide bone imaging as a means of differentiating loosening and infection in patients with a painful total hip prostesis. Radiology 133:723, 1979.

7. Wagner J, Schoutens A, Crockaert F et al, Intérêt du scannin au citrate de Gallium-67 dans la chirurgie de la hanche suspecte d'infection. Acta orthop. belg. 44:841, 1978.

8. Thakur ML, Coleman RE, Welch MJ, Indium-111 labelled leucocytes for the localization of abscesses: preparation, analysis, tissuedistribution and comparison with Gallium-67 citrate is dogs. J. Lab. clin. Med. 89:217, 1977.

9. McAfee JG, Gagne GM, Subramanian G et al, Distribution of leucocytes labelled with In-111 oxine in dogs with acute inflammatory lesions. J. nucl. Med. 21:1059, 1980.

10. Thakur ML, Lavender JP, Arnot RN et al: Indium-111 labeled autologous leucocytes in man. J. nucl. Med. 18:1012, 1977.

11. Ascher NL, Ahrenholz DH, Simmons RL et al, Indium-111 autologous tagged leucocytes in the diagnosis of intra-peritonea sepsis. Arch. Surg. 114:386, 1979.

12. Coleman RE, Black RE, Welch DM et al, Indium-111 labeled leucocytes in the evaluation of suspected abdominal abscesses. Amer. J. Surg. 139:99, 1980.

13. Rövekamp MH, Hardeman MR, Van der Schoot JB et al, ^{111}Indium labelled leucocytes scintigraphy in the diagnosis of inflammatory disease- First results. Brit. J. Surg. 68:150, 1981.

14. Rövekamp MH, Van Royen EA, Koning J et al, Indium-111 leucocyte scintigraphy. A new method in diagnosis of infected vascular prosthetic grafts. Preliminary results. In: Cardiovascular Surgery 1980. Bircks W, Ostermeyer J, Schulte HD (eds), Springer-Verlag, Berlin, Heidelberg, pp 573-579, 1981

15. Rövekamp MH, Indium-111 labelled leucocyte scintigraphy in the diagnosis of inflammatory disease - a clinical study. Ph.D. Thesis pp 17-37, 1982.

16. Serota AI, Williams RA, Rose JG et al, Uptake of radiolabeled leucocytes in prosthetic graft infection. Surgery 90:35, 1981.

17. Segal AW, Arnot RN, Thakur ML et al, Indium-111 labelled leucocytes for localisation of abscesses. Lancet 13:1056, 1976.

18. Goodwin DA, Doherty PW, McDougall IR, Clinical use of Indium-111 labeled white cells: an analysis of 312 cases. In: Indium-111 labelled neutrophils, platelets and lymphocytes. Thakur ML, Gottschalk A (eds), Trivirum Publish. Comp. New York City, New York, pp 131-145, 1980.

31 RADIATION DOSIMETRY OF ^{111}IN-OXINATE LABELLED LEUCOCYTES

E. BUSEMANN-SOKOLE, D. HENGST, M.H. RÖVEKAMP

INTRODUCTION

Since the labelling of leucocytes with Indium-oxinate was introduced by McAfee and Thakur in 1976, scintigraphy with ^{111}In-labelled autologous leucocytes has been shown to be a useful non-invasive method for the identification and localization of inflammatory processes (1-4). Labelling methods continue to undergo refinement in order to improve cell isolation and cell labelling, the retention of cell viability being of the utmost importance. The quality of the labelled cells and the composition of the labelled cell suspension reinjected will influence the in-vivo distribution of the labelled cells, and hence also the absorbed radiation dose.

Non-circulating ^{111}In-labelled leucocytes distribute mainly in liver, spleen and bone marrow (5). In-vivo quantitation of radioactivity in the liver and spleen is reasonably straightforward. However, in-vivo quantitation of bone marrow activity present difficulties due to its distribution throughout the body and there is no reliable method of quantitating this activity. Little ^{111}In is excreted and we have therefore assumed that bone marrow activity is equal to the total injected activity minus the activity measured in the total circulating blood, liver and spleen (2,4). This assumption will give the maximum estimate of bone marrow activity, and hence its absorbed radiation dose.

Various methods for the in-vivo quantitation of radioactivity in an organ have been described (6,7). It is generally accepted that for discrete organs, such as the liver and spleen, the geometric mean counts obtained from anterior and posterior measurements give a value that is approximately independent of the geometry of the organ within the body, but is dependent on the cross section of the patient. Converting this geometric mean count value into units of activity (MegaBq or microCi) requires knowledge of the attenuation of the radiation in the body and of the efficiency of the measuring instrumentation. In addition organ size will play a role. We have used phantoms closely resembling the liver and the spleen in both size and shape in order to determine conversion factors from geometric mean counts into MegaBq of activity for each patient cross-section (8-10).

The redistribution of ^{111}In in liver, spleen and circulating blood was measured during a period of 4 days after administration of ^{111}In labelled leucocytes. These data were used for the calculation of the absorbed radiation dose and somatic effective dose equivalent (11-13).

In order to assess whether interindividual differences in liver and spleen concentrations could be related to differences in the composition of the labelled cell suspension administered, the individual cell type and their associated activity were also evaluated.

Materials and methods

The patients studied were referred for routine abscess localization with ^{111}In-labelled autologous leucocytes. A series of 9 patients was studied between 4 hours and 4 days after reinjection of labelled cells.

The leucocytes were isolated by a gravity sedimentation method and labelled with ^{111}In-oxinate according to methods described by Rövekamp and co-workers (4,14). The labelled cell suspension administered to the patient contained between 11 and 15 MegaBq (300-400 microCi) of ^{111}In.

^{111}In-concentration in the liver and spleen was quantitated using a Siemens Gammasonics LFOV (T.M.) scintillation camera and a DEC GAMMA-11 computer system. A medium-energy parallel-hole collimator was used, and 20% energy windows set over both 171 keV and 245 keV energy peaks of ^{111}In. The stability of the scintillation camera/computer system was checked each time patient measurements were made, by measuring a known quantity of ^{111}In under constant scatter conditions using the same aquisition parameters as for the patient studies. For measurement of geometric mean counts, the same aquisition time was used to obtain anterior and posterior images of liver and spleen. With the patient remaining supine, the cross-section of the patient was measured from a lateral view by the distance between radioactive sources placed along the contours of the chest and the back.

From the digitized data in the anterior and posterior views, regions of interest were selected (wheneven possible by an automatic edge algorith, otherwise by eye) over the liver and spleen activity, and also over background activity just below each organ (fig 1).

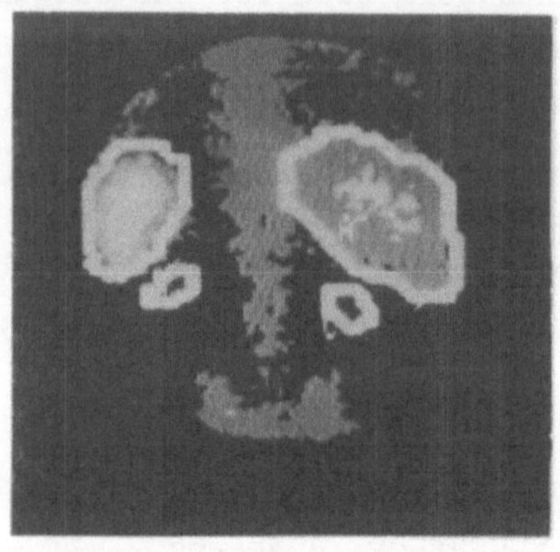

Fig. 1. Regions of interest selected over liver, spleen and background in the posterior view.

For both views, the net counts in liver and spleen regions were obtained by subtracting the averaged background counts corrected for region size. The geometric mean counts were then calculated for each organ using the anterior and posterior net counts.

Phantom studies were carried out to obtain conversion factors of geometric mean counts per MegaBq of activity for different cross-sections (9). For the liver conversion factors, a phantom was used that resembled the size and shape of a standard liver (fig 2); for the spleen conversion factors, a plastic sack was used that had dimensions similar to a standard size spleen (10). Each phantom was filled with a known quantity of ^{111}In and measur at different depths in a water bath. Conversion factors were determined for each organ as a function of various attenuation

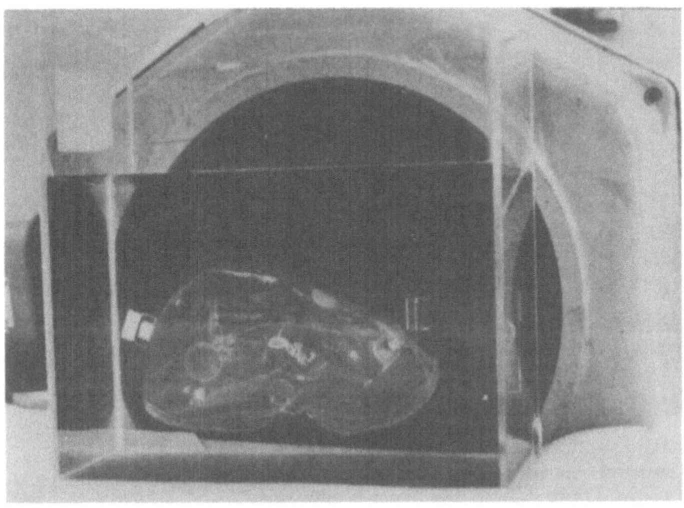

Fig. 2. Liver phantom in water bath as viewed by the scintillation camera.

thicknesses. Using the conversion factors appropriate for the particular patient cross-section the patient's liver and spleen activity was calculated. Measurements were corrected for physical decay of ^{111}In and expressed as a percentage of the administered activity.

Additionally, the total circulating blood-activity was determined at various intervals between 1 hour and 4 days (4). No active inflammatory processes were demonstrated scintigraphically in these patients, so that a maximum estimate of bone marrow activity could be made at each time interval using the basic assumption that the total administered activity was distributed solely between liver, spleen, circulating blood and bone marrow.

Using the data obtained from these source organs, the absorbed radiation dose to various target organs was calculated in each patient using the MIRD methods and tables (11). Using weighting factors according to the ICRP Publication no. 26 the somatic effective dose equivalent was also calculated for each patient (12,13).

The composition of the cell suspension administered was evaluated and the activity associated with each cell type was determined.

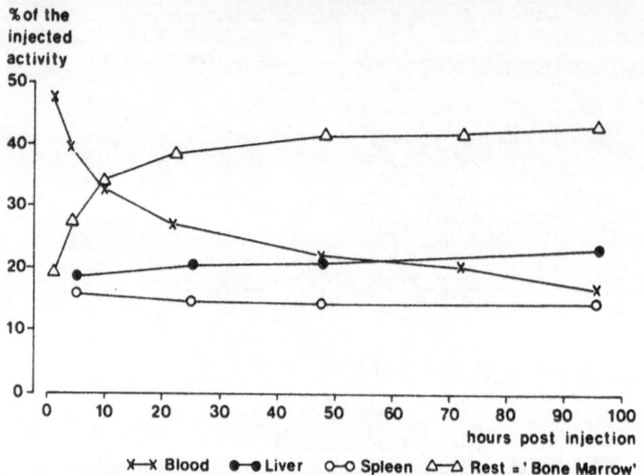

Fig. 3. Average distribution of ^{111}In in liver, spleen, circulating blood and "bone marrow" up to 4 days after reinjection of ^{111}In-oxinate labelled leucocytes, obtained from 9 patients.

Results and discussion

The average distribution of ^{111}In measured in liver and spleen and circulating blood, and the estimated bone marrow activity, is shown in fig 3. In each patient, the spleen activity remained constant, and the liver activity increased very slightly over the 4-day observation period. The blood-activity showed an initial rapid decline followed by a slower decrease. With our cell isolation and labelling methods, labelled thrombocytes and erythrocytes form, to a varying degree, part of the cell suspension reinjected. The blood-curve reflects these labelled cells in the circulation. The initial decline in activity is probably due to the removal of labelled leucocytes from the circulation.

The liver and spleen activity measured at 1 day after reinjection of labelled cells was, respectively (21.6% +/-4.3% SD)and (15.2% +/-4.9% SD). In another group of 15 patients, liver and spleen activity was on average, respectively (15.6% +/-5.6% SD) and (11.6% +/-3.7% SD) at a day after reinjection of labelled leucocytes. Although slightly lower, these latter values supported those obtained in the present series of patients. A wide inter-individual variation in activity distribution was found. This variation has been omitted in fig 3 only to avoid obscuring the basic pattern of redistribution in each organ over the period of

4 days, which was similar in each patient regardless of the actual amount of activity measured.

The ^{111}In-activity injected was not bound solely to leucocytes, but was divided amongst the various cell suspension components as follows: (49% +/- 19% SD) in leucocytes, (10% +/- 4%) in thrombocytes, (21% +/- 12%) in erythrocytes, and (20% +/- 12%) as "free" ^{111}In, that is, non-cell bound. No connection could be found between the various cell components reinjected and the amount of activity measured in liver, spleen and circulating blood. The liver and spleen activity is probably dependent not only on the natural pooling of viable cells but also on the amount of damaged cells reinjected. The blood-activity was high when a large percentage of the injected activity was bound to erytrocytes in the labelled cell suspension. This was especially noticeable in one patient who had 46% injected activity associated with the erythrocytes and a proportion high blood-activity curve.

Because of the large interindividual variation in organ distribution, we calculated both the absorbed radiation dose to various organs and the somatic effective dose equivalent for each individual patient. The average and range of these values are given in table 1. Per organ, a wide range in absorbed doses was found. Nevertheless, when taking into account the total effect of the absorbed radiation dose to the various organs of the body, and the different radiosensitivities of the various organs and tissues, thereby obtaining the somatic effective dose equivalent, these values showed a much narrower range. This implies that, although the radiation doses to individual organs from ^{111}In-labelled leucocytes will vary considerably from patient to patient, the overall somatic risk will be similar.

Bjurman and co-workers have reported on the increased radiation dose from ^{114m}In-contamination of ^{111}In-radiopharmaceuticals (15). ^{114m}In has a physical half-life of 49.5 days, compared to 2.81 days of ^{111}In. On the basis of our distribution data, Johanssen has calculated the absorbed dose from ^{114m}In to be 760 milliGy/MegaMq (281 rads/milliCi) for spleen, 130 milliGy/MegaBq (481 rads/MilliCi) for liver and 330 milliGy/MegaBq (1221 rads/mCi) for bone marrow; the somatic effective dose equivalent would be 99 milliGy/MegaBq

Table 1. Absorbed radiation dose from ^{111}In-oxinate labelled leucocytes (n=9)

Organ	microGy/MegaBq		rads/milliCi	standard deviation
	mean	(range)	mean	(%)
Muscle	111	(107-123)	0.4	4
Lungs	151	(142-161)	0.6	4
Bone marrow	836	(649-1058)	3.1	18
Bone	190	(166-211)	0.7	8
Thyroid	57	(48-76)	0.2	15
Spleen	3790	(2410-5358)	14.0	28
Liver	961	(562-1343)	3.6	24
Pancreas	423	(338-526)	1.6	15
Adrenals	302	(278-328)	1.1	6
Kidneys	301	(265-341)	1.1	8
Ovaries	133	(116-145)	0.5	9
Testes	40	(34-62)	0.1	24
Somatic effective dose	652	(527-770)	2.4	12

(366 rads/mCi (16). Assuming the presence of 0.04% ^{114m}In in the ^{111}In-product at reference time, the effective dose equivalent from ^{111}In-labelled leucocytes used at reference time will be increased by approximately 6%. This increase in radiation dose to the effective dose equivalent is similar to that reported by Bjurman and co-workers (15).

The absorbed radiation doses from ^{111}In to liver and spleen obtained with our labelling methods in our series of patients is of the same order of magnitude as those reported by other authors. Thakur and co-workers report for ^{111}In-labelled leucocytes contaminated with erythrocytes a radiation dose to liver of between 1 and 5 rads/milliCi (270 and 1351 microGy/MegaBq) and to spleen of between 6 and 18 rads/milliCi (1622 and 4865 microGy/MegaBq) (2). Goodwin and co-workers report for ^{111}In-labelled white cells (mainly neutophils) an absorbed radiation dose of 2.4 rads/

milliCi (649 microGy/MegaBq) to liver, 17 rads/milliCi (4595 microGy/MegaBq) to spleen and 4.6 rads/milliCi (1243 microGy/MegaBq) to bone marrow (5).

According to Thakur and co-workers, increased ^{111}In activity in the lungs clears by 4 hours after reinjection of labelled cells (2). In the present series of patients we observed no increased lung activity at 4 hours compared to later time intervals, and have not taken early lung activity into consideration with our absorbed dose calculations.

Conclusion

For a scintigraphic study using 13 MegaBq (350 microCi) of ^{111}In-labelled leucocytes, the patient will receive a somatic effective dose equivalent in the order of 8.5 milliGy (0.84 rads). This radiation dose is high compared to other scintigraphic procedures (12). The presence of the long-lived nuclide ^{114m}In will further increase the radiation dose. The application of these labelled cells for diagnostic scintigraphy must therefore be carefully considered. Moreover, cell isolation and labelling techniques are important factors in the in-vivo activity distribution and should be carried out with care.

Acknowledgements

We wish to express our sincere thanks to the valuable contribution of Mrs. E.G.J. Eitjes-van Overbeek and Mrs. A.J.M. van Velzen. Our thanks are also due to Dr M.R. Hardeman and Dr E.A. van Royen. We are indebted to Dr H. Beekhuis for his advice and assistance in the calculation of the absorbed radiation doses from ^{111}In.

REFERENCES

1. McAfee JG, Thakur ML, Survey of radioactive agents for in-vitro labeling of phagocyte leukocytes I. Soluble Agents. J. nucl. Med. 17:480, 1976.
2. Thakur ML, Lavender JP, Arnot RN, Silvester DJ, Segal AW, In-111 labeled autologous leukocytes in man. J. nucl. Med. 18:1012, 1977.
3. Goodwin DA, Doherty PW, McDougall PW, Clinical use of In-111 labeled white cells: An analysis of 312 cases. In: Indium-111 labeled neutrophils, platelets and lymphocytes. Thakur ML, Gottschalk A (eds), Trivirum Publ. Comp. New York, pp 131-145, 1980.
4. Rövekamp MH, Indium-111 labelled leucocyte scintigraphy in the diagnosis of inflammatory disease - a clinical study. Ph.D. Thesis, University of Amsterdam, 1982.
5. Goodwin DA, Finston RA, Smith SI, The distribution and dosimetry of In-111 labeled leukocytes and platelets in humans. In: Proceedings of 3rd International Radiopharmaceutical Dosimetry Symposium, HHS Publication FDA, 81-8166, Oak Ridge, Tennessee, pp 88-101, 1981.
6. Fleming JS, A technique for the absolute measurement of activity using a gamma camera and computer. Phys. in Med. Biol. 24:176, 1979.
7. Myers MJ, Lavender JP, De Oliviera JB, Maseri A, A simplified method of quantitating organ uptake using a gamma camera. Brit. J. Radiol. 54:1062, 1981.
8. Mould RF, A liver phantom for evaluating camera and scanner performance in clinical practice. Brit. J. Radiol. 44:810, 1971.
9. Sokole-Buseman E, Hengst D, Schatting van de stralingsdosis in de lever en milt t.g.v. met In-111 oxinaat, gelabelde leucocyten. Vangnet 4-13, 1981.
10. International Commission on Radiological Protection, Report on the task group on reference man. ICRP Publication no. 23, Pergamon Press, 1975.
11. Snyder WS, Ford MR, Warner GG, Watson SB, "S" absorbed dose per unit accumulated activity for selected radionuclides and organs. MIRD Pamphlet no. 11, Soc. Nucl. Med. New York, 1975.
12. International Commission on Radiological Protection. Recommendations of the International Commission on Radiological Protection. ICRP Publication no. 26, Pergamon Press, 1977.
13. Roedler HD, Radiation dose to the patient in radionuclide studies. In: Medical radionuclide imaging. Internat. Atomic Energy Agency, Vol. 1, Vienna, pp 527-542, 1981.
14. Rövekamp MH, Hardeman MR, Van der Schoot JB, Belfer AJ, In-111 labelled leucocyte scintigraphy in the diagnosis of inflammatory disease - first results. Brit. J. Surg. 68:150, 1981.
15. Bjurman B, Johansson L, Mattson S, In-114m in In-111 radiopharmaceuticals and its contribution to the absorbed dose in the patient at investigations with In-111 labeled blood cells. In: Nuclear Medicine and Biology. Proc. of the 3rd World Congress of Nuclear Medicine and Biology, Vol.3, Paris, pp 2403-2406, 1982.
16. Johansson L, Private communication, 1982.

LYMPHOCYTES

32 THE LYMPHOCYTE IN HODGKIN's DISEASE: HAS IT LOST ITS WAY?

J. WAGSTAFF, Ch. GIBSON, D. CROWTHER

Hodgkin's disease (HD) is a progressive disorder of the lymphoid system which provides a peculiar medical paradox. On the one hand there is often lymphopenia and deficits in cell mediated immunity (CMI) and on the other "reactive cells" are frequently observed in the peripheral blood suggesting that stimulation of the immune system may be occurring. The lymphopenia is frequently present in patients with stage I and II disease where the tumour is localized to one or two lymphnode groups, but does become increasingly more common as the disease advances. The defect in CMI includes an inability to reject skin grafts, anergy to in vivo challenge with antigens and a failure to respond normally to T cell mitogens (1,2,3). Several hypotheses have been advanced to explain these perturbations including an intrinsic lymphocyte abnormality, the presence of serum blocking factors or an alteration in the normal migratory properties of lymphocytes. The first two explanations both fail to account for all the observed facts and can only be regarded as partial answers. The third hypothesis has been entertained because of evidence from several authors suggesting that there are increased numbers of T lymphocytes in the spleen and lymphnodes of HD patients (4,5,6). De Sousa (7) has called this altered distribution of lymphocytes in disease states "ecotaxopathy". To date there have been no in vivo studies of lymphocyte migration in HD patients which confirm this hypothesis. Lavender et al (8) studied the migration of autologous lymphocytes in normal subjects and patients with HD using an attractive new radioisotopic cell namely ^{111}In-oxine. However, they failed to demonstrate a preferential uptake of cells by involved as opposed to normal nodes.

Recently we have developed techniques which make the study

of lymphocyte migration in man a viable proposition and subsequently turned our attention to the study of this intriguing and enigmatic disease. The methodology which we use has been published in full elsewhere (9,10). Briefly, peripheral blood lymphocytes were obtained from patients with HD using a Hemonetics cell separator. Yields of approximately 10^9 have been obtained and this allows a sufficient quantity of radioactivity to be injected without exceeding the critical lymphocyte specific activity of 20-40 μCi per 8 cells which has been shown to alter their recirculation in experimental animals. The residual red cells, granulocytes and platelets are then removed and the lymphocytes resuspended in saline. They are then labelled with ^{111}In obtained from the Radiochemical Centre, Amersham, England. The cells are then reinjected into the patient and their subsequent fate determined by use of serial blood-sampling and gamma camera imaging.

7 Patients with HD have now been studied and the results are proving consistent. The blood-clearance curves show either a more rapid clearance than normal individuals or one similar to them. There are too few patients to be certain whether this represents variation in proportion to the extent of the disease. The percentage of cells found within the spleen again shows patient to patient variation but neither the pattern nor degree of uptake are significantly different from normals. The lymphnodes however show dramatic sequestration of labelled reinjected cells. In all patients studied there was a considerable accumulation of lymphocytes in the involved nodes. This amounted to 5 to 10% of the injected cells in one lymphnode group.

It seems clear from both De Sousa's work and our own that there is an increased traffic of lymphocytes to lymphnodes involved with HD. The phenomenon appears extensive enough to cause a redistribution of lymphocytes from the blood to the extra-vascular recirculating lymphocyte pool. This could easily result in the peripheral blood lymphopenia which is seen in all stages of disease (11). If cells were trapped in one particular compartment there would be fewer available to recirculate through other areas. This might explain the anergy to cutaneous hypersensitivity recall antigens which commonly occurs in HD.

Few direct measurements have been made of lymphocyte outputs in the lymphatics of patients with HD but those that have been performed show that lymphocyte levels in the lymph parallel those found in the blood. However, the numbers of large (activated) lymphocytes are increased. These "activated" lymphocytes have also been found in the blood of HD patients and similar cells have been observed in the blood of infected or immunised individuals (12). Serum immunoglobulin levels are frequently elevated and circulating immune complexes have been found (11). All of these events have been interpreted as representing the activation of the immune system and a search has ensued to find the antigen responsible. Viral infection of cells is known to alter their antigenic nature such that the host no longer recognizes them as "self" and mounts an immune response against them. Indeed antigen "trapping" has been shown to occur in the regional lymphnodes and spleens of mice bearing virally induced tumours (13). Despite some epidemiological evidence that HD may be caused by an infective agent the belief that the disease is virally mediated is not generally accepted. Others have suggested that iron proteins particularly ferritin, may be responsible and siderosis of lymphnodes and spleen of HD patients lends support to this idea. These authors also describe a number of other diseases where perturbation of lymphocyte traffic may be occurring and where iron proteins are also normal.

The neoplastic cell of HD have antigenic proporties which the host does not recognize as self thus resulting in immune situation. There is evidence implying that lymphocytes in close proximity to Reed-Sternberg cells are engaged in cytotoxic activities. But others have disputed this. Although it seems feasible that the lymphocytes seen in the affected tissues of HD patients may be engaged in an immunological insult the evidence is not entirely consistent with this view. Further one would expect the output of lymphocytes in the lymph draining the affected sites to be increased as occurs in lymphdrainage of the cell mediated immune lesions or rejecting allografts. It almost seems as if the immune response has "got stuck" in the "trapping" phase. This anomaly could be explained if the cell which had undergone neoplastic transformation in HD was the same cell involved in the modulation of lymphocyte traffic through the tissues. As we have suggested earlier there is a certain amount of evidence to suggest that the Interdigitating Reticulum Cell (IDRC) is important in this regard. The possibility that the Reed-Sternberg or Hodgkin Cell is derived from the IDRC is therefore raised. If this were the case then it is possible that the some of the normal functions of the IDRC could be "switched on" inappropriately resulting in both the lymphocyte trapping response and the production of "mitotic" stimulators causing the appearance of the reactive lymphocytes which are seen in the lymph and blood.

Other types of neoplastic cell are well known for inappropriately producing substances (e.g. ectopic hormone production) and it is possible that IDRC may behave in a similar manner. Since IDRC are found in sites other than lymphnodes and spleen (although in much smaller numbers) it is possible that HD could originate in these sites also (although much less frequently) and this is in fact the case. IDRC have been described in afferent lymph as "veiled cells" but have not been seen in the blood. This would be consistent with the findings in HD where clinical patterns of disease have been thought to suggest that the major route of dissemination is by lymphatic spread between contiguous lymphnodes. This view does not preclude the possibility of haematogenous but it would suggest that splenic and liver involvement, if this occurred via the blood, would be more likely when lymphnodes with more direct drainage to the thoracic duct and thence to the vena cava were involved. This is in fact the case. In HD it has been suggested that the numbers of lymphocytes in the lymphnodes and spleen are increased even when histological criteria are not sufficient to diagnose involvement of these tissues by the disease. This may only be explained by mechanisms which have perturbed the normal migratory patterns of the lymphocytes concerned. The important point for students of HD to realize is that a histological section of a lymphnodes or spleen is not a static picture; it is more like looking at one frame of a cine film. Many of the cells seen in the sections may have recently come from the blood and are destined to return there. It is therefore of paramount importance that we have a clear grasp of the factors which control the continuous flow of lymphocytes through the tissues and that attention is paid to the perturbations in their migration that may occur in disease.

Indeed it is true to say that we do not know whether the perturbation of lymphocyte traffic which seems to be occurring in HD are beneficial or detrimental to the patient and much further work needs to be done.

REFERENCES

1. Kelly WD, Laneb DL, Good RA, Investigation of Hodgkin's disease with respect to problems of homotransplantation. Ann. N.Y. Acad. Sci. 87:187, 1960.

2. Aisenberg AC, Studies of delayed hypersensitivity in Hodgkin's disease. J. clin. Invest. 41:1964, 1962.

3. Levy R, Kaplan HS, Impaired lymphocyte function in untreated Hodgkin's disease. New Engl. J. Med. 290:181, 1974.

4. Aisenberg AC, Long JC, Lymphocyte surface characteristics in malignant lymphoma. Amer. J. Med. 58:300, 1975.

5. Grifoni V et al, Lymphocytes in the spleen in Hodgkin's disease. Lancet 1:332, 1975.

6. Hunter CP et al, Increased T lymphocytes and Ig MEA-receptor lymphocytes in Hodgkin's disease spleens. Cell. Immunol. 31:193, 1977.

7. De Souse M et al, Ecotaxis. The principle and its application to the study of Hodgkin's disease. Clin. Exp. Immunol. 27:143, 1977.

8. Lavender JP et al, Kinetics of Indium-111 labelled lymphocytes in normal subjects and patients with Hodgkin's disease. Brit. med. J. 2:797, 1977.

9. Wagstaff J et al, A method for followinq human lymphocyte traffic using Indium-111 labelling. Clin. Exp. Immunol. 43:435, 1981.

10. Wagstaff J et al, Human lymphocyte traffic assessed by Indium-111 oxine labelling: clinical observations. Clin. Exp. Immunol. 43:443, 1981.

11. Kaplan HS, Hodgkin's disease. 2nd ed. Harvard Univ. Press Ch. 6:236, 1980.

12. Crowther D, Hamilton Fairley G, Sewell R, Significance of the changes in the circulating lymphoid cells in Hodgkin's disease. Brit. med. J. 2:473, 1969.

13. Zatz MM, White A, Goldstein AL, Alterations in lymphocyte populations in tumorigenesis. I. Lymphocyte trapping. J. Immunol. 3:706, 1974.

33 LABELLING OF HUMAN LYMPHOCYTES WITH ^{111}IN-OXINATE

R.J.M. TEN BERGE, A.T. NATARAJAN, S.L. YONG, M.R. HARDEMAN,
E.A. VAN ROYEN, P.Th.A. SCHELLEKENS

INTRODUCTION

Recently, several investigators have advocated the use of the Indium radionuclide ^{111}Indium (used as ^{111}Indium-oxinate) for labelling of lymphocytes, to study their homing and recirculation (1-4). In fact, this method has already been applied in man (5-9). However, data on the functional properties of ^{111}In-labelled human lymphocytes are sparse (10). The present study was undertaken to measure the spontaneous release of ^{111}In from labelled cells and the effect of ^{111}In labelling on the proliferative capacity of human peripheral blood lymphocytes. As a parameter for radiation-induced cell damage, the chromosomal pattern of the cells was studied.

Materials and methods

Freshly drawn blood from healthy volunteers was defibrinated and diluted 1:1 with Earle's balanced salt solution (BSS). Lymphocytes were isolated by Ficoll-Isopaque density-gradient centrifugation, washed three times, pelleted and resuspended in 300 µl serum-free medium RPMI-1640. In our hands, the labelling was more efficie under serumfree conditions, compared with labelling in RPMI-1640-containing serum. Labelling was performed with an aqueous preparation of the ^{111}In-oxinate complex, purchased from Byk-Mallinkrodt CIL B.V. (Petten, The Netherlands). At activity reference time, the specific activity was 1 mCi per 25 µg 8-hydroxyquinoline (oxine). The cells were incubated with varying doses of ^{111}In-oxinate, ranging from 2 to 20 µCi/10^7 lymphocytes, for 30 min at roomtemperature. In control experiments, decayed ^{111}In-oxinate was used a well, to determine the effect of various concentrations of oxinat itself on the lymphocyte cultures. After three washings with RPMI containing 5% human serum, the ^{111}In-labelled cells were resuspended in RPMI containing 10% human serum, counted and resuspended at the required concentrations. After labelling of lymphocytes wit ^{111}In-oxinate, several parameters were measured:

1) Spontaneous and maximal release in-vitro; maximal release from the cells was determined upon treatment with 2,5% saponin. The cell suspensions were incubated for varying times at 37°C in a humidified atmosphere of 5% CO_2 in air.
2) Viability of the cell suspension was determined by trypan-blue exclusion both before labelling with ^{111}In-oxinate and several times after the labelling procedure.
3) Lymphocyte cultures of both unlabelled cells and cells from the same donor labelled with varying doses of ^{111}In-oxinate were performed as previously described (11). The total ^{3}H-thymidine counts were corrected by subtraction of ^{111}In cross-over, which averaged about 2 to 5% of the counts present.
4) Cytogenetic studies following stimulation with PHA. The lympho cytes were harvested for cytological studies at 72 hours follo ing initiation. The cells were blocked at mitosis by colcemid for 2 hours and further subjected to hypotonic shock (0.56% NaCl) before fixation in acetic acid methanol. Standard air-dry preparations were made. The slides were stained with aqueous Giemsa solution and, wherever possible, 100 well-sprea metaphases were scored for the presence of chromosomal abberations.

Results

When 10^7 lymphocytes were incubated with ^{111}In-oxinate at increasing concentrations in the range of 2 to 20 μCi, the incorporated radioactivity was linearly dependent on the added dose. Initial studies revealed a rather high spontaneous release of ^{111}In-oxinate from human lymphocytes, i.e. about 25% at 24 hours labelling. Several modifications in experimental conditions did not result in a lower spontaneous release. Additional washings or prolonged incubation of the labelled cells did not affect the subsequent spontaneous release from the cells, which was always about 25% at 24 hours after labelling. Yet, cell viability, as measured

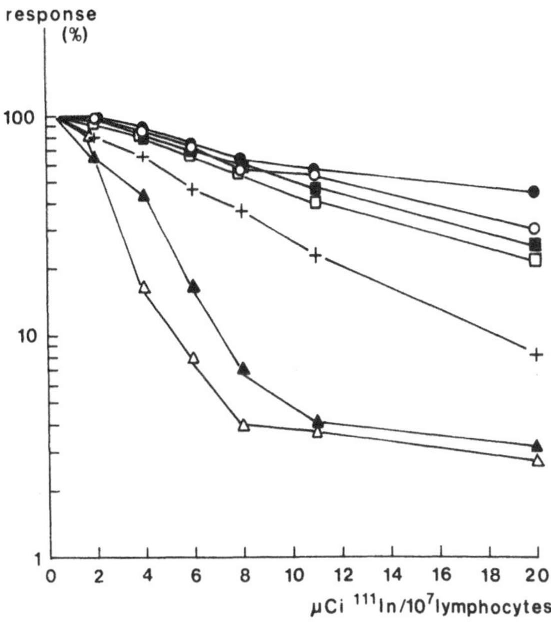

Fig. 1. Relative responses of lymphocytes to several stimuli after labelling with varying concentrations of ^{111}In-oxinate plotted on a semi-logarithmic scale. H-3-thymidine incorporation of unlabelled cells is expressed as 100%. Absolute values of the cells are expressed in cpm x 10^{-3}; Anti-lymphocyte serum (ALS), •20.7±3.2; phytohaemagglutinin (PHA), ■12.7±2.5; Concanavalin A (ConA), ○10.1±3.0; pokeweed mitogen (PWM), □9.1±3.7; antigen cocktail (a mixture of PPD, varidase, mumps, trichophyton and candida), Δ4.1±2.8; tetanus toxoid, ▲7.1±4.9; mixed lymphocyte culture (MLC) responder capacity, +7.9±1.6. All values represent the mean ± SD of 4 donors.

by trypan-blue exclusion, remained high. Neither changes in the concentration of serum nor variation of the cell number during incubation improved the spontaneous release. To assess the effect of ^{111}In-labelling on the proliferative capacity of lymphocytes, dose response curves were performed. From fig. 1, it is evident that the proliferative capacity of lymphocytes in response to all stimuli is affected, although to a different extent, even when cells have been labelled with rather low doses of ^{111}In-oxinate. Control experiments revealed that decayed ^{111}In-oxinate did not have a deleterious effect on the cultures, when tested in amounts of about 0.10 to 2 µg per 10^7 lymphocytes, which is in the same order of magnitude as the quantity of oxinate present during labelling. Chromosome preparations of the ^{111}In-labelled cells revealed several aberrations, viz. gaps, breaks and exchanges were encountered. Most of the aberrations were of chromosome type, indicating that they were induced in the G_0 or G_1 stage of the cell cycle. The frequency of chromosomal aberrations was dependent on the labelling dose. Labelling with high doses (from 8 μCi/10^7 lymphocytes) resulted in a lower proportion of cells in division (see table).

Table 1. Frequencies of chromosomal aberration in human lymphocytes labelled with ^{111}Indium-oxinate (results from 2 individuals are shown).

Dose of ^{111}In-oxinate per 10^7 lympfocytes	Number of cells analyzed	% of abnormal cells	Aberrations / 100 cells gaps	breaks	exchanges
Donor A					
0 μCi	100	3	0	2	1
3.6 μCi	100	54	5	82	12
9.4 μCi	100	90	16	211	55
14.9 μCi	73	93	24.7	354.8	102.7
29.2 μCi	8	100	62.5	600.0	87.5
Donor B					
0 μCi	100	14	5	10	0
2.2 μCi	100	15	5	14	3
8.2 μCi	71	91.5	16.9	190.1	59.2
14.8 μCi	46	93.5	13.0	233.9	52.2
29.2 μCi	61	100	13.1	537.7	162.3

Breaks : include both chromatid breaks and chromosome breaks; 60 to 80% of breaks were chromosome-type.
Exchanges: include both chromatid and chromosome exchanges; more than 90% of exchanges were chromosome-type.

Discussion

In the present study, humer peripheral blood lymphocytes were labelled with several concentrations of ^{111}In-oxinate. The extent of spontaneous release from the labelled cells was measured at several time-points and the labelled cells were tested of their proliferative capacity in-vitro as well as for possible chromosomal damage. Although a low spontaneous release is generally mentioned to be one of the advantages of ^{111}In labelling, we found a rather high spontaneous release, which could not be diminished by varying the experimental conditions. According to Frost et al (4), the released ^{111}In cannot be re-utilized by lymphocytes. Recent studies in rats have revealed that the label is probably transferred to non-recirculating cells, presumably macrophages (12). In interpreting data from in-vivo studies on lymphocyte migration, one should be aware of this rather high spontaneous release of the ^{111}In label. Indeed, after infusion of ^{111}In labelled lymphocytes, detected radioactivity could be associated with other cells. Labelling with ^{111}In-oxinate is clearly detrimental for the proliferative capacity of human lymphocytes. This effect occurs already at relatively low doses. In control cultures, a possibly toxic effect of oxinate on the lymphocyte cultures was excluded. Cytogenetic analysis revealed that ^{111}In-oxinate is a powerful inducer of chromosomal aberrations. After labelling with 9.4 μCi/10^7 cells, lymphocytes with damaged chromosomes were observed in a frequency similar to that observed after 200 to 250 rad of X-rays (13). This indicates a very high efficiency of this nuclide to induce chromosomal aberrations. Although most of the aberrations were of chromosome type, some 20% appeared as chromatic aberrations, indicating that the radioactivity persists and is capable of including lesions even in S and G_2 stages of the cell cycle.

From this study, it is clear that ^{111}In-oxinate, even in low doses (1 to 4 μCi/10^7 lymphocytes), has detrimental effects on human lymphocytes, especially on the structure of their chromosomes. Such labelled cells are still able to proliferate, although to a lower extent. Thus, infusion of ^{111}In-labelled lymphocytes may lead to the presence, in the circulation, of long-lived lymphocytes with cytogenetic abnormalities, which are aparently still capable to proliferate. One could envisage a possibility that, by infusing labelled lymphocytes, a stable transformed clone is introduced, and that this may cause a malignant process. These findings pose the question whether labelling with ^{111}In can be safely used in-vivo to monitor homing and recirculation of lymphocytes.

Acknowledgements

The investigations were financially supported in part by the Foundation for Medical Research FUNGO, which is subsidized by the Netherlands Organization for the Advancement of Pure Research (ZWO), The Hague, The Netherlands (grant no. 13-29-42), and in pa by the Queen Wilhelmina Fund (grant no. SG 81.91).

REFERENCES

1. Thakur ML, Indium-111: a new radioactive tracer for leucocytes. Exp. Hemat. 5:145 (supplement), 1977.
2. Rannie GH, Thakur ML, Ford WL, An experimental comparison of radioactive labels with potential application to lymphocyte migration studies in patients. Clin. Exp. Immunol. 29:509, 1977.
3. Goodwin DA, Cell labelling with oxine chelates of radioactive metal ions: techniques and clinical implications. J. nucl. Med. 19:557, 1978.
4. Frost Ph, Smith J, Frost H, The radiolabelling of lymphocytes and tumor cells with 111-Indium. Proc. Soc. Exp. Biol. Med. 157:61, 1978.
5. Lavender JP, Goldman JM, Arnot RN et al, Kinetics of Indium-111 labelled lymphocytes in normal subjects and patients with Hodgkins disease. Brit. med. J. 2:797,1977.
6. Miller RA, Coleman CN, Fawcett HD et al, Sézary syndrome: a model for migration of T lymphocytes to skin. New Engl. J. Med. 303:89, 1980.
7. Wagstaff J, Gibson C, Thatcher N et al, A method for following human lymphocyte traffic using Indium-111 oxine labelling. Clin. Exp. Immunol. 43:435, 1981.
8. Wagstaff J, Gibson C. Thatcher N et al, Human lymphocyte traffic assessed by Indium-111 oxine labelling: clinical observations. Clin. Exp. Immunol. 43:443, 1981.
9. Wagstaff J, Gibson C. Thatcher N, Crowther D, The migratory properties of Indium-111 oxine-labelled lymphocytic leukaemia. Brit. J. Haemat. 49:283, 1981.
10. Segal AW, Deteix P, Garcia R et al, Indium-111 labelling of leucocytes: a detrimental effect on neutrophil and lymphocyte function and an improved method of cell labelling. J. nucl. Med. 19:1238, 1978.
11. Van Oers MHJ, Pinkster J, Zeijlemaker WP, Cooperative effects in mitogen- and antigen-induced responses of human peripheral blood lymphocyte subpopulations. Int. Arch. Allergy 58:53, 1979.
12. Sparshott SM, Sharma H, Kelly JD et al, Factors influencing the fate of 111-Indium-labelled lymphocytes after transfer to syngeneic rats. J. Immunol. Methods 41:303, 1981.
13. Van Buul PPW, Natarajan AT, Chromosomal radiosensitivity of human leukocytes in relation to sampling time. Mutation Res. 70:61, 1980.

ERYTHROCYTES

34 Tc^{99m} LABELLING OF RED BLOOD-CELLS AND THEIR CLINICAL APPLICATION

J.B. VAN DER SCHOOT, E. BUSEMANN-SOKOLE, E.A. VAN ROYEN, C. THOMAS, A. VYTH

INTRODUCTION

Radioactive labelled red blood-cells (RBC) were originally used for haematological investigations and, when heat damaged, for spleen scintigraphy (1,2). The major current use of labelled RBC is in cardiac blood-pool scintigraphy, and a further recent application is in the identification and localization of gastro-intestinal bleeding sites. This paper compares various methods of labelling RBC and presents some clinical results in the diagnosis of bleeding sites.

In-vivo labelled RBC

In-vivo labelling of RBC with Tc^{99m} was first observed in patients who underwent brain scintigraphy a few days after bone scintigraphy. In these patients, a higher than normal blood background in the brain images was observed (3). This was attributed to labelling of RBC with Tc^{99m}-pertechnetate due to the stannous ions from the bone imaging agent. This observation led to the development of the method of in-vivo labelling of RBC (4,5). With this labelling method, stannous pyrophosphate, or another stannous compound, is injected intravenously and followed 15-20 min later b Tc^{99m}-pertechnetate. The stannous ions enter the erythrocyte and, when later Tc^{99m}-pertechnetate also enters the erythrocyte, the technetium pertechnetate is reduced and bound to the heme, simila ly to the binding of Cr^{3+} to the beta-polypeptide chain. The labe ing efficiency is dependent on the amount of stannous ion adminis ed (6-8).

Approximately 70% of the Tc^{99m} is bound to the circulating R (9,10). The remainder is distributed throughout the body and is taken up in part by gastric mucosa and colon (11). Gastric activ will be excreted in the gastric juice and will mask or imitate gastrointestinal (GI) bleeding. If in-vivo labelling of RBC is us for the detection of GI bleeding sites, then constant removal of gastric juice by suction through a nasogastric tube is necessary (11).

In-vitro labelling of RBC

A totally in-vitro method of labelling RBC with Tc^{99m}-pertech netate was first decribed by Fischer and co-workers in 1967 (2). This method was unreliable and had a poor labelling efficiency as well as unstable binding of the label (12). A higher labelling efficiency of 50-60% with only negligible elution was achieved by reducing the pertechnetate with stannous chloride after incubatio of the RBC with Tc^{99m}-pertechnetate (13). An even higher labellin efficiency was achieved by adding stannous chloride before the incubation of RBC with Tc^{99m}-pertechnetate (14-16). It has been demonstrated that the labelling efficiency depends on the amount of stannous ion present: too few or too many stannous ions will reduce the labelling efficiency. An excess of stannous ions in the plasma will reduce the pertechnetate which inhibits its entrance into the cells so that removal of excess stannous ions by washing is necessary before pertechnetate is added (15). Maximal binding of 97% will be obtained when 0.5-1.0 microgram of stannous ions is added per 3 ml of whole blood (16). Such small quantities of reduced stannous chloride cannot be easily kept on store, and this method has, therefore, not gained general acceptance.

Semi in-vitro labelled RBC

For routine use, the in-vivo labelling method appears attractive, due to its simplicity of only two successive intravenous injections and no manipulations of blood-samples in-vitro. However the recovery in the circulation of Tc^{99m} approximates only 70%. A method that maintains an uncomplicated labelling procedure, but offers a higher Tc^{99m} recovery in the circulation, is desirable.

We have, therefore, developed a semi in-vitro method of labell ing RBC: the RBC are pretinned with Tc^{99m} in-vivo and a RBC pellet obtained from a sample of pretinned blood is labelled by incubatio with Tc^{99m}-pertechnetate (9). For the pretinning a 1 ml solution of a stannous DTPA solution containing 1 mg of stannous ion is used. This product is prepared in house and sealed in 1 ml ampoules under nitrogen. After 1 year of storage, the amount of bivalent stannous ions is still 75% of the original quantity, as measured by a developed colorimetric method (17).

The labelling procedure is as follows. The stannous DTPA solution is injected intravenously and 15 min later 4,5 ml of whole blood is withdrawn into a 5 ml syringe containing 0.5 ml of a 3.2% sodium citrate solution and mixed well. After cutting off the protruding bar of the plunger of the syringe, this syringe now stimulates a centrifuging tube. After centrifuging the content at 300xg for 10 min, the plasma and buffy coat are removed. The remaining RBC are then added to a volume of about 1 ml saline containing 550 MBq (15 mCi) of Tc^{99m}- pertechnetate. After incubating for 10 min at room temperature, the percentage cell bound activity is usually approximately 97% and the labelled cells are intravenously reinjected.

Semi in-vitro labelled whole blood

A similar semi in-vitro labelling method was recently published (11,18). Using this method, 0.5 mg of stannous ion as stannous pyrophosphate is injected intravenously for pretinning the RBC. 20 min later, 3 ml of whole blood is withdrawn into a shielded syringe containing Tc^{99m}-pertechnetate and allowed to incubate for 10 min. The content of the syringe is then injected.

Comparison of labelled RBC

Since the use of in-vivo labelled RBS is widespread and both semi in-vitro methods of labelling RBC offer apparent advantages with regard to a higher percentage of circulating Tc^{99m}, we have compared the in-vivo and two semi in-vitro methods of labelling RBC in patients undergoing routine cardiac gated blood-pool studies. In each case, pretinning of the RBC was achieved with 1 ml of our in-house prepared stannous DTPA solution.

Circulating Tc^{99m}-activity was compared between 10 and 60 min after injection of activity. It was found to decrease only slightly for each labelling method; 4% for in-vivo, 5% for semi in-vitro

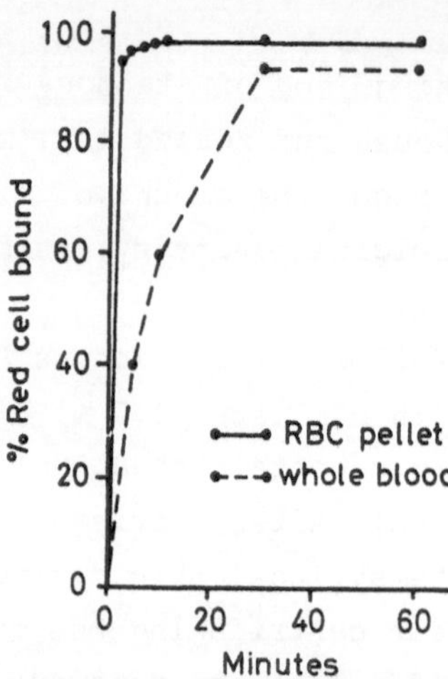

Fig. 1. RBC labelling efficiency measured at various times after administration of Tc^{99m}-pertechnetate to a pretinned RBC pellet and a whole blood sample.

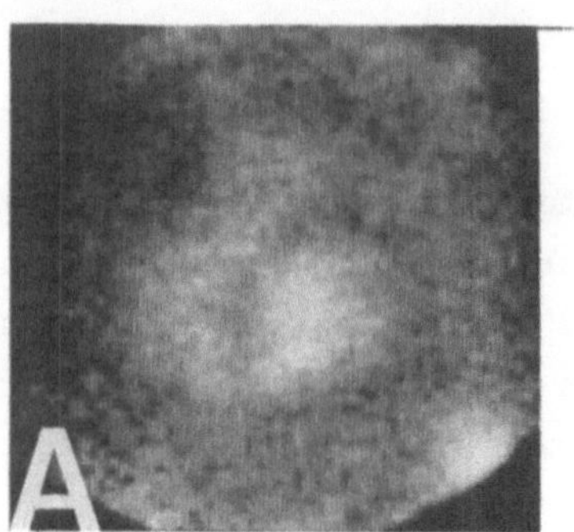

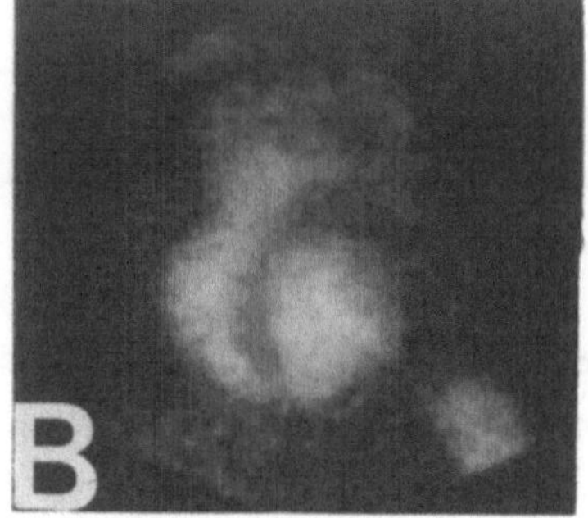

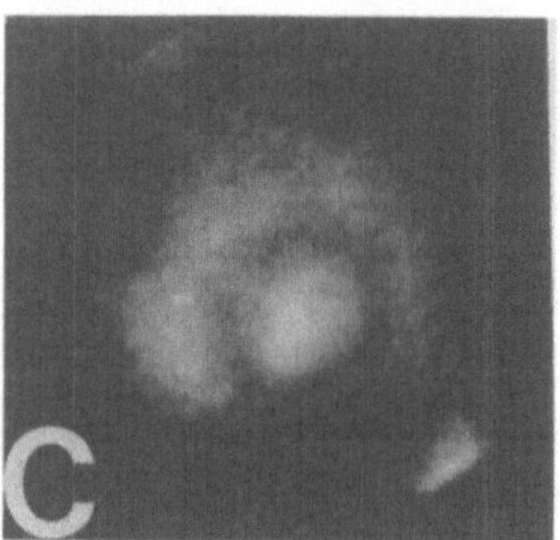

Fig. 2. Gated blood pool images obtained in the same patient using 3 labelling methods. The left anterior oblique 45° and diastolic images are shown without any contrast enhancement. A: in-vivo labelled RBC. B: semi in-vitro labelled whole blood and C: semi in-vitro labelled RBC.

whole blood and 5% for semi in-vitro RBC labelling.

The labelling velocity of Tc^{99m} when added to a RBC pellet and a whole blood-sample was also compared. For the RBC pellet the labelling efficiency was approximately 98% by 5 min, whereas for the semi in-vitro whole blood-sample labelling reached only 40% at 5 min and increased to a plateau of 93% by 30 min (fig. 1). This latter finding was in agreement with that reported by others (18).

More importantly, the mean recovery of Tc^{99m} in the circulation was found to be only 71.3% +/- 3.5% (SEM) for in-vivo labelling, whereas this was found to be 91.5% +/- 2.9% (SEM) for semi in-vitro labelled whole blood and 92.6 +/- 3.6% (SEM) for semi in-vitro labelled RBC (19). These values were determined for each labelling method in 10 patients from blood-samples taken at 10 min after injection of activity and using blood-volumes read from a nomogram based on patient weight. This 20% lower circulating activity for the in-vivo labelled RBC implied a higher concentration of activity in surrounding tissue so that the in-vivo labelled RBC could be expected to give lower contrast scintigraphic images than those produced by the semi in-vitro labelling methods.

Comparison of labelled RBC in cardiac blood-pool studies

The difference in image quality could readily be perceived in gated cardiac blood-pool images as is indicated in the cardiac images of fig. 2. In order to quantitate this difference in image quality, the left ventricular activity was compared with the surrounding background activity. Quantitation was carried out in 32 cardiac studies for in vivo labelled RBC in 49 studies for semi in-vitro labelled RBC and in 35 studies for semi in-vitro labelled whole blood. The end diastolic image of the left anterior oblique view was used. A left ventricular contour was defined using an automatic edge detection algorithm and square regions of interest of 4 pixels were positioned over the maximum left ventricular activity within this contour, and also directly adjacent to this contour. A target to non-target ratio was then calculated from the counts within these regions of interest to be the ratio of the maximum left ventricular activity to the average background activity adjacent to the left ventricular between 4 and 6 o'clock. The

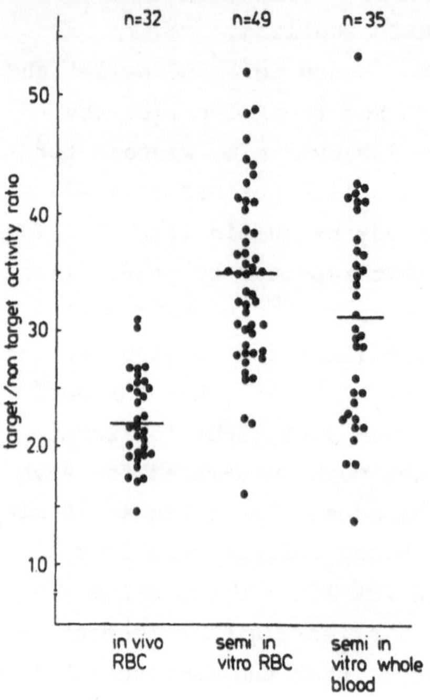

Fig. 3. Comparison of the target to non-target ratios obtained with different RBC labelling methods.

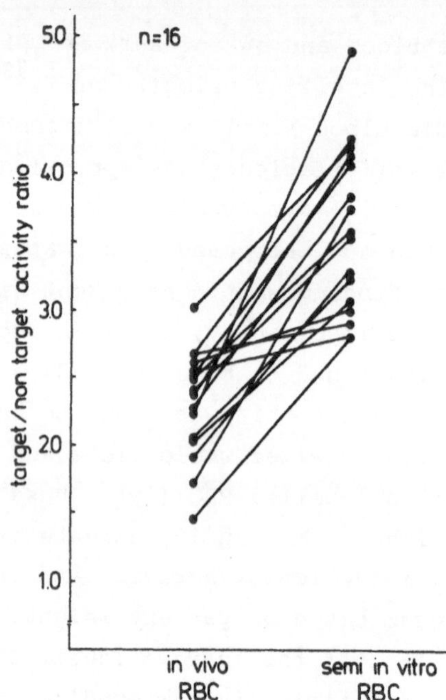

Fig. 4. Comparison of the target to non-target ratios in repeated cardiac blood-pool imaging using in-vivo labelled RBC on the one occasion and semi in-vitro labelled RBC on the other occasion.

latter counts represented an average background activity. Fig. 3 shows the results of this ratio obtained for the three labelling methods. The spread in values reflected in part the labelling and in part the heart geometry. Nevertheless, the in-vivo labelling gave a lower average ratio of 2.4 compared to an average ratio of 3.2 for semi in-vitro labelling of whole blood and 3.5 for semi in-vitro labelling of RBC.

In 16 patients both in-vivo and semi in-vitro labelled RBC were used for cardiac blood-pool scintigraphy on different occasions. In this group quantitation using these labelling methods could be compared in the same patient, and results are shown in fig.4. In each patient a higher ratio was obtained with the semi in-vitro labelled RBC (average 3.6) than with the in-vivo labelled RBC (average 2.2).

When the contribution of background activity to the gross left ventricular end diastolic counts was calculated assuming that the

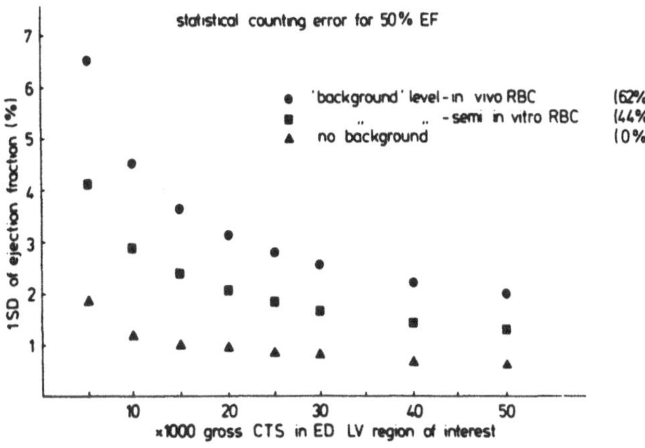

Fig. 5. Standard deviation, in ejection fraction units, expected in the calculation of a 50% ejection fraction at different levels of counts in the left ventricular region. A background subtraction of 62% of the total left ventricular counts represents the situation encountered using in-vivo labelled RBC; a background subtraction of 44% represents that encountered using semi in-vitro RBC; a background subtraction of 0% represents the ideal situation when no background contributes to the left ventricular counts.

background in the left ventricular region was constant and was represented by the average background activity between 4 and 6 o'clock, it was found that the background was on average 62% of the total left ventricular counts for in-vivo labelled RBC and only 44% for semi in-vitro labelled RBC.

A diminished background activity using semi in-vitro labelled RBC will not only improve image quality but will also offer more reliability in quantitative evaluation of cardiac images. It is well known that the choice of a background region and subtraction algorithm will influence the results of an ejection fraction calculation. The higher the background, the greater will be the influence of the net counts from variations in the background. In addition, the counting statistics will be influenced. Fig. 5 illustrates the effects of background subtraction on the statistical accuracy of an ejection fraction measurement. Below 10,000-15,000 counts in the left ventricular region the background subtraction starts to play an important role. It is this lower count region that is encountered in stress cardiac studies, in which often a single exercise measurement is compared with a resting measurement.

In conclusion, we have found that semi in-vitro labelled RBC has advantages over both in-vivo labelled RBC and semi in-vitro labelled whole blood: a higher recovery of Tc^{99m} in the circulation is obtained; the labelling is complete prior to reinjection of labelled cells resulting in more consistant imaging; and the volume reinjected is smaller than for semi in-vitro labelled whole blood which is important in first pass studies. We are now routinely using semi in-vitro labelled RBC as the method of choice for all blood-pool imaging.

Use of labelled RBC in the detection of GI bleeding

In addition to cardiac studies, a diagnostic application of labelled RBC has been the detection and localization of bleeding sites in the gastrointestinal (GI) tract (11,20,21). An active bleeding site in the upper GI tract can readily be detected by modern fiber optic endoscopy. However, it is more difficult to visualize an active bleeding site in the lower GI tract, due to the necessity of proper bowel preparation. Angiography has a high sensitivity and precision for localizing a bleeding site but has the disadvantage that it will not show any extravasation of contrast material, and will mostly be negative when the patient is not acutely bleeding. Due to its short biological half-life in plasma the latter argument also holds for Tc^{99m} labelled colloid that has been advocated by others (22).

Detection and localization of bleeding sites when a patient exhibits intermittent bleeding is problematic. In order to detect intermittent GI bleeding sites we have therefore applied our method of semi in-vitro labelled RBC, because they produce a high retention of Tc^{99m} in the circulation, no hampering gastric or colonic activity, and imaging may be carried out until 24 hours after injection. The examination is started directly after injection of the labelled cells, and continues for approximately 45 min. Repeated images are obtained between 2 and 24 hours after injection, dependent on the clinical indication and scintigraphic findings (fig.6). Initial results in 14 patients have been reporte by Van Royen and co-workers (20). In 9 patients a bleeding site was demonstrated (table 1). As also found by others, the scintigraphic images often became positive only after 1 hour. This

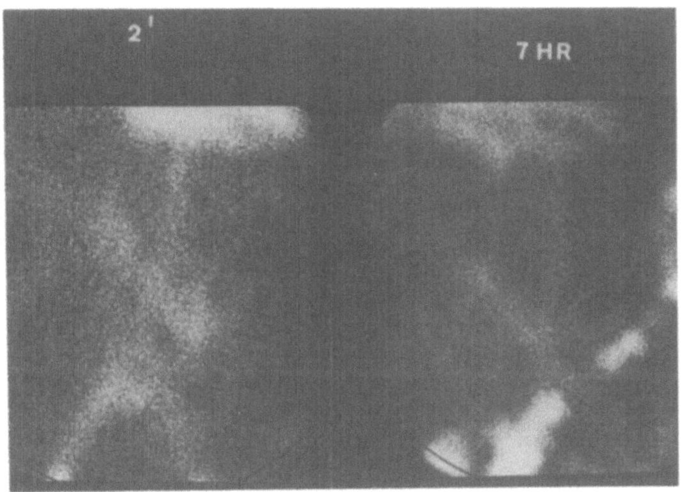

Fig. 6. Bleeding lesion in the descending colon demonstrated 7 hours after injection of Tc^{99m}-labelled RBC.

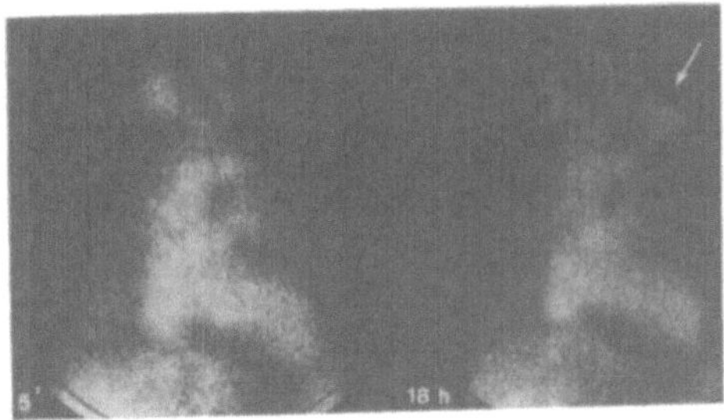

Fig. 7. Bleeding site demonstrated in the upper left lobe of the left lung (arrow).

indicates that an intravascular tracer with a fast plasma disappearance, such as Tc^{99m} labelled colloid, will probably give negative results (21). Scintigraphy with labelled RBC allows follow-up images to be obtained up to 1 day and may therefore provide positive results where other "one-shot" procedures fail. When the patient is not acutely bleeding, scintigraphy with labelled RBC seems to be the method of choice in detecting GI bleeding sites. Scintigraphy may also assist in determining an optimal time for endoscopy or angiography, and direct selective angiography.

Table 1. Results of scintigraphy with semi in-vitro Tc^{99m}-labelled RBC

Patient	Bleeding site	Scinti-graphy	Gastro-scopy	Colono-scopy	Angio-graphy	Diagnosis
1	upper GI	–	–	–	–	hiatus hernia
2	"	+	+			hemorrh. gastritis
3	"	–	–			stomach ulcer
4	"	+	–			esoph. varices
5	lower GI	+	–	–	–	ileum diverticle
6	"	+		–	–	thrombopathy
7	"	+	–	–		jejunal venectasies
8	"	+			–	?
9	"	+		–	–	colon carcinoma
10	"	+	–	–	–	angiodysplasia colon
11	"	+		+	–	angiodysplasia colon
12	?	–	–	–	–	?
13	?	–	–	–		?
14	?	–			–	?

In addition to GI bleeding, we have been able to detect a bleeding site in a case of chronic intermittent pulmonary bleeding. This could not be localized by bronchoscopy, but was clearly demonstrated as an accumulation of activity in the left upper lung lobe 18 hours after injection of labelled cells (fig. 7). On surgery a chronic aspergillus infection was found.

Conclusion

Semi in-vitro labelled RBC produce a lower background than other labelling methods and no complicating gastric activity. This results in improved image quality for cardiac blood-pool scintigraphy and detection of bleeding sites in the body.

REFERENCES

1. Gray SJ, Sterling K, The tagging of red blood cells and plasma proteins with radioactive chromion. J. clin. Invest. 29:1604, 1950.
2. Fischer J, Wolf R, Leon A, Technetium-99m as a label for erythrocytes. J. nucl. Med. 11:229, 1967.
3. Walker AG, Effect of Tc-99m bone agents on subsequent pertechnetate brain scans. J. nucl. Med. 16:579, 1975.
4. Stokely EM, Parkey RW, Bonte FJ et al, Gated blood pool imaging following Tc-99m stannous pyrophosphate imaging. Radiology 120:433, 1975.
5. Pavel DG, Zimmer AM, Patterson VN, In vivo labelling of red blood cells with Tc-99m: a new approach to blood pool visualization. J. nucl. Med. 18:305, 1977.
6. McRae J, Sugar RM, Shipley B, Hook GR, Alterations in tissue distribution of Tc-99m-pertechnetate in rats given stannous tin. J. nucl. Med. 15:151, 1974.
7. Jones AG, Davis MA, Uren RF, Shulkin P, In vivo red blood cell labelling with Tc-99m. J. nucl. Med. 18:637, 1977.
8. Hamilton RG, Alderson PO, A comparative evaluation of techniques for rapid and efficient in vivo labelling of red cells with (Tc-99m) pertechnetate. J. nucl. Med. 18:1010, 1977.
9. Vyth A, Raam CFM, Van der Schoot JB, Semi in vitro labelling of red cells with Tc-99m: a comparison with the in vivo labelling. Pharm. Weekblad 116:1302, 1981.
10. Hegge FN, Hamilton GW, Larson SM, Ritchie JL, Richards P, Cardiac chamber imaging: comparison of red blood cells labeled with Tc-99m in vitro and in vivo. J. nucl. Med. 19:129, 1978.
11. Winzelberg GG, McKusik KA, Strauss HW, Waltman AC, Greenfield AJ, Evaluation of gastrointestinal bleeding by red blood cells labelled in vivo with Technetium-99m. J. nucl. Med. 20:1080, 1979.
12. Weinstein MB, Smoak WM, Technical difficulties in Tc-99m-labeling of erythrocytes. J. nucl. Med. 11:41, 1970.
13. Eckelman W, Richards P, Hauser W, Atkins H, Technetium-labeled red blood cells. J. nucl. Med. 12:22,1971.
14. Hennig K, Francke WG, Woller P, Berger R, Johanssen B, Eine neue Methode zur Markierung roter Blutkörperchen mit Tc-99m und ihre Klinische Bedeutung. In: Proceedings 7 Jahrestagung Gesellschaft für Nuklearmedizin, Zürich, 1969.
15. Bardy A, Fouyé H, Gobin R, Beydon J, De Tovar G, Pannecière C, Hégésippe M, Technetium-99m labelling by means of stannous pyrophosphate: application to bleomycin and red blood cells. J. nucl. Med. 16:435, 1975.
16. Smith TD, Richards P, A simple kit for the preparation of Tc-99m labeled red blood cells. J. nucl. Med. 17:126, 1976.
17. Vyth A, Colorimetric determination of Tin(II) levels in Tc-99m labelling kits. Pharm. Weekblad 4:79, 1982.
18. Callahan RJ, Froelich JW, McKusik KA, Leppo J, Strauss HW, A modified method for the in vivo labeling of red blood cells with Tc-99m: concise communication. J. nucl. Med. 23:315, 1982.

19. Busemann-Sokole E, Vyth A, Raam CFM, Van der Wieken LR, Van der Schoot JB, Improved image quality in cardiac blood pool scintigraphy with semi- in vitro labelled red blood cells. J. nucl. Med. 22:10, 1981.

20. Van Royen EA, Van der Schoot JB, Vyth A, Detection of GI bleeding by an improved red blood cell (RBC) labeling technique. J. nucl. Med. 22:32, 1981.

21. Winzelberg GG, McKusik KA, Froelich JW, Callahan RJ, Strauss HW, Detection of gastrointestinal bleeding with Tc-99m labeled red blood cells. Sem. Nucl. Med. 12:139,1982.

22. Alavi A, Detection of gastrointestinal bleeding with Tc-99m sulfur colloid. Sem. Nucl. Med. 12:126, 1982.

SUBJECT INDEX